Contents

Introduction		iv
1	Adolescence	1
2	Adolescent Psychiatry	17
3	Causes of Disorder and Influences on Development	30
4	Disorders : Classification and Prevalence	50
5	The Clinical Interview : Assessment and Diagnosis	57
6	Educational and Developmental Problems and Mental Handicap	73
7	Emotional Disorders and Depression	84
8	Conduct Disorders and Delinquency	111
9	Enuresis and Encopresis	124
10	Problems of Sexual Identity, Experience and Behaviour	130
11	Misuse of Drugs and Other Substances	140
12	Anorexia Nervosa, Bulimia and Obesity	151
13	Tics	161
14	Autism and Other Major Disorders of Personality Development	165
15	Schizophrenic Disorders	179
16	Depressive and Manic Depressive Illness	192
17	Physical and Psychosomatic Problems	204
18	An Outline of Management	216
Index		270

Introduction

This book is intended primarily for undergraduate and postgraduate students in the health and care fields who have a basic grounding in their own field, but to whom the subject of adolescent psychiatry is relatively new. I hope it will be useful for psychiatrists, psychologists, social workers and nurses beginning specialized training in work with adolescents, and for others, too, who want to make sense of the issues raised in clinical meetings, case conferences and in child and adolescent psychiatrists' letters and reports.

It is a diverse field. To borrow a point made in an earlier book, adolescent psychiatry, as a sub-speciality of a sub-speciality, could be regarded as rather narrow and esoteric. In fact it has a wide span, encompassing all of the general psychiatry and psychotherapy of young people, from eleven-year-olds at school to young adults in work or further education. Because of this age range, it involves aspects of life which do not feature so prominently in adult psychiatry or general medicine – such as matters to do with school and family life. It also requires working across professional boundaries. The trainee in adolescent psychiatry therefore finds a field in which, for example, family therapy and paediatrics, developmental science and psycho-analytic theory, neurophysiology and art therapy, general psychiatry, consultative work, ethical questions and the law come together in a field which is complex, challenging and stimulating.

Given this variety, what constitutes a basic book? The approach I have taken is to try to cover everything, or nearly everything, however briefly, and to provide as full a guide as possible to further reading; in particular, where to find key books, chapters and clinical and research review articles. I hope I have conveyed the sort of questions being asked in the field, and shown that much more needs to be discovered, particularly about preventive work and management. However, given that we have to work with major gaps in our knowledge, I have also devoted space to issues of practical management : what we actually do. This is discussed in relation to each group of problems and disorders, and outlined as a general overview in the last chapter.

It will come as no surprise to hear that there is a good deal of disagreement in the field. I have tried to represent the controversies fairly, and to make it clear when I am giving my own points of view or practice. This approach, I hope, will help those still taking examinations, those institutions much valued by the professions but for which the more respectable books are not supposed to be written.

I cannot acknowledge all those colleagues from whom I have learned and with whom I have worked over the years, but I do want to thank, as I have thanked them before, my friends and colleagues at the Adolescent Unit at Bethlem Royal Hospital, whose skills and style make difficult work a delight. And on the subject of hard labour, now that the book is in print I feel able to thank Richard Miles of Blackwell Scientific Publications who first suggested it should be written, and helped see it through; and my thanks too to Gill, my wife, for her work on the index.

Derek Steinberg
The Adolescent Unit,
Bethlem Royal Hospital,
Beckenham, Kent

Chapter 1

Adolescence

Definitions and developmental milestones : physical

Puberty means the onset of adolescence. It usually begins between 11 and 16 years in boys and between 9 and 16 years in girls. In boys it begins with enlargement of the testes, the first growth of downy pubic hair at the base of the penis, and the ability to ejaculate both spontaneously and by masturbation. In girls the breast buds enlarge to form a small mound, the areolar diameter widens, there is a fine growth of downy hair along the labia and the first menstruation occurs : this is known as the menarche.

Adolescence refers to the period from puberty to adulthood. The latter is defined by several different criteria : in general terms, by achieving independence from parents; more specifically, by reaching the age of legal majority, at present 18 years in the United Kingdom. The body marks the end of the dramatic period of growth that began at puberty by the completion and ossification of the clavicle (collar bone) between 18 and 25 years. This occurs earlier in young women than in young men.

Figure 1.1 shows the sequence of events between puberty and adolescence in boys and girls. Both androgen and oestrogen hormones are influential in both sexes; in both boys and girs small amounts of androgens and oestrogens are produced by the adrenals during childhood.

The first endocrine event in puberty in both sexes is a rise in the level of pituitary gonadotrophins, leading to the development of the ovarian follicles in girls and the testicular tubules in boys, leading to the release of the sex hormones oestrogen and androgen in both sexes. In boys androgen production markedly exceeds oestrogen production as adolescence proceeds, and in girls oestrogen production exceeds androgen

Figure 1.1   Physical changes in adolescence.

Boys	Girls
Testes enlarge. Pubic hair appears. First ejaculation. Some gynaecomastia, usually transient. N.B. Onset of puberty 2 years (mean) later than in girls.	Breast buds enlarge, areola widens. Pubic hair appears. Menarche. N.B. Onset of puberty 2 years (mean) earlier than in boys.
Axillary and facial hair appear about 2 years after puberty. Sweat gland development and enlargement of facial pores more marked in boys.	Appearance of axillary hair, earlier than in boys. Sweat gland and pore development less marked than in boys.
Growth spurt in height and weight, and laryngeal growth (voice 'breaks'), with the maximum velocity of change at 14 (range 12–17). Most height change comes later in boys than girls.	Growth spurt in height and weight about 2 years earlier in girls than in boys. Less post-pubertal gain in height in girls than in boys.
Pubic hair spreads vertically up abdomen and to medial surfaces of thighs. Increase in shoulder breadth.	Pubic hair spreads horizon-tally across lower abdomen and onto the medial surfaces of thighs. Nipple projects from pigmented areola.

production. During adolescent development periods of hormonal imbalance are not uncommon, and may become clinically apparent, as in the case of the gynaecomastia in boys which usually disappears after a year or so (Tanner, 1962).

Delay in puberty is usually constitutional, and may be familial, though this is not always evident. Klinefelter's syndrome (XXY chromosomal abnormality) in boys, and Turner's syndrome (XO abnormality) in girls, pituitary and gonadal disorders interfere with the onset of normal puberty.

Psychological changes (cognitive)

There is considerable cognitive development throughout adolescence. General intellectual development appears to be able to continue into the twenties, with environmental factors (such as intellectual stimulation) appearing to be very influential in determining the peak achieved of scored intelligence quotient (IQ; i.e. performance on standardized tests compared with the performance of children of comparable age in the same tests). Boys seem to be at an advantage over girls in the development of visuo-spatial ability and mathematical ability, and girls' language development appears to begin earlier. The differences are small, and the degree of environmental influence uncertain.

The Swiss psychologist Jean Piaget (1955, 1972) described cognitive changes in a way that related them to emotional and social development, as follows:

Sensorimotor development (up to 2 years)
The child is stimulation-seeking and object manipulating and begins to build up a picture of the outside world.
Pre- operational thinking (2–7 years)
The child develops elementary ways of classifying what is perceived.
Concrete operations (7–11 years)
In this stage, the child perceives the relations between things so that organization and classification become more logically developed.
Formal operations (adolescence)
This is characterized by the ability to think in abstract terms, construct hypotheses, use ideas and imagination, and distinguish from each other fantasies, ideas, beliefs, probabilities and possibilities.

Emotional and ethical development

At about 14–15 years adolescents begin to develop abstract conceptions of social, ethical and political matters. For example they become able to consider questions from a wider perspective and think in terms of balanced rather than only authoritarian solutions to problems, and seem more able to think empathically of others.

The many psychodynamic theories of emotional development in adolescence have much in common, despite differences in emphasis and terminology. A useful common thread is found by regarding the adolescent as someone who is able to contemplate achieving in reality a number of goals that in earlier life were largely fantasy. For example, the sexual drive that is central to Sigmund Freud's theories (e.g. Freud, 1922) and which is represented in talk and play during childhood, becomes more powerful and charged with more potential for individual and shared sexual activity during adolescence, partly because of physical development, partly because of the shared sexual interest of peers, and partly because of social expectations and opportunities. This drive is directed in adolescence towards genital sexuality (masturbation, inter-course) but also towards the establishment of relationships with other people. These necessarily recapitulate the child's learned experience of love so far, namely within his or her own family.

Peter Blos has described the adolescent's move towards independence from the family as a second step in what he terms the individuation process. In the first step, the young child aged 3 or 4 develops an internal picture or model of the mother, and having this 'portable' mother can be more adventurous in achieving physical distance from her. The second step, in adolescence, involves abandoning this internal representation in order to seek and use real, loving relationships with other people. Powerful sexualized, loving, dependent and angry feelings, and the mixed feelings about autonomy *versus* independence, once safely 'held' within the immature child in the containing family, now become social and behavioural realities, near the surface if not 'over the top'. Thus to achieve freedom of action and movement, i.e. independence, appears to the adolescent to risk inappropriately assertive, aggressive and sexual behaviour, and the retribution, abandonment and loss that may be its consequence. It is as if the adolescent is old enough to want to experiment in these ways, but not sufficiently mature to conduct his or her experiments confidently with completely new people, well away from the family either emotionally or in reality. As a result there can be a certain amount of confusion and blurring about roles, a good deal of ambivalence about what he or she actually wants, and a lot of resultant anxiety (Blos, 1962, 1970, 1979).

D.W. Winnicott has described development and maturation in terms of imaginative play. A secure parental environment – i.e. good, or what he termed 'good enough' parenting – enables the young person to explore possible ways of being and behaving; he or she can conduct experiments in this safe play area or 'laboratory'. In adolescence the fantasy is about independence, which means doing *without* the parents, and which in turn has implications of doing *away with* the parents: hence 'I could kill you' is said and felt (Winnicott, 1971, 1972).

A further dimension is added by an aspect of Melanie Klein's theory (Brown, 1961). Here, in early childhood, the helpless infant, at the mercy of external 'good' and 'bad' forces, is said to experience powerful idealizing and hating (paranoid) feelings. With the maturation of perception, and the realization that the 'good' and the 'bad' are not located in separate places, but are aspects of the same parent, the infant becomes sadder and wiser and experiences guilt. The move from the paranoid to depressive stages, or positions, is regarded as an essential maturational step, and one which can be recapitulated in either direction when infantile feelings are reactivated, as in a disturbed, anxious adolescent having difficulties with the developmental moves described earlier.

Anna Freud described these and other powerful competing feelings, and proposed that the developing ego, or sense of self, dealt with them by psychologically defensive manoeuvres – the mechanisms of defence (Freud,A,1936,1958,1966). These included denial of strong feelings (e.g. denial to oneself or to others); self-isolation (e.g. within the family); idealization, i.e. seeing as unequivocally good, a person, group, movement or attitude; and ambivalence, in which strong and opposing feelings (e.g. love and hate) are held at the same time towards someone or something. For example, an adolescent in difficulties may want to be treated by his parents as an adult and as a child at the same time.

One of the achievements of Anna Freud's account is in describing psychodynamic mechanisms in terms of their dealing with the outside as well as with internal psychic reality. Erik Erikson (1965,1968) has taken this further by relating emotional development to both social and cultural opportunities and expectations. His epigenetic model of development describes a sequence of stages from infancy through adolescence and adulthood to old age and death. Each stage is described in terms of the resolution of a conflict or crisis between competing alternatives. Thus in adolescence the key conflict is between the establishment of personal identity on the one hand and role confusion on the other, with each successive challenge having the possibility of a favourable or unfavourable outcome. This 'good outcome', in adolescence, would be what Erikson calls devotion, fidelity, a capacity for commitment. The next stage, young adulthood, is a conflict between intimacy and isolation, with a capacity for affiliation and love as the positive outcome. Erikson's model is a dynamic one, and the eight stages he describes in *Childhood and Society* (Erikson, 1965) should not be taken as too self-contained. Rather, each stage is a dynamic balance, rather like the outcome of a parallelogram of forces, itself dependent on the state of balance of the stages passed, and providing the foundation for the achievement of balance in the stages still to come.

These models and theoretical positions use different terms and concepts, but have in common the idea that emotional development from dependence (being totally looked after) to independence is not an easy path, but is full of challenges and possible sources of anxiety, depression and confusion. These challenges may be coped with more or less well, depending on the many influences that form the basics of aetiological theories (Chapter 3). How well they have been managed will strongly influence the individual's experience and management of future relationships – with friends, with the future family, and for that matter with therapists too. All being well the adolescent becomes an independent young adult able to form mature relationships with other adults, and with the capacity to look after children. The core of this aspect of healthy and normal development is in the maturation of the ego, that conscious sense of self, i.e. the 'I'. The ego performs a balancing act between three sets of demands or expectations : those of the instincts, those of the conscience, and those of external reality. With a mature ego we can modify or suppress primitive impulses, behave reasonably, postpone gratification of one sort or another, plan things and organize ourselves, deal with practical choices and dilemmas and cope with changes in how we feel; in short, act sensibly and make sense of things.

Psychodynamic theory in practice

It is important to remember that the different schools of thought all deal with the same organism, albeit in different language, and with different emphases which reflect the different personalities, experience and circumstances of their authors. If you do not become too concerned with the fine print of each theoretical position, you will find that, taken together, the psychodynamic models throw light on the less rational aspects of thinking and behaviour that we see in our patients and, if we are honest and conscientious observers, in ourselves.

A patient may make you angry, anxious or in some other way upset; or you may see people in a family or group affecting each other in a way which defies rational explanation. Psychodynamic concepts help illuminate what people do to each other, and why, and provide clues about how best to proceed. 'Insight' means in psychodynamic terms having some grasp of the motives and feelings that lie behind supposedly purely rational thinking and actions.

Adolescent patients are not generally very enthusiastic about their therapists' flashes of insight, although the more courteous or compliant boys and girls may express polite interest. Denial (i.e. of feelings about self and others) is commonly evident in psychotherapeutic work with adolescents. Ambivalence, the possession of powerful but conflicting feelings (e.g. an immature person's hostile rejection of someone on whom he or she is determinedly dependent) is a phenomenon also commonly seen, and often denied.

Rapid changes in mood, and up and down the scale of emotional maturity, will be seen, so that an adolescent may be sober and reflective on one occasion, and childish and impulsive on another. A boy or girl may, for example, blame everything on others, perceiving other people as being hostile and destructive and the cause of all the trouble, i.e. he or she will adopt a 'paranoid' position; or he or she will unreasonably take all the blame and feel guilty to the point of self-destruction (the 'depressive' position). Again, a young person who is too immature to cope with ambiguity (e.g. right and wrong on both sides) will cope with this uncomfortable dual message by 'splitting'. Thus, a child who is unable to grasp the 'good' and 'bad' in individual members of his family, or among his teachers or the therapeutic team, will decide that some of them are 'good' and the others are 'bad.'

These and other shifts in attitude, according to psychodynamic theory, are powerfully influenced by unconscious, non-rational feelings, and can be behind conscious feelings which are inappropriate or extreme, and behind behaviour which is unsociable, unpleasant, unpredictable or to a greater or lesser extent destructive : for example, inability to settle down to schoolwork at one extreme, violent behaviour at the other. Such vicissitudes of feeling and behaviour, if not too severe or disabling, or if transient, can fall within the broadly normal range of behaviour. When more marked, they can underlie conduct and emotional disorders, as these problems are termed in children and younger adolescents, or conduct problems and neuroses as they may be called in older adolescents.

Often these emotional problems will operate around a reasonably stable base, so that the boy or girl has sufficient strenths (ego capacity and social skills) to manage for most of the time. Such young people have their problems, but they are not totally chaotic; their problems are described further in Chapters 7 and 8.

Some young people, however, develop such major problems in the way they feel, the attitudes they develop, and in their capacity to form relationships, that the type of problems outlined above pervade most or all aspects of their personality development. Then, instead of finding ourselves treating an adolescent who is for the most part functioning normally, we find we are dealing with a young person who seems quite chaotic, and whose whole personality structure seems vulnerable to disorder. Their problems are discussed in Chapter 14.

Good introductions to psychodynamic principles in general will be found in Brown (1961) and Brown and Pedder (1979).

Adolescent turmoil and identity crisis

Is adolescence a time of life marked by emotional turbulence? Does it amount to a crisis of identity? It depends on what is meant by these terms.

'Crisis' does not necessarily mean a dramatic, head-clutching event, and we must differentiate between (a) the notion of crisis as a normal critical period, i.e. a time of change and the resolution of opposing pressures, as described by Erikson; and (b) crisis as an acute period of distress and disorder, for example as described in the International Classification of Diseases (ICD9; World Health Organization, 1975) as an *adjustment reaction*: i.e. a few months of anxiety, depression or behaviour problems without previous mental disorder, and closely related in time to an identifiable stressor. It is described in the American classification system (the Diagnostic and Statistical Manual DSM III; American Psychiatric Association 1979) in similar terms. The latter is a description of a clinical state, the former an expected stage of emotional development. In psychiatry, however, it is too much to hope that the one can be precisely delineated from the other. For example, failure of parents to help a teenager negotiate an essentially normal critical phase of development may result in the boy or girl being referred to a psychiatric clinic, and identified there as a patient (for a fuller account of the referral process in relation to adolescent psychiatry see Steinberg, 1983).

Two psychodynamic points of view are worth noting here. First, Anna Freud (1958; 1966) described adolescent turbulence in terms that suggested it was a normal *period of abnormality*, a contradiction in terms likely to cause muddle rather than illumination, but which drew attention to the depth of turmoil she perceived as happening at this stage of development.

Second, Erikson (1968) spoke of identity crisis in terms of identity confusion. Identity confusion resulted from a failure to integrate various senses of self, for example the personal senses of self as one is and as one would like to be (which includes notions of selves abandoned and selves anticipated), and the sense of self acquired from social roles.

For example, a girl may feel herself to be the most responsible and grown-up of her brothers and sisters, and she may be encouraged in this role by her parents because, as everyone believes, this helps her be adult and independent. Far from facilitating independence, however, the role she fulfils only operates while she is being a conscientious, compliant child who does things for her family. When an opportunity for really independent action comes along, for example in the shape of a boyfriend or an opportunity to leave home, she finds this does not feel right, and she doesn't know how to act her new 'part'. The explanation given here of her dilemma may be clear to the psychiatrist or family worker but far from clear to her. She does not perceive her problem in terms of taking on too much at home, or her independence being compromised, but rather in terms of muddle, anxiety and perhaps depression about mixed loyalties and real uncertainty about what she herself wants.

In a study of the feelings of younger adolescents (aged around 14) as part of the Isle of Wight epidemiological study (Rutter *et al.*, 1976), distressing feelings were quite common among this normal (i.e. non-clinical) population. Over 40 per cent reported feelings of misery, 30 per cent ideas of reference, 20 per cent feelings of self-deprecation and just under 8 per cent suicidal ideas. The adults in contact with these young people tended not to know about these feelings. Note that this is likely to be a low estimate as far as adolescents in general are concerned, because the incidence of a wide range of emotional and behavioural problems tends to increase through the teenage years (see, for example, the review by Graham and Rutter, 1985). Moreover, there is evidence of greater disturbance in inner city areas compared with areas like the Isle of Wight (e.g. see Rutter and Madge, 1977; Rutter, 1979).

Does all this mean that 'most' adolescents are likely to be disturbed? The answer is no; in Graham and Rutter's account the authors draw attention to the various problems in interpreting statistics. To take one example, delinquency does indeed rise in adolescence; but delinquency is a legal term, and younger children cannot be convicted and therefore do not enter the statistics. Further, while a large number of adolescents do report problems in their feelings (some 10–40 per cent, as described above) more than half do not. In drawing conclusions it is therefore important to distinguish between anomalies in the reporting of problems, as in the delinquency statistics; and problems of definition, e.g. when do troubled feelings become persistent enough or disabling enough to become a disorder? Moreover, the processes involved in referring adolescents are likely to have an arbitrary effect on which adolescents with problems become identified as patients (Steinberg *et al.*, 1981; Steinberg, 1981).

Finally, in addition to the effect of definition and referral patterns, and the effect on prevalence of age and location, there is also variation with sex. Before puberty, emotional problems in general occur equally in boys and girls, while depressive disorders are more prominent in boys. After puberty, girls are more strongly represented for both types of problem. Prevalence is discussed further in Chapter 4.

Storm and stress

Sturm und Drang, the name of the radical movement in eighteenth century Germany, captures a common conception, or myth, about the adolescent period. It is worth separating one notion from the other.

Are adolescents, in general, stormy, aggressive and rebellious? Is there a so-called generation gap? A series of studies from the United States, Europe and the United Kingdom have shown that most adolescents and their parents get on well with each other, although of course there are occasional rows (part of normal family functioning) and recurring disagreements about such matters as personal style, friends and habits. Delinquency, including vandalism and violence, is increasingly reported among young people, although it is important when interpreting statistics to bear in mind that an increase in reported incidents is not necessarily a precise reflection of a general increase in this behaviour. However, there does seem to be a real increase in violence and vandalism, with boys far outnumbering girls. Girls, however, now show twice the rate of increase compared with boys; i.e. they are catching up. It is important to note that these alarming trends are still confined to a minority of adolescents and are particularly related to problem areas of large towns and cities. Studies of adolescent 'rebelliousness' in general and delinquency in particular are very helpfully reviewed in Rutter (1979) and Rutter and Giller (1983).

What about sexual attitudes? Again, there have been changes but they are not so striking as is sometimes imagined. Sexual relations before marriage is more widely accepted as 'all right', and more widely practised, but there has not been a dramatic shift away from loving and stable relationships and towards casual sexual behaviour among the majority of young people (Rutter, 1979), and although there is a real increase in sexual relationships it does not always amount to coition, and nor does it seem that very much of the increase in premarital sexual activity is promiscuous in the sense of involving several casual partners (Chilman, 1986). In view of the dangerousness of acquired immune deficiency syndrome (AIDS) it will be important to see if this view is sustained.

It is interesting to see that the findings of scientific surveys are matched by the occasional informal enquiries newspapers conduct among young people, who emerge for the most part as rather conservative in everything except fashion, and at least as responsible and compassionate as the young of previous generations, if not more so.

Turning from storm to stress, there is adequate evidence that many young people, perhaps a third to half, often experience sad, anxious and muddled feelings, as discussed previously in this chapter. Why should there be such a discrepancy between the findings of surveys which suggest that it is a real but minority phenomenon (Rutter *et al.*, 1976) and the reports of so many psychodynamic writers (e.g. A. Freud, 1958; Erikson, 1965, 1968; Blos, 1970; Winnicott, 1971; Hyatt Williams, 1975)? Were they all misguided? The answer is that the epidemiological investigators of measurable behaviour, and the psychodynamic clinicians who draw inferences from what they hear and see in their clinical experience, are describing two quite different sets of material. The epidemiologists report the outcome : observed or reported mood, like a measure of an individual's blood sugar at a particular time. The psychodynamic clinicians report their understanding of the various components (e.g. anger, anxiety, defence mechanisms) of a psychodynamic system, sometimes in balance and sometimes not balanced, and which results in the phenomena which the epidemiologists measure. The heat in the disputes between the two sorts of workers owes more to their differences in feelings and personality than to faulty thinking.

Adolescent development in the family

The normally functioning family helps prepare its adolescent members for independence over a number of years, and then goes on to encourage each young person actually to leave.

We have seen how the child develops inner capacities from his experience of parents over the years, and in adolescence actually tries them out, not always with comfortable results (e.g. Winnicott, 1971; Blos, 1979). Family functioning can be viewed from the psychodynamic (psychoanalytic) perspective or from the perspective of general systems theory (Bruggen and Davies, 1977). These two ways of understanding family functioning and family development contribute to each other but are essentially different. The psychoanalytic perspective is concerned with feelings, attitudes, perceptions and beliefs which individuals may possess or which the family as a group may share, and the family therapist will tend to use interpretation, i.e. communicating to the family what the therapist understands they are feeling. The systems approach derives from Von Bertalanffy's *General Systems Theory* (1968) which describes how the different sub-systems of any organization interact with each other, each affecting the functioning of the other parts, and of the whole, and the whole affecting each part. Dare (1986) has provided an interesting and clear account of the development of different approaches to the understanding of families, drawing attention to a number of fundamental aspects of family theory, including (a) the importance of how roles are attributed, allocated and accepted (e.g. the sick or symptomatic role, sex roles, the 'responsible' member of the family, the 'failure' etc.)' (b) the ways in which patterns of behaviour develop (coalitions, alliances, conflicts) which maintain or resist the way the system is operating; (c) the ways in which power, authority and control operate; and (d) how communication and co-operation take place. Other helpful accounts of family theory and family therapy will be found in Skynner (1976), Hinde (1980), Gorell Barnes (1984), Skynner and Cleese (1984) and Barker (1986).

For the family that contains adolescent members a number of delicate moves need to be negotiated. Parent-child affection, including its physical expression, has to be modulated in the light of the adolescent's sexual development. The adolescent must achieve independence and autonomy by adopting some strategies through which he wants to be like one or other parent, some strategies through which he wants to demonstrate that he is different, and some strategies about which he is ambivalent. The adolescent will have mixed feelings about how much he or she wants to be left alone and how much to be looked after, and this is reciprocated by parental uncertainty about being underprotective or overprotective. When social experiments go wrong, the dilemma on both sides is still sharper, and each move, for better or worse, necessitates a further adjustment of the homeostasis achieved so far. The challenge of these and other pressures, which are physical, psychological and cultural as well as deriving from the family, will also be affected by the adolescent's siblings, whose current roles will be influential: for example, there may be a successfully near-independent older sister, a younger brother who is still enjoying his position as a child, and so on. Meanwhile the parents of the adolescent will themselves be entering or be well into middle age with the self-doubts and self-reappraisal that go with it. Moreover, the two people who started the family, and negotiated the development of their own relationship with their childrens' participation, now have the prospect of facing life without them, a post-parenting phase described by Dare (1982) as the empty nest syndrome. Dare (1986) has pointed out that this (like other) complications in the family life-cycle can be protected against by the adolescent developing symptoms that keep the boy or girl in a dependent position, so that the question of leaving home is postponed. It is important to appreciate that this doesn't mean that the family pattern has necessarily 'caused' the disorder; but it may be playing a part in perpetuating it.

Social and sexual development

The young child's social relationships tend to be with family members, parents' friends and the children of parents' friends. With developing confidence and competence and the emergence of wider social activities. (e.g. through school) the child can begin to pick friends for himself. Before adolescence these friendships tend to be with others of the same sex, although this is not exclusively so, and there is considerable interest in sexual matters before puberty. In pre-adolescence, intense friendships with children of the same sex occur, and there may be sexual experimentation between them, especially between boys, although the relationship between this and the future choice of a homosexual style of life is not clear. Masturbation is normal and common if not universal in adolescence, though reported with more confidence as a male predilection, but it is a private activity or one shared with a few friends. Public, disinhibited masturbation is likely to be a sign of a major problem in social development. The boundary between sexual experimentation and sexual and gender choice is discussed in Chapter 10.

There is a tendency in the adult Western world to attribute to adolescents considerable sexual disinhibition, confidence and opportunity, an ambivalent attitude perhaps tinged with envy. In fact adolescents are often quite troubled about their sexual and social fantasies, wishes and experiments, and this deserves adult understanding and tactful help. Without adult guidance adolescents do make many mistakes, particularly when they try to establish 'permanent' relationships (for example, marriage) too early.

For further reading on sexual and social development in adolescence, Farrell and Kellaher (1978), Coleman (1980), and Graham and Rutter (1985) are recommended.

Concluding note

What may be considered 'normal' in terms of developing life styles must take account of an individual's and a family's wishes, choices and cultural background. Psychiatrists, social workers, psychologists and others should be seen in their proper light as helpers and, if necessary, advisers. They should not be presented as authorities on normal living, on which for the most part they are not outstandingly well qualified.

There are specific areas, however, where knowledge of normal adolescent development should guide clinical practice and the sort of advice we give. Delayed physical development, which can become chronic in anorexia nervosa, requires careful evaluation in terms of age, weight and height, and in relation to the growth history of the adolescent's parents. A paediatrician's advice will be needed if normal growth is not quickly re-established by psychiatric treatment, because physical stunting of growth can become permanent when, in mid to late adolescence, normal joint fusion occurs.

Moderate problems in relationships and transient misbehaviour are universal but, as we have seen, normal adolescence is not marked by persistent aggressiveness, promiscuousness or chaotic relationships with parents, peers and others. Such problems are not always psychiatric in nature, but they do deserve concern and attention, and where there is a distressing, handicapping problem in adolescence it must not be assumed that the young person will 'grow out of it', particularly where disturbed conduct is concerned. Moreover, even when a condition seems self-limiting (e.g. mild or moderate emotional disturbances), the difficulty caused to social relationships and education should not be underestimated.

References and further reading

American Psychiatric Association (1979) *Diagnostic and Statistical Manual* (DSM III), 3rd edition. Washington, D.C.: American Psychiatric Association

Barker, P. (1986) *Basic Family Therapy*, 2nd edition. London: Collins Professional Books.

Blos, P. (1962) *On Adolescence: A Psychoanalytical Interpretation*. New York: Free Press.

Blos, P. (1970) *The Young Adolescent : Clinical Studies*. London: Collier-Macmillan.

Blos, P. (1979) *The Adolescent Passage : Developmental Issues*. New York: International Universities Press.

Brown, D. and Pedder, J. (1979) *Introduction to Psychotherapy*. London: Tavistock.

Brown, J.A.C. (1961) *Freud and the Post Freudians*. Harmondsworth: Penguin Books.

Bruggen, P. and Davies, G. (1977) Family therapy in adolescent psychiatry. *British Journal of Psychiatry* **131**, 433–47.

Chilman, C. (1986) Adolescent heterosexual behaviour. *In* Feldman, F.A. and Stiffman, A.R. (Eds), *Advances in Adolescent Mental Health*, Volume 1, part A, pp 205–75.

Coleman, J.C. (1980) *The Nature of Adolescence*. London: Methuen.

Dare, C. (1982) The empty nest: families with older adolescents and the models of family therapy. *In* Bentovim, A., Gorell-Barnes, G. and Cooklin, A. (Eds), *Family Therapy 2*, pp 353–60. London: Academic Press.

Dare, C. (1985) Family therapy. *In* Rutter, M. and Hersov, L. (Eds), *Child and Adolescent Psychiatry : Modern Approaches*, pp 809–25. Oxford: Blackwell Scientific Publications.

Dare, C. (1986) Family therapy and an adolescent in-patient unit. *In* Steinberg, D. (Ed), *The Adolescent Unit : Work and Teamwork in Adolescent Psychiatry*, pp 83–95. Chichester: John Wiley and Sons.

Erikson, E. (1965) *Childhood and Society*. London: Hogarth Press; and Harmondsworth : Penguin Books.

Erikson, E. (1968) *Identity, Youth and Crisis*. London: Faber.

Farrell, C. and Kellaher, L. (1978) *My Mother Said: The way young people learn about sex and birth control*. London: Routledge and Kegan Paul.

Freud, A. (1936) *The Ego and the Mechanisms of Defence*. London: Hogarth Press.

Freud, A. (1958) Adolescence.*Psychoanalytic Study of the Child* **13**, 255–78.

Freud, A. (1966) *Normality and Pathology in Childhood*. London: Hogarth Press.

Freud, S. (1922) *Introductory Lectures on Psychoanalysis*. London: George Allen and Unwin.

Gorell-Barnes, G. (1984) *Working with Families*. London: Macmillan.

Graham, P. and Rutter, M. (1985). Adolescent disorders. *In* Rutter, M. and Hersov, L. (Eds), *Child and Adolescent Psychiatry : Modern Approaches*, pp 351–67. Oxford: Blackwell Scientific Publications.

Hinde, R.A. (1980) Family influences. *In* Rutter, M. (Ed), *Scientific Foundations of Developmental Psychiatry*, pp 47–66. London: William Heinemann Medical Books.

Hyatt Williams, A. (1975) Puberty and phases of adolescence. *In* Meyerson S. (Ed), *Adolescence : The Crises of Adjustment*, pp 27–40. London: George Allen and Unwin.

Klein, M. (1932) *The Psycho-Analysis of Children*. London: Hogarth Press.

Klein, M. (1950) *Contributions to Psychoanalysis*. London: Hogarth Press.

Piaget, J. (1955) *The Child's Construction of Reality*. London: Routledge and Kegan Paul.

Piaget, J. (1972) Intellectual evolution from adolescence to adulthood. *Human Development* **5**, 1–12.

Rutter, M. (1979) *Changing Youth in a Changing Society : Patterns of Adolescent Development and Disorder*. London: Nuffield Provincial Hospitals Trust.

Rutter, M. (1980) (Ed) *Scientific Foundations of Developmental Psychiatry*. London: William Heinemann Medical Books.

Rutter, M. and Giller, H. (1983) *Juvenile Delinquency : Trends and Perspectives*. Harmondsworth: Penguin Books.

Rutter, M. Graham, P., Chadwick, O. and Yule, W. (1976) Adolescent turmoil : fact or fiction? *Journal of Child Psychology and Psychiatry* **17**, 35–56.

Rutter, M. and Madge, N. (1977) *Cycles of Disadvantage : A Review of Research*. London: Heinemann.

Skynner, A.C.R. (1976) *One Flesh – Separate Persons*. London: Constable.

Skynner, R. and Cleese, J. (1984) *Families and How to Survive Them*. London: Methuen.

Steinberg, D. (1983) *The Clinical Psychiatry of Adolescence. Clinical work from a social and developmental perspective*. Chichester: John Wiley and Sons.

Steinberg, D. (1981) *Using Child Psychiatry. The functions and operations of a speciality*. London: Hodder and Stoughton.

Steinberg, D., Galhenage, D.P.C. and Robinson, S.C. (1981) Two years' referrals to a regional adolescent unit : some implications for psychiatric services. *Social Science and Medicine* **15E**, 113–22.

Tanner, J.M. (1962) *Growth at Adolescence*. Oxford: Blackwell Scientific Publications.

von Bertalanffy, L. (1968) *General Systems Theory*. New York: George Brazillier.

Winnicott, D.W. (1971) *Playing and Reality*. London: Tavistock.

Winnicott, D.W. (1972) *The Maturational Process and the Facilitating Environment*. London: Hogarth Press.

World Health Organisation (1975) *A Multi-Axial Classification of Child Psychiatric Disorder*. Geneva: WHO.

Wyss, D. (1966) *Depth Psychology : A Critical History*. London: George Allen and Unwin.

Chapter 2

Adolescent Psychiatry

The day's work in adolescent psychiatry

It should be said at once that there are many different ways of being an adolescent psychiatrist, or becoming one. Some psychiatrists work exclusively with adolescents, others combine it with work with older or younger patients, or both, and the training and experience of different clinicians vary too. In general, training in the psychiatry of younger children is to be encouraged, because adolescence is developmentally part of the childhood move from total dependence to independence, and best understood from that perspective.

A psychiatrist working with adolescents may work in an in-patient unit with a large team of colleagues from different professions, as is described in *The Adolescent Unit* (Steinberg 1986). He or she may work with a smaller team in the out-patients' department of a general or specialist hospital, or in a child psychiatric clinic (also known as child and family psychiatric units or clinics). Some psychiatrists' clinical work is conducted largely by themselves, rather than in a team, for example in private practice or when their work is largely psychotherapeutic.

Diversity is an important characteristic of the field. It is a deceptively vast area of practice, deceptive because by all appearances it is a rather narrow speciality. In practice, and in common with paediatrics and child psychiatry, it deals with a very wide range of problems albeit in a relatively narrow age band. The truly holistic clinician in the field would be something of a general psychiatric practitioner, interested in helping with major and minor mental illness, having some knowledge of the cause and effects of brain damage, mental handicap and the epilepsies, and able to advise parents, teachers and residential care workers. Some understanding of families, schools and other organizations is important, and the ability to use (personally, or in collaboration with others)

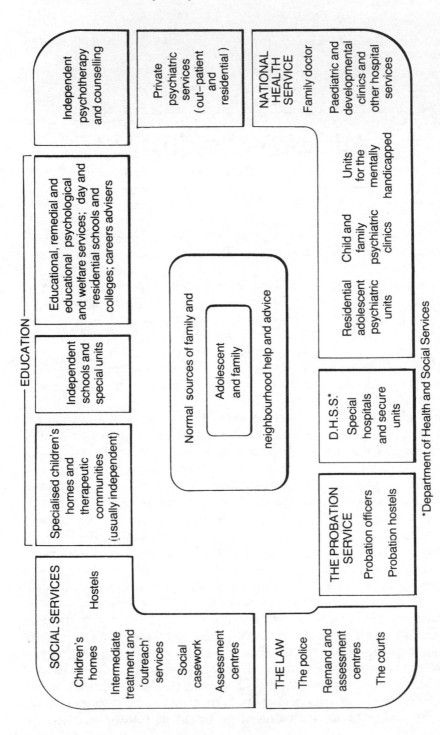

SOCIAL SERVICES

Children's homes   Hostels

Intermediate treatment and 'outreach' services

Social casework

Assessment centres

Specialised children's homes and therapeutic communities (usually independent)

Independent schools and special units

Educational, remedial and educational, psychological and welfare services; day and residential schools and colleges; careers advisers

—— EDUCATION ——

Independent psychotherapy and counselling

Private psychiatric services (out–patient and residential)

NATIONAL HEALTH SERVICE

Family doctor

Paediatric and developmental clinics and other hospital services

Normal sources of family and

Adolescent and family

neighbourhood help and advice

Units for the mentally handicapped

Child and family psychiatric clinics

Residential adolescent psychiatric units

THE LAW

The police

Remand and assessment centres

The courts

THE PROBATION SERVICE

Probation officers

Probation hostels

D.H.S.S.*

Special hospitals and secure units

*Department of Health and Social Services

Figure 2.1

psychological, psychodynamic, biological, family and social approaches in assessment and management. Many adolescent psychiatrists will have developed special areas of interest so that as well as the 'general practitioners' there are also those who are primarily family therapists, individual psychotherapists or who work with residential communities.

Many will have teaching and training functions, and for some there will be the time or expectation for conducting research. All will have administrative and organizational responsibilities, great or small, and most will divide the 'service' aspect of their work into direct clinical work with patients, the supervision of colleagues in training, and consultative work. Consultative work (see Chapter 18) means helping other professionals with their own work with young people, rather than taking on the latter as patients.

Adolescent psychiatrists, then, work in many different ways and divide their time between a number of settings. Figure 2.1 is a reminder of where and with whom adolescent psychiatrists may work in the course of a day or in the course of a career. It is also a reminder of the different settings to which adolescents may be sent or attend for help, training or custody of one sort or another.

How do adolescents become psychiatric patients?

The prevalence of psychiatric disorder among adolescents in the community is discussed in Chapter 4. It will be seen that some 20-40 per cent of young people could be said to be in need of some help for minor or major emotional, behavioural, educational, social and psychiatric problems. Who provides that help, and whether psychiatric help will be needed, tends to operate on an arbitrary basis, and an understanding of the factors involved helps define the limits and role of adolescent psychiatry.

For example, suppose a 15-year-old girl becomes depressed because of problems at school. Her parents may be perceptive enough, available enough and competent enough to help her effectively by themselves. This says something about their skills as parents, and about relationships in the family as a whole.

If they can't help, their perception of what is wrong (which is likely to be a subjective judgement and determined by past experience) will influence what action they take next. They might see the problem in 'normal' terms, to do with growing up in general and school in particular, and talk to their daughter's teacher. This may prove a helpful step which resolves the problem. Alternatively they might be more influenced by the girl's symptoms, and this plus a tendency to use, or

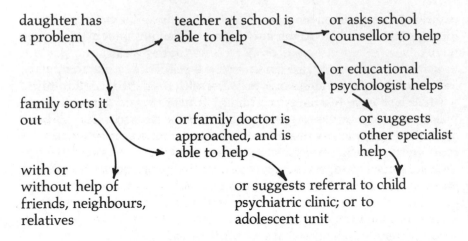

Figure 2.2   Routes to psychiatric and other help.

trust, medical services in general, or their family doctor in particular, may result in an approach to their general practitioner.

Let us suppose a teacher is approached, but can't help sufficiently. It may then be decided that the girl should see the school counsellor. Or, there may not be a school counsellor, but the educational psychologist may happen to have an interest in helping young people with emotional problems, and his or her assistance might be sought.

Let us suppose that she is very distressed indeed, perhaps with ideas of injuring herself. The educational psychologist may have the experience, personality and skills to see the girl through this difficult time, and does so successfully. Another educational psychologist, however, might have suggested the girl's referral to a child psychiatric clinic.

Had the girl seen the family doctor, he or she might have treated her successfully by talking things over once or twice with the girl and the family, separately or together; or the health visitor or community psychiatric nurse might have been asked to help in a similar way; or the doctor might have prescribed tranquillisers or antidepressant drugs. At any point, early or late, the family doctor might have decided on a referral to the child psychiatrist at the local clinic or adolescent unit.

It takes little imagination to think of the other permutations of personalities and circumstances which could take an adolescent through every conceivable route in Fig. 2.2, coming across an adolescent psychiatrist early, late, not at all, or even more than once. And note that the alternative sequences described above do not necessarily mean that successive helpers have tried, failed and then referred. The referral routes are as much guided by adults' perceptions and attitudes as by 'success' or 'failure' in helping. Some grasp of this network of possible pathways from person to person will help the adolescent psychiatrist understand not only how the perceived problem has built up, but who is still available to help.

Elsewhere I have discussed more fully the influences on the referral of young people to adolescent psychiatrists (Steinberg, 1981, 1982, 1983), and Bruggen and Westland (1979) have discussed the question of 'hard to place' young people. Meanwhile, it is fundamental to appreciate that when an adolescent becomes a psychiatric patient, external factors (e.g. in school, family and elsewhere) contribute as much to the 'psychiatric problem' as do factors within the young person's *soma* and *psyche*. Hence the adolescent psychiatrist and his colleagues are prepared to respond partly with diagnosis and treatment of the adolescent, and partly with help, advice and consultation for the other people in the adolescent's life.

Schools of thought

With so many different types of problem and presentation, professional workers can 'go in', as it were, at any level, and correspondingly have developed quite different ways of working, different training programmes and qualifications, and a whole range of schools of thought. Suffice it to say that the professional work likely to be encountered in the field will include individual counselling; individual psychotherapies of many different types; creative therapies such as art and drama; work in groups, sometimes focussed on family activities, sometimes on vocational training programmes and sometimes in the form of group therapy; residential educational or therapeutic programmes, often combining both; various types of behaviour therapy; and physical treatment. The latter will usually be drugs for psychiatric symptoms or physical disorder, but may also include general attention to physical health (as in acne, malnutrition or self-injury) and, although rarely, electroconvulsive treatment.

Few treatments are the province of only one sort of worker. Although only registered medical practitioners can prescribe officially listed drugs, anybody else can legally undertake the various psychotherapies and social and behavioural therapies. In practice the newcomer to the field will find that there is much variation in who does what, this depending on individual workers' training, skill and experience and the policy of the unit or department. Thus it is not unusual in psychiatric settings for a psychologist to conduct family therapy, a nurse to run a behaviour training programme or for a social worker to be an individual psychotherapist.

Commonly, more than one approach to overall management is taken. It sometimes happens that an adolescent may attend for regular individual out-patient sessions and for the rest of the 167 hours of the week lead his or her ordinary life. But it is common in adolescent psychiatry for some other work to be necessary too. For example, work with the parents and school may go in parallel with the adolescent's psychotherapy. Adolescents with more than one problem may have combinations of treatment, especially in clinics which are regarded as eclectic, i.e. willing to try anything that may help. Thus a boy or girl might be treated with both individual and family psychotherapy, or family therapy and a behaviour programme, or any of these plus medication.

Eclecticism is by no means universally admired, on the grounds (which I consider dubious) that if a clinician is truly 'committed' to a particular way of seeing an adolescent's problems, his or her purity or vision and practice is compromised by considering another perspective. A more serious criticism of eclecticism, in my view, is when a clinician or team purports to consider the whole range of approaches, but in practice has a hidden ranking system prejudiced in favour of a limited number of approaches. Thus a psychiatrist may believe firmly that, for example, drugs or individual psychotherapy is in general the best approach but 'allows' a colleague to conduct family therapy too; or vice versa. A better form of eclecticism is holism: i.e. a comprehensive, holistic (or 'wholistic') view is taken of the problems adolescent and family bring, and the whole range of possibly helpful responses considered. The different conceptual models used in psychiatric diagnosis and treatment in general are discussed elsewhere (Tyrer and Steinberg, 1987). Also considered elsewhere are the range of different professional contributions to adolescent psychiatry and the problems and opportunities of working together (Steinberg, 1986).

The development of adolescent psychiatry

Child and adolescent psychiatry has its roots in the child guidance movement. This began in the United States with the Judge Baker Guidance Centre in Boston in 1917, and the Boston Habit Clinic in 1921. A number of earlier developments had produced a climate in which such developments were possible.

First, in Europe and the United States, there had in the nineteenth century been a growth of the State taking an interest in children and their education, as opposed to the Church and purely private institutions. New possibilities in psychological assessment contributed to this.

Second, again on both sides of the Atlantic, and partly due to the Industrial Revolution with its vast movement of populations from the country into the towns, governments became more aware of how many rootless and neglected boys and girls there were, and set out to improve the law and the facilities for young people and families. No doubt they were driven by the need for competent, fit recruits to industry as well as by humanitarian aims. Thirdly, there had been major developments in psychiatry, psychology and education, notably the work of Pavlov (1849-1936) on physiological conditioning, Watson (1978-1958) on behaviourism, and Freud (1856-1939) on psychoanalysis; and the work of therapist-educationalists such as Montessori (1870-1952), Froebel (1782-1852) and Steiner (1861-1925). Children came to public attention as young people to whom the community had serious responsibilities, their deprivation and problems were perceived a little more clearly, and there now seemed to be radical new means for assessing and helping them.

This new atmosphere was partly due to the influence of the psychiatrist Adolf Meyer (1866-1950) who saw disorder in terms of interacting physical, psychological and environmental factors. It was the influence of Meyer and his followers which led to the development of child guidance, as it was called, in the United States, in which psychiatrists, psychologists and social workers operated together in the interests of disturbed children. Similar clinics were set up in England in the 1920s. Among the first was the East London Child Guidance Clinic, later named the Emmanuel Miller Clinic after its first director. By 1939 there were forty-six clinics in Great Britain.

Some of the children seen in these clinics were adolescents, but two groups of particularly disturbed or handicapped adolescents were meanwhile receiving attention elsewhere. Since the nineteenth century there had been special hospital units for severely retarded children and adolescents, and mentally ill young people were among those admitted to the general psychiatric hospitals. Two hospitals in particular were able, from the 1930s, to admit voluntary patients and not only those who were certified insane. They were St Ebba's Hospital in Epsom, Surrey, and Bethlem Royal Hospital in South London. Both hospitals began to accumulate a number of adolescent patients, and this led to the first adolescent psychiatric units being founded at St Ebba's in 1948 (Sands, 1953) and Bethlem Royal Hospital in 1949 (Warren 1952). The St Ebba's unit later moved to Long Grove Hospital. Soon after this, Beech House adolescent unit, near Canterbury, was opened (Turle, 1960). This was followed by an expansion in the number of in-patient

Table 2.1   Some developmental milestones in child and adolescent care.

1890–1920	Development of psychoanalysis and behavioural psychology. Development of intelligence tests (Stanford-Binet test, 1916). Establishment of special educational methods by Montessori and Steiner.
1883	Foundation of National Society for the Prevention of Cruelty to Children.
1909	Chicago Juvenile Psychopathic Clinic founded.
1917	Judge Baker Guidance Centre, Boston, founded.
1921	Boston Habit Clinic founded.
1920s	First child guidance clinics in Britain established.
1870–1944	Successive Education Acts, raising school leaving age first to 14, then higher.
1913–1927	Mental Deficiency Acts, legislating for the care of the mentally handicapped of all ages.
1930	Mental Treatment Act enabled voluntary treatment as well as compulsory treatment 'under certificate'.
1927–1935	Development of children's clinics at the Maudsley Hospital, and the opening of the Children's Department in 1939.
1933	First of a long series of Children's and Young Persons' Acts.
1942	Beveridge Report: Abolition of the Poor Law.
1948	National Assistance Act, based on the new concept of general social welfare; foundation of the National Health Service.
1949	First Adolescent Psychiatric Units opened in England.
1959	Mental Health Act, and new Act in 1983.

adolescent units, and a number of papers have described their functioning (e.g. Evans and Acton, 1972; Bruggen *et al.*, 1973; Framrose, 1975; Perinpanayagam 1978; Wells *et al.*, 1978; Bedford and Tennent, 1981; Steinberg *et al.*, 1981; Steinberg, 1982; Parry-Jones, 1986; Pyne *et al.*, 1986; Steinberg 1986).

From the 1960s on there was a degree of excitement about adolescent services, accompanied by a degree of concern. Adolescent psychiatry, and particularly the in-patient units, were breaking new ground in multidisciplinary work; in helping bring family therapy, community therapy and psychotherapy into the work of mental hospitals; and in trying to deal with a flood of particularly demanding young patients, whose crises could not always be readily resolved by those old psychiatric standbys of sedation, detention under the Mental Health Act or discharge.

The vicissitudes of multidisciplinary work generated interest and also some concern for staff, as did their need for encouragement and support and the need for proper training and supervision in a developing field. Such discoveries, (and they had some characteristics of the results of experiments) led to the foundation in 1969 of the Association for the Psychiatric Study of Adolescents. Its journal, the *Journal of Adolescence*, appeared in 1978, and should be known to people in the field. So also should the *Journal of Child Psychology and Psychiatry*, the organ of the Association for Child Psychology and Psychiatry. Serious students of adolescent psychiatry should find out what both organizations have to offer, in their meetings and through their journals.

Controversies

There are a number of important debates about the type of adolescent service to be preferred and encouraged. One argument is that the emphasis should be on treating the 'majority consumer group' – conduct problems – rather than the less common psychoses (Wells, 1986) while Steiner (1986) in a similar vein argues against adolescent units being 'eclectic' on the grounds that units with a limited but coherent approach are more successful, although he provides neither evidence nor anecdote to substantiate this. My own argument, by no means generally accepted, is that a psychiatric service for adolescents should be primarily a *general* psychiatric service, helping all those it can and conducting teaching and research about the generality of adolescent problems. (Steinberg 1983, 1986). The dual grounds for this view are that (a) this is the proper use of expensive, complex hospital units, whose historical and intellectual credentials and social justification are based on dealing with problems which have a strong biological component; and (b) that there is every reason to think that problems with a primarily social or psychosocial component can and should be the province of facilities whose framework is primarily psychosocial rather than medical – i.e. social, educational and psychotherapeutic services

(Steinberg 1981, 1982, 1983). In order to help adolescents and their families both sorts of service and expertise are needed, and they should collaborate closely. It is also important that medically based units, i.e. those run primarily by doctors and nurses, should be genuinely holistic, incorporating all aspects of life, including psychodynamic understanding, in their approach. But it is hard to see why any psychiatric unit should be founded or developed on an exclusively socially therapeutic or psychotherapeutic basis.

This, however, is one point of view among many. The trainee will need to be acquainted with the arguments, and make sure that he or she achieves a thorough and balanced experience.

An encouraging development has been the emergence of child and adolescent psychiatric nursing as an increasingly strong and professional group among the disciplines, although not invariably with the full support and encouragement of the nursing hierarchy within the hospitals. In the 1970s and 1980s, postgraduate training for nurses in the speciality has developed too (Wilkinson 1983, 1986). Child and adolescent psychiatric nurses expect (and are expected by their colleagues) to involve themselves in supervised therapeutic work, to take time for learning and teaching, to attend courses for their professional development, and to be involved in clinical and administrative decision-making meetings. It is only fairly recently that senior nursing administrators have come to accept these moves, and to see them as a model for wider aspects of nursing too, but they remain vulnerable to the Health Service's major economic problems.

During 1985 the National Health Service's Health Advisory Service conducted a major survey of adolescent services in parts of England, Scotland and Wales (Health Advisory Service 1986). They found a great deal of work going on, an impressive amount of commitment to the needs of young people, but also considerable muddle and overlap of services, many gaps in provision, much distrust between health, social services and education departments, and poor co-ordination – particularly at the higher managerial levels which controlled the financing of services. They found managers often lacking in a grasp of what was needed for young people, and tending to underestimate the types of problems and the expertise needed to deal with them. Further, insufficient account seemed to be taken of the views of the consumers of services. In psychiatry there was a lack of academic posts, and while child and adolescent psychiatric training was of a high standard, there was concern about the lack of psychiatrists with primarily adolescent experience. A particular need was recognized for better services for older adolescents, for those with brain damage, mental handicap, autism and other major disorders, and for greater emphasis on advisory and consultative work with other professions and agencies. In some respects the report makes sorry reading, and not everyone was in agreement with all the HAS findings nor indeed with the way the survey was conducted. For all its deficiencies, however, it drew attention to some major questions about adolescent services and adolescent psychiatry.

Concluding note

What conclusions can be drawn for clinical practice from the story of adolescent psychiatry's development so far? The field is still developing, and there is still no general agreement about the best way to organize services, or about the most appropriate roles for the people involved. There is also a lack of research, particularly about the effectiveness of different forms of intervention and management. Important emerging trends include a growing experience in psychological and social methods of management among professions other than psychology and psychiatry, and, part of the same process, the development of family work (including family therapy).

Three important effects of these trends can be predicted. First, there is the possibility of more work being conducted in homes and schools (the 'community') instead of in institutions; second, a 'pushing back' of help for troubled adolescents away from highly technical specialists and towards parents and teachers, though with the specialists' help on a consultative basis where needed; and, thirdly a reappraisal of the core functions of psychiatric practice with young people (Steinberg, 1981).

Finally, the history of the position of children in society is an important subject and puts developments in adolescent psychiatry into perspective. *The History of Childhood* (de Mause, 1980) and *Centuries of Childhood* (Aries, 1962) are both excellent. Warren's account of the development of child psychiatry at the Maudsley Hospital (Warren, 1975) and of adolescent services (Warren, 1971) are well worth reading, as is Barker on residential treatment (1974). The brief outline of adolescent psychiatry's history in this chapter is given a little more fully elsewhere (Steinberg, 1983). Finally, Millham and his colleagues have written excellent accounts of the community's clumsy attempts to deal with troublesome young people (Millham *et al.*, 1978; Millham, 1981).

References and further reading

Aries, P. (1962) *Centuries of Childhood*. New York: Vintage.

Barker, P. (1974) History. *In* Barker, P. (Ed), *The Residential Psychiatric Treatment of Children*. London: Crosby Lockwood Staples.

Bedford, A.P. and Tennent, T.G. (1981) Behaviour training with disturbed adolescents. *News of the Association for Child Psychology and Psychiatry* **7**, 6–12.

Bruggen, P., Byng-Hall, J. and Pitt-Aikens, T. (1973) The reason for admission as a focus of work in an adolescent unit. *British Journal of Psychiatry* **122**, 319–29.

Bruggen, P. and Westland, P. (1979) Difficult to place adolescents: are more resources required? *Journal of Adolescence* **2**, 245–50.

de Mause, L. (1980) *The History of Childhood*. London: Souvenir Press.

Evans, J. and Acton, W.P. (1972) A psychiatric service for disturbed adolescents. *British Journal of Psychiatry* **120**, 429–32.

Framrose, R. (1975) The first seventy admissions to an adolescent unit in Edinburgh : general characteristics and treatment outcome. *British Journal of Psychiatry* **126**, 380–9.

Health Advisory Service (1986) *Bridges Over Troubled Waters*. London: Department of Health and Social Security.

Millham, S. (1981) The therapeutic implications of locking up children. *Journal of Adolescence* **4**, 1, 13–26.

Millham, S., Bullock, F. and Hosie, K. (1978) *Locking Up Children: Secure Provision within the Child Care System*. Farnborough: Saxon House.

Parry-Jones, W.L. (1986) Multidisciplinary teamwork: help or hindrance? *In* Steinberg, D. (Ed), *The Adolescent Unit*, pp 193–208. Chichester : John Wiley and Sons.

Perinpanayagam, K.S. (1978) Dynamic approach to adolescence: treatment. *British Medical Journal*, **1**, 563–6.

Pyne, N., Morrison, R. and Ainsworth, P. (1986) A consumer survey of an adolescent unit. *Journal of Adolescence* **9**, 1, 63–72.

Sands, D.E. (1953) A special mental hospital unit for the treatment of psychosis and neurosis in juveniles. *Journal of Mental Science* **99**, 123–9.

Steinberg, D. (1981) *Using Child Psychiatry : the Functions and Operations of a Speciality*. London and Sevenoaks: Hodder and Stoughton.

Steinberg D. (1982) Treatment, training, care or control? The functions of adolescent units.*British Journal of Psychiatry* **141**, 306–9.

Steinberg, D. (1983) *The Clinical Psychiatry of Adolescence*. Chichester: John Wiley and Sons.

Steinberg, D. (ed) (1986) *The Adolescent Unit : Work and Teamwork in Adolescent Psychiatry*. Chichester: John Wiley and Sons.

Steinberg, D., Galhenage, D.P.C. and Robinson, S.C. (1981) Two years' referrals to a regional adolescent unit: some implications for psychiatric services. *Social Science and Medicine* **15E**, 113–22.

Steiner, J. (1986) Bridges over troubled waters. *Bulletin of the Royal College of Psychiatrists*, **10**, 9, 246 (correspondence).

Turle, G.C. (1960) On opening an adolescent unit. *Journal of Mental Science* **106**, 1320–6.

Tyrer, P. and Steinberg, D. (1987) *Models for Mental Disorder : Conceptual models in psychiatry*. Chichester: John Wiley.

Warren, W. (1952) In-patient treatment of adolescents with psychological illness. *Lancet* **i**, 147–50.

Warren, W. (1971) You can never plan the future by the past. The development of child and adolescent psychiatry in England and Wales. *Journal of Child Psychology and Psychiatry* **11**, 241–57.

Warren, W. (1975) Child psychiatry and the Maudsley Hospital: an historical survey. *In Institute of Psychiatry, 1924–1974*, pp 70–75.

Wells, P.G. (1986) Cut price adolescent units that meet all needs and none? *Bulletin of the Royal College of Psychiatrists*, 10.9, 231–232.

Wells, P.G., Morris, A., Jones, R.M. and Allen, D.J. (1978) An adolescent unit assessed: a consumer survey. *British Journal of Psychiatry* **132**, 300–8.

Wilkinson, T.R. (1983) *Child and Adolescent Psychiatric Nursing*. Oxford: Blackwell Scientific Publications.

Wilkinson, T.R. (1986) Education for nurses: support, supervision, training. *In* Steinberg, D. (Ed), *The Adolescent Unit*, pp 155–67. Chichester: John Wiley and Sons.

Chapter 3

Causes of Disorder and Influences on Development

Problems, disorders and causes : some general principles

First, the referral of an adolescent to a psychiatric clinic does not make the boy or girl the repository of disorder. This may seem an obvious point to make but in fact psychiatrists tend to be reluctant to diagnose 'no psychiatric abnormality'. That the referral has been made at all indicates a problem somewhere, and this needs a helpful response in the form of explanation or advice to adolescent and family, and perhaps consultation with the referring agent (see Chapter 18); but a diagnosis and treatment may both be unnecessary.

Second, where there is disorder, it should be remembered that aetiology in psychiatry is a complex matter. Many important factors are associated with the development of disorder in the sense that statistically they cluster with it, but that does not mean they *cause* disorder in the individual's case. Where such factors do lead more or less directly to disorder, they may act by:

(1) Predisposing to disorder (e.g. genetic vulnerability to a schizophrenic illness)
(2) Precipitating disorder (e.g. adverse circumstances)
(3) Perpetuating disorder (e.g. a pattern of behaviour in a family)

Note also that protective factors may operate, so that disorder does not always develop even when adverse factors are present. Furthermore, several different factors may operate (i.e. aetiology may be multifactorial), they are likely to affect each other (i.e. they are interactional) and that this interaction happens over time (it is developmental).

Third, competent management in adolescent psychiatry requires recognition of the different possible components of disorder. Disorder may be manifested in any or all of the following ways:

(1) Distress – felt by the patient.
(2) Disability – something the patient should be able to do but cannot.
(3) Disturbed behaviour about which others are concerned, whether or not the patient is also distressed or disabled.
(4) Diagnostic symptoms and signs – whether or not accompanied by any of the above.

This categorization of the 'disorder' allows for both a statement of *problems* being experienced by all concerned, and a *clinical diagnosis*. It is always helpful to attempt both. Even when a definite disorder cannot be identified, a simple statement of who is concerned about what is an immediate guide as to how to proceed helpfully. When a clinical diagnosis can be made, there is still a need to clarify how the adolescent and family are affected. This discussion is taken further in Chapter 5.

Fourth, it should be recognized that family therapists give priority to an account by the family of the family's problems, rather than to the individual diagnosis of the identified patient. Some never concern

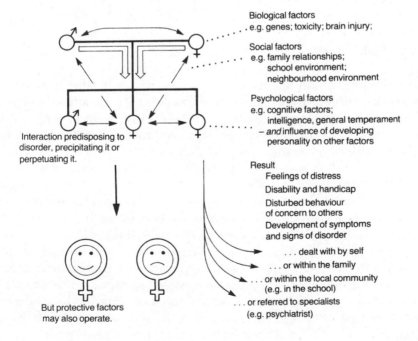

Biological factors
e.g. genes; toxicity; brain injury;

Social factors
e.g. family relationships;
school environment;
neighbourhood environment

Psychological factors
e.g. cognitive factors;
intelligence, general temperament
– *and* influence of developing
personality on other factors

Interaction predisposing to
disorder, precipitating it or
perpetuating it.

Result
Feelings of distress
Disability and handicap
Disturbed behaviour
of concern to others
Development of symptoms
and signs of disorder

. . . dealt with by self
. . . or within the family
. . . or within the local community
(e.g. in the school)
. . . or referred to specialists
(e.g. psychiatrist)

But protective factors
may also operate.

Figure 3.1 Schema for interaction of factors.

themselves with individual clinical diagnosis at all; others allow for the individual diagnosis while concentrating on family issues (see Chapter 18). However, the concept of disorder given above, and outlined in Fig. 3.1 incorporates both internal (individual) and external (family and social) systems and can be adapted to both approaches.

Fifth, disorder may be more or less circumscribed, or more or less pervasive, i.e. involving personality development. In childhood and adolescence it is not always easy to tell which is the case. Thus enuresis, for example, or a psychotic illness, may occur in an adolescent who has so far developed normally and who after the illness is over will continue to develop normally. Alternatively, a disorder may be part of longer standing problems in psychological, neurophysiological and social development, and in turn contribute to further developmental problems. An adolescent who needs only a short period of counselling to help him over a crisis may be launched upon several years of open-ended psychotherapy in the belief that his problem is more pervasive or profound than it actually is. Conversely, an adolescent's symptoms may be treated without sufficient attention being paid to longer standing, more pervasive factors in his personality or family which have sustained the disorder and will very likely lead to relapse. A proper understanding of the nature of disorder and good clinical practice should allow for both possibilities.

Aetiological factors

It is the interaction between aetiological factors as time goes by that makes a *developmental* conceptual model necessary in child and adolescent psychiatry. Thus depression in a mother, alcoholism in a father and poor parenting skills in both may lead to conduct problems in their child, and these become steadily worse as child and parents distress each other further and habits become established. Again, social and cultural circumstances, similar to those which made the parents what they are, may now lead the misbehaving young person into a school or children's home environment in which even worse behaviour, more distress and despair and more deficient social skills develop. It takes little imagination to appreciate how deprived social circumstances may lead to brain damage (see Chapter 17) through injury, malnutrition or toxic effects, and add another dimension to the complex spiral of cause and effect. While keeping in mind this interaction over time, and its effect on development, it is possible nonetheless to separate out the following factors in the origins of abnormal development and disorder:

- Genetic and chromosomal factors;
- Neurological factors;
- Constitutional and temperamental factors;
- Family and social influences.

Genetic factors

The concept of genetic influence upsets those who like to believe that environmental management can achieve an ideal normality for all. This political view assumes that geneticists believe that our genes predetermine everything important about us, which of course they do not. Leaving aside major diseases clearly transmitted by genes, such as Huntington's chorea, genetic influences in psychiatry are characterized by (a) the inheritance of traits or tendencies rather than specific abnormalities; (b) polygenic inheritance, that is to say more than one gene being influential; (c) the concept of threshold effects (i.e. the presence of particular genes does not mean that the characteristic they represent will be exhibited). Furthermore, the end-effect of genes is to fix what Gottesman (1963) called a reaction range, the *possibilities* (e.g. of intellectual level, or of an illness like schizophrenia) which require particular other influences (biological, psychological or social) to operate for their full expression.

In an extended family the particular characteristic or anomaly may be fully expressed or only partially expressed. Thus an adolescent may develop a schizophrenic illness while a parent, for example, may show schizoid traits. If this is the case in a particular family, schizoid characteristics such as oddness, social withdrawal and difficulties in relationships on the part of a parent may contribute to the anxieties and confusion of the child. In this way the developing young person may be on the receiving end of both internal and external factors leading to the development of disorder. Conversely, it is not difficult to see how the absence of one factor may mean that the *potential* problem of having an odd gene or an odd parent never becomes an *actual* problem.

Schizophrenia is used as an example because its genetics have been widely studied (see Chapter 15) but this model of family genes and family patterns of behaviour interacting may well apply to other conditions, including minor personality traits as well as major disorders. For an excellent account of genetic influences in child and adolescent psychiatric disorder see McGuffin and Gottesman (1986).

Genes are carried on chromosomes, and chromosomal abnormalities therefore increase genetic abnormalities and their effects. Human cells contain twenty-three pairs of chromosomes – twenty-two pairs of autosomes and one pair of sex chromosomes. The latter are identified as XX in the female and XY in the male. Chromosomes are studied by microscopical examination of white blood cells or cells scraped from the buccal mucosa. Abnormalities of the autosomes have profound effects and where the foetus survives cause major physical abnormalities and severe degrees of mental retardation. Such problems will not present for the first time in adolescence, although it is important to remember that there are adolescents with such abnormalities in various institutions; in general the problems of these young people and their families do not attract the interest and resources devoted to adolescents with other mental problems.

Before considering sex chromosome anomalies it is worth noting Shield's point (1980) that the most far-reaching influence on social and emotional development, including predisposition to different types of disorder, is the inheritance of an XX (i.e. female) or XY (i.e. male) chromosomal constitution. It is the presence or absence of the Y chromosome that determines the formation and maturation of testes or ovaries, the primary sex characteristics, which in turn produce the hormones which lead to exhibition of the secondary sex characteristics in adolescence. Sex chromosome abnormalities such as Klinefelter's syndrome (for which the notation is 47,XXY or alternatively XXY, i.e. an extra X chromosome) and Turner's syndrome (45,X or alternatively XO) widely affect development. The term for the technical notation for describing the chromosomes in this way is the karyotype. For an account of chromosomal anomalies and their effects see Gath (1985) and Kirman (1985).

Neurological factors

Four main areas of disorder should be considered separately:

Brain damage: various degrees of injury to the brain.
Mental retardation: various degrees of intellectual deficit and general mental handicap.
Epilepsy: This may or may not be associated with brain damage, mental handicap and psychiatric problems.
Neurological disorder: brain disorder, including neurodegenerative disorders.

Some of these, such as the neurodegenerative disorders, are extremely rare, but can present in adolescence with all the appearances of primarily psychiatric disorders. Hepatolenticular degeneration

(Wilson's desease) is an example. Other conditions are relatively common, e.g. the epileptic disorders, but their contribution to an adolescent's problems can be extremely varied. For example, a boy or girl may suffer from the direct effect of the epilepsy on his or her behaviour; from the side effects of medication; or from parental anxiety or social stigma. The effect of mental retardation can be similarly complex and variable. These conditions and their significance for clinical practice are described in Chapter 17.

Fuller reading in this area requires familiarity with neurology and developmental paediatrics. The investigation of the neurodegenerative disorders represents several growing points of research and is not readily summed up in the textbooks. Shaffer (1985) provides a good guide to brain injury in general, and Ebels (1980) to underlying principles of central nervous system maturation. Lishman's *Organic Psychiatry* (1978) is excellent as a guide to neuropsychiatry despite containing little specific to adolescence. Again not specific to adolescence, but useful nonetheless, is Neville's account (1979) of neuropsychiatric investigation. A good guide to paediatric neurology is provided by Brett (1983).

Constitutional and temperamental factors.

If by *personality* we mean that more or less characteristic, coherent and enduring set of ways of thinking and behaving that develop through childhood and adolescence, then by *constitution* we mean those inherited (genetic) and acquired physiological qualities that underlie personality.

The intervening variable, the link between constitution and personality, is described as the *temperament*. Temperament is difficult to define or even describe (see, for example, Berger 1985); the individual qualities to which it refers are such things as emotional style and responsiveness, sociability, adaptability and activity levels, in so far as these are attributes of the developing individual rather than occasional reactions to circumstances. Until these complicated concepts are defined more tidily, one may say that constitution is essentially physical; that temperamental characteristics grow out of this physical substrate, for example as activity levels, sociability and a tendency to various moods; and that personality represents the integration of temperament with prevailing ideas, attitudes and ways of behaving.

There is no doubt that children's individuality in these respects is identifiable early in life, and that temperamental characteristics can predict later problems, e.g. at school (Graham *et al.*, 1973). Such characteristics seem to operate largely by making the child vulnerable to external (e.g. parental) influences, which themselves may make a passing problem into a persisting one. By the time of adolescence, distinguishing between primarily individual factors and primarily family (and other environmental) factors is to a large extent a matter of conjecture. What is important for clinical practice is that the evidence points to a complex interaction between individual and environmental influences as already described.

Family and social influences

Important areas which have been studied include:

- the effects of separation and loss
- effects of parental care and control;
- effects of parental mental disorder;
- effects of parental criminal behaviour;
- effects of family structure
- effects of family patterns of behaviour;
- effects of adoption and fostering;
- effects of school;
- social group influences;
- cultural and transcultural influences;

Attachment, separation and loss

Attachment theory (in fact it is a conceptual model incorporating a number of observations and theories) developed from studies of infants and young children (Bowlby, 1969, 1973, 1980). It proposes that social competence and normal emotional development depend on the experience of secure emotional attachments in earlier life.

There is, for example, some evidence of emerging social confidence in young children who had experienced good mother-infant relationships (Campos *et al.*, 1983) and of self-reliance and courage in adverse conditions among young men from families which had achieved the right balance between protection and exposure (Ruff and Korchin, 1967; Bowlby, 1973). What is not clear from the various studies is how far such positive experiences in childhood help in later life because of a development in emotional development, in social skills (e.g. capacity to recruit and use help) or in the persistence of a series of supportive relationships; all three could of course operate. Attachment theory can provide a conceptual model for the successful integration of good experience throughout life, so that the indiviual who has been competently cared for in turn becomes a competent care-giver (Steinberg, 1983), and this is of course crucial for adolescence, where dependent child becomes potential parent. However, the theory is wide-ranging and its many facets have yet to be explored empirically.

It is known that early experience of disrupted or discordant family relationships, or lack of parental affection, increases the incidence of emotional and personality problems later (Brown *et al.*, 1985; Quinton and Rutter, 1984; and review by Wolkind and Rutter, 1985a).

Studies of bereavement and depression suggest that the death of a parent in childhood, especially around the age 3 or 4, and especially if the parent was of the same sex, increases the likelihood of psychiatric disturbance in later childhood or adolescence. Loss of a parent by separation or divorce carries a greater risk, which may be accounted for by the influence of the problems leading up to and perhaps following the actual separation. (Rutter, 1966). Emotional reality has no less an impact than objective reality : loss of a parent by separation can be felt by the child as at least as great a trauma as loss by death – perhaps even greater, depending on circumstances leading up to and following the loss. The way both parents handle a separation of any sort can profoundly influence how the child copes with it. It is important to remember the wider effects of loss on the family : the loss of one parent may depress, preoccupy and incapacitate the other to an extent that it is as if the child has lost both parents. Careful history-taking almost invariably demonstrates what many studies show : that it is not the single tragic event that profoundly disturbs children, but the accumulation and interaction of sequences of linked and interacting events.

Shorter term studies show that depressed mood and school problems are common in the first year after bereavement, but severe adult-type depressive illness appears to be less common. When it does occur it is particularly seen in adolescent boys who have lost their fathers (Van Eerdewegh *et al.*, 1982).

Parental care and control

It is the extremes of parental behaviour, e.g. excessive permissiveness, negligence, overprotectiveness and rigid discipline which tend to be associated with many of the problems in child and adolescent development. However, studies have shown that it is the details of parental behaviour rather than the general approach which are the most formative. For example, the parents of impulsive, aggressive children tend to be less controlling, less demanding and less well organized than other groups; while the parents of anxious and insecure children tend to be overcontrolling in a way that generates anxiety and fails to provide emotional support (see review by Rutter and Cox, 1985).

In adolescence there is an important degree of reciprocity between what the young person experiences in the family and what goes on outside. If relationships and experiences are satisfactory in the home, the adolescent is likely to use parents as well as peers as guides to behaviour. If relationships are unsatisfactory, it is more likely that peer behaviour will be sought which is in opposition to parental influence. (Brittain, 1968; Larson, 1975; Parry-Jones, 1985). In this respect the degree to which the adolescent is able to use a parent as a role model is important (Conger, 1977; Coleman, 1980).

In clinical work the parental behaviours often associated with adolescent disturbance, and which when modified can help put things right include:

(1) lack of confidence about being adult and weakness at limit-setting;
(2) parental and marital distress;
(3) inability to provide the model of a reasonably competent adult who enjoys life;
(4) difficulty in maintaining appropriate roles and boundaries so that, for example, it may not be clear whether parents, grandparents or the children are in charge;
(5) difficulty in getting the balance right between being too protective and intrusive on the one hand or negligent and uninterested on the other;
(6) giving in too readily to adolescent demands, on the one hand, or not listening to the adolescent's point of view on the other;
(7) becoming so upset by adolescent demands that the parent becomes childishly angry and vulnerable. This can lead to parents saying hurtful, undermining things to their children; every bit as bad is the loss of confidence on the part of the adolescent, who gets the impression (sometimes accurately) that the adults are scared of them, dislike them, cannot look after them and don't know what to do.

It is all a matter of balance between one extreme and the other, and most parents get it sufficiently right (including of course the balance between making mistakes and being perfect). However, where parents are in real difficulties the clinician should look in particular at three areas: *first*, the parents' experience of their own adolescence and their own parents at the time; *second*, the family's capacity for new learning and change; *third*, the possibility that individual disorder in the adolescent is the primary destabilizing factor.

Parental mental disorder

The systematic studies of the effects of parental mental illness on children are largely concerned with the very young, and in general they show a real but variable risk. It is at its greatest when the effect of the illness is to undermine parental skills and confidence as outlined above, and particularly when both parents are unwell (see Rutter and Cox, 1985).

In clinical practice parental mental illness can have impact in three main ways: (1) When it has been a feature of family life and interacting with the child's problems for several years past; (2) when it interferes with the developmental tasks of adolescence, for example when a depressed parent is thereby too vulnerable to the adolescent's challenges; and (3) when it interferes with treatment. This may happen in many ways, for example when the parent is quite unable to change his or her pattern of parenting, or when a distressed parent becomes envious of the care and attention the adolescent is receiving, and begins to compete for it.

Parental criminal behaviour

There is a strong association between delinquency in the child and criminality in the parent, and where both parents are criminal the association is even stronger (Rutter and Giller, 1983). There has been much speculation on the reasons for this, and poverty and large family size seem influential but are by no means the whole story (West and Farrington, 1973). Again, poor parenting skills and family discord may be important linking factors. Modelling may be another factor, except that by the time delinquency appears in young people their parents tend to have ceased active engagement in crime (West and Farrington, 1973).

Family size and structure

Children from large families (more than 5 children) tend to show a greater incidence of conduct problems, delinquency, lower verbal intelligence and lower reading attainment (Rutter and Mittler, 1972; Rutter and Madge, 1976). The risk of antisocial behaviour is higher when the children are all or mostly boys (Robins et al., 1975; Jones et al., 1980). First-born (i.e. eldest) children tend to have higher levels of achievement (Rutter and Madge, 1976) and higher incidence of emotional disorder (Rutter et al., 1970).

Family patterns of behaviour

There have been a very large number of intriguing studies of ways in which the family system and its mode of communication might cause mental disorder; most of them are inconclusive. Thus there is no evidence that family behaviour can cause autism or schizophrenia (although it can precipitate episodes of the latter illness). On the other hand confused or conflicting communication in families, problems in resolving arguments or making decisions, and the generation of high levels of tension do seem to be associated with child disturbance in general (see review by Rutter and Cox, 1985) An interesting finding by Blakar and his colleagues was that 'pseudodialogue', a mutual retreat from the task of useful communication, was evident in families with schizophrenic members. In the same study, families with borderline members were characterized by a preoccupation with misunderstanding and its use as a form of conflict (Blakar, 1980).

Other ways in which family behaviour may influence the emergence and resolution of disorder are described in Chapter 18.

Adoption, fostering and institutional care

There is an increased rate of psychiatric disorder among adopted children, with conduct disorder among adopted boys being most prominent. The reasons for this may include whatever factors led to adoption; the fact of adoption itself; parental attitudes, expectations and style of upbringing; the adolescent's image of natural and adoptive parents; and the effect of this on self-image (Hersov, 1985). A recurring impression in the cases of disturbed young people who have been adopted, is that the adolescent cannot seem to take his belonging to the family for granted in the way that another boy or girl can. Similarly, there is a real or imagined vulnerability on the part of the parents to the adolescent's challenges. This vulnerability, with the consequent feeling of being on thin ice when the adolescent becomes really difficult, may be a factor in the aetiology of some problems and a complicating factor in others.

A number of studies have shown, however, that even though the rate of problems in adopted children is higher than for the general population, it is lower than for children brought up in institutions. Further, most adoptions have a good outcome, including children adopted 'late' (between the ages of 5 and 12). (See Hersov's review, 1985; and also Tizard, 1977 and Triseliotis and Russell, 1984.).

The term fostering causes confusion. In the United States it includes care in institutions, while in Britain it may mean anything from daily minding at one extreme to the provision of a long-term home (and which, incidentally, it can be hard for the adolescent to distinguish from adoption). Most studies of fostering show quite a high failure rate (Parker, 1966) and an increased rate of emotional, conduct and educational problems (Prosser, 1978). A more encouraging picture has come from the Kent Special Family Placement Project with reports of high levels of success with difficult and disturbed teenagers placed with foster families (Hazell, 1980; Kent Family Placement Project, 1980).

Institutional care, the placement of children and adolescents in children's homes, is associated with a higher rate of disturbance than in the general population and than among adopted children, with antisocial behaviour being prominent (Wolkind, 1974). In a long-term study, women who had been in residential care in childhood showed a high incidence of psychosocial problems including family breakdown in adult life. Nevertheless, one third of the women studied were doing well, and among those who weren't their current problems seemed as influential as their past ones (Rutter and Quinton, 1984; Quinton and Rutter, 1984).

The outcome of institutional care is marked by problems through childhood and adolescence and into adult life, though it is important to remember that the circumstances that led to such care in the first place are likely to be influential too. Rutter (1982), Rutter and Quinton (1984) and Quinton and Rutter (1984) report the high level of personality problems, criminal behaviour, marital discord and disruption and major problems in parenting shown by women who had been brought up in children's institutions. These studies show that current circumstances are as important as their early childhood experiences. Correspondingly it has been shown in many studies that good experiences in early adulthood can counteract bad earlier experiences (e.g. Koluchova, 1976; Birtchnell and Kennard, 1983; Parker and Hadzli-Pavlovica, 1984); but the pattern tends to be one of adverse childhood experiences making the subsequent obtaining of 'protective' support less likely (Wolkind and Rutter 1985a).

There are, of course, many types of institutional care, and it may be assumed that children's homes vary in their successes with different children. The various specialized therapeutic communities, which are often selective, highly staffed with people with special skills, and correspondingly expensive, tend to report good results (e.g. Rose, 1986; Lampen, 1978) but this is a difficult field to study systematically. This type of setting is discussed further in Chapter 18.

The effects of schools

In Quniton's and Rutter's study (1984), girls brought up in institutions and who had a good school experience had a better outcome in adult life. It does seem that schools can have an influence on young people's achievements and behaviour that is not attributable simply to how the pupils were on entry (Rutter *et al.*, 1979). Wolkind and Rutter (1985b) have listed features of schools which have a positive effect on their pupils: high expectations for work and behaviour; good models of behaviour from teachers; respect for the children, with opportunities for them to take responsibilities in the school; good discipline, with appropriate praise and encouragement and sparing use of punishment; a pleasant working environment with good teacher-pupil relationships; and a good organizational structure that enables staff to work together with agreed academic and other goals. These findings perhaps come as no great surprise, yet there is no doubt that large numbers of adolescents are in schools which either do not acknowledge the above characteristics as desirable, or are unable to provide them.

The way in which the school has impact on the child is complex. It is mediated through the social group as a whole, and in particular through the peer group (Wolkind and Rutter, 1985b). The influence of the wider community, and in particular the standing of the school and its teachers in the community, are likely to be influential since we know that adolescents are influenced by a balance between what their peers think and what their parents think.

It is a common clinical experience that many behaviour problems, particularly of the less entrenched kind, can often be helped considerably when both parents are encouraged to go with their child to meet a key teacher. The young person's experience of all the adults being together in agreeing goals, setting limits and noting achievements seems helpful in many cases, and surprisingly often it hasn't been attempted before in the individual adolescent's case.

Social, cultural and transcultural influences

Life in inner city areas seems in general to increase the rate of behaviour problems compared with small towns and rural areas. For example, the prevalence of psychiatric disorder among young teenagers in rural areas seems to be about 10 per cent in studies in England (Rutter *et al.*, 1976; Graham *et al.*, 1973), and 8 percent in Norway (Lavik, 1977), with a rise to 20 per cent or more in towns (Leslie, 1974; Lavik, 1977). The possible reasons for this association are unclear and complicated; it is obvious that city life does not universally cause problems in adolescence, nor does rural life entirely protect against them. In inner cities there is more crowding, more general excitement and opportunities for a wide repertoire of behaviour, good and bad, and higher incidences of family discord, poor living conditions and parental mental illness. In some cities and some areas of cities there will be less social cohesion, poorer facilities of every sort and poorer schools/ For detailed reviews of this subject see Rutter and Madge (1976), Rutter (1979) and Wolkind and Rutter (1985b).

Similar influences, plus the effects on the family of immigration, unemployment and prejudice affect adolescents belonging to ethnic minority groups. The effect of such factors on the incidence of psychiatric disorder is not clear, but certainly there are a number of intercultural differences. For example, what have been described as hysterical pseudopsychotic states are more common among adolescents from some non-European cultures, conduct disorder and delinquency more common among black girls than white (Rutter and Giller, 1983), and anorexia nervosa is rare among black adolescents (Halmi *et al.*, 1977). The somatic expression of emotions is more common among black and Asian families (Katon *et al.*, 1982). For a general review of this subject from the point of view of general adult psychiatry, see Littlewood and Lipsedge (1982), and see p. 183.

What social circumstances do adolescents themselves worry about? In a survey by Porteous of 775 fifteen- year-olds in the north of England, anxiety about employment was prominent, especially among girls, as were worries about feeling adequate and confident and able to cope with the expectations at school; anxiety about examinations was common (Porteous 1979).

It now seems established that unemployment among adolescents is associated with an increase in psychiatric problems (Banks and Jackson, 1982) and in distress, lowered self- esteem and feelings of disillusion about using their own abilities and having any influence on their wider circumstances (Furnham, 1985). Conversely, young people with con- duct problems when at school are more likely than others to lose early any job they get (Rutter, 1982). Few studies mention the effect on adolescents of being members of a family where the father is out of work.

The effects of film and television violence have now been widely studied. There seems to be a modelling and imitative effect, particularly in younger children and among adolescents who already show conduct problems and delinquency, and the effects are more marked in boys. However, it is not clear how often the aggressiveness induced is translated into delinquent behaviour, and the greatest problems occur when exposure to this material is part of general exposure to violence, social problems and domestic chaos in the home. (Brody, 1977; Belson, 1978).

Concluding note

What are adolescents like, given these many and powerful influences acting on their development in a time of strain and change? Most people nurture their favourite stereotypes. In a British survey of newspapers' impressions (Falchikov, 1986), the 'typical adolescent' of 1985 was a criminally inclined, sporting boy or girl who is likely to be the victim of a wide variety of crimes and accidents, and likely also to be unemployed.

Williams (1986) reported on a more systematic survey of young people aged from 'under 14' to 'over 19' in which 15000 were contacted and a random sample of 2417 questionnaires studied. Most respondents were taking exams. For the most part they weren't cynical about governments, and most believed that politicians had influence and power; most also believed that in a technological age unemployment was inevitable. Nearly half, especially those from Asian or West Indian backgrounds had no views they regarded as political. Most thought premarital sexual relationships were acceptable but disapproved of extramarital sexual relationships. Over half the boys but well under half the girls thought homosexual relationships wrong. There was a high level of fear that riots and lack of safety on the streets would be increasingly common, but violent revolution was the prediction of only a small minority. Only a minority thought alcohol and drugs harmful. Most (70 per cent) believed in a deity 'at least some of the time', and over half believed in horoscopes. Racial prejudice was admitted by 42 per cent of whites and those from West Indian backgrounds; three-quarters of Asian background said they weren't racially prejudiced at all.

It is important to have an overall picture of the social and cultural influences on young people's lives, particularly because it throws light on alternative ways of helping those in difficulty, and on possible preventive measures. It also helps us ask the right questions in the individual adolescent's case. But it is also crucial to remember the essential individuality of the adolescent and family referred to the clinic, and not to make premature assumptions, whether based on simple prejudice or on the results of even the most sophisticated theory or respectable of surveys. It is particularly important to be aware of the great gulf between professional worker and 'patient' or 'client'. This divide is sometimes far greater, in my view, than any 'generation gap', or than the gap between some other cultural differences.

References and further reading

Banks, M.H. and Jackson, P.R. (1982) Unemployment and risk of minor psychiatric disorder in young people: cross-sectional and longitudinal evidence. *Psychological Medicine* **12**, 789–98.

Belson, W.A. (1978) *Television Violence and the Adolescent Boy*. Farnborough: Saxon House.

Berger, M. (1985) Temperament and individual differences. *In* Rutter, M. and Hersov L. (Eds), *Child and Adolescent Psychiatry: Modern Approaches* pp 3–16. Oxford: Blackwell Scientific Publications.

Birtchnell, J. and Kennard, J (1983) Marriage and mental illness. *British Journal of Psychiatry* **142**, 193–8.

Blakar, R.M. (1980) *Studies of Familial Communication and Psychopathology. A Social-Developmental Approach to Deviant Behaviour*. Oslo: Universitetsforlaget.

Bowlby, J. (1969) *Attachment and Loss. Volume 1: Attachment*. London: Hogarth Press.

Bowlby, J. (1973) *Attachment and Loss. Volume 2: Separation: Anxiety and Anger*. London: Hogarth Press.

Bowlby, J. (1980) *Attachment and Loss. Volume 3: Loss*. London: Hogarth Press.

Brett, E.M. (1983) (Ed) *Paediatric Neurology*. London: Churchill Livingstone.

Brittain, C.V. (1968) An exploration of the basis of peer-compliance and parent-compliance in adolescence. *Adolescence* **2**, 445–58.

Brody, S. (1977) Screen violence and film censorship – a review of research. *Home Office Research Study No 40*. London: Her Majesty's Stationery Office.

Brown, G.W., Harris, T.O. and Bifulco, A. (1985) Long-term effects of early loss of parent. *In* Rutter, M., Izard, C. and Read, P. (Eds), *Depression in Childhood: Developmental Perspectives*. New York: Guilford Press.

Campos, J.J., Barrett, K.C., Lamb, M.E., Goldsmith H.H. and Stenberg, C. (1983) Socioemotional Development. *In* Haith M.M. and Campos J.J. (Eds) *Infancy and Developmental Psychobiology Volume 2, Handbook of Child Psychology Edition 4*, pp 783–915. Chichester: John Wiley and Sons.

Coleman, J. (1980) *The Nature of Adolescence.* London: Methuen.

Conger, J.J. (1977) *Adolescence and Youth.* New York: Harper and Row.

Ebels, E.J. (1980) Maturation of the central nervous system. *In* Rutter, M. (Ed), *Scientific Foundations of Developmental Psychiatry*, pp 25–39. London: William Heinemann Medical Books.

Falchikov, N. (1986) Images of adolescence: an investigation into the accuracy of the image of adolescence constructed by British newspapers. *Journal of Adolescence* **9**, 167–80.

Farrell, C. and Kellaher, L. (1978). *My Mother Said: The Way Young People Learn About Sex and Birth Control.* London: Routledge and Kegan Paul.

Furnham, A. (1985) Youth unemployment : a review of the literature. *Journal of Adolescence* **8**, 109–24.

Gath, A. (1985) Chromosomal Abnormalities. *In* Rutter, M. and Hersov, L. (Eds), *Child and Adolescent Psychiatry : Modern Approaches.* 118–28. Oxford: Blackwell Scientific Publications.

Gottesman, I.I. (1963) Genetic aspects of intelligent behaviour. *In* Ellis, N. (Ed), *The Handbook of Mental Deficiency : Psychological Theory and Research*, pp 346–7. New York: McGraw-Hill.

Graham, P., Rutter, M. and George, S. (1973) Temperamental characteristics as predictors of behaviour disorders in children. *American Journal of Orthopsychiatry* **43**, 328–39.

Halmi, K.A., Goldberg, S.C., Eckert, E., Casper, R. and Davis, J.M. (1977) Pretreatment evaluation in anorexia nervosa. *In* Vigersky, R.A. (Ed), *Anorexia Nervosa*, pp 43–54. New York: Raven Press.

Hazell, N. (1980) Normalization or segregation in the care of adolescents. *In* Triseliotis, J. (Ed), *New Developments in Foster Care and Adoption*, pp 101–17. London: Routledge and Kegan Paul.

Hinde, R.A. (1980) Family Influences. *In* Rutter, M. (Ed), *Scientific Foudations of Developmental Psychiatry*, pp 47–66. London: William Heinemann Medical Books.

Hersov, L.A. (1985) Adoption and Fostering. *In* Rutter, M. and Hersov, L. (Eds), *Child and Adolescent Psychiatry : Modern Approaches*, pp 101–17 Oxford: Blackwell Scientific Publications.

Jones, M.B., Offord, D.R. and Abrams, N. (1980) Brothers, sisters, and antisocial behaviour. *British Journal of Psychiatry* **136**, 139–45.

Katon, W., Kleinman, A. and Rosen, G. (1982) Depression and somatisation : a review. *American Journal of Medicine* **72**, pp 127–35 and 241–7.

Kent Family Placement Project (1980) *Fourth Report*. Maidstone, Kent: Social Services Department.

Kirman, B. (1985) Mental retardation : medical aspects. *In* Rutter, M. and Hersov, L. (Eds), *Child and Adolescent Psychiatry : Modern Approaches*, pp 650–60. Oxford: Blackwell Scientific Publications.

Koluchova, J. (1976) Severe deprivation in twins : a case study. *In* Clarke A.M. and Clarke A.D.M. (Eds) *Early Experience : Myth and Evidence*, pp 45–55. London: Open Books.

Lampen, J. (1978) Drest in a little brief authority : controls in residential work with adolescents. *Journal of Adolescence* **1**, 163–75.

Larson, L.E. (1975) The relative influence of parent-adolescent effect. *In* Conger J.J. (Ed), *Contemporary Issues in Adolescent Development*. New York: Harper and Row.

Lavik, N.J. (1977) Urban-rural differences in rates of disorder. A comparative psychiatric population study of Norwegian adolescents. *In* Graham, P.J. (Ed), *Epidemiological Approaches in Child Psychiatry*, pp 223–51. London: Academic Press.

Leslie, S.A. (1974) Psychiatric disorder in the young adolescents of an industrial town. *British Journal of Psychiatry* **125**, 113–24.

Lishman, W.A. (1978) *Organic Psychiatry*. Oxford: Blackwell. Scientific Publications.

Littlewood, R. and Lipsedge, M. (1982) *Aliens and Alienists : Ethnic Minorities and Psychiatrists*. Harmondsworth: Penguin Books.

McGuffin, P. and Gottesman, I.I. (1986) Genetic influences on normal and abnormal development. *In* Rutter, M. and Hersov, L. (Eds), *Child and Adolescent Psychiatry : Modern Approaches* pp 17–33. Oxford: Blackwell Scientific Publications.

Neville, B. (1979) Progresive and static pathology in paediatric neurology. *Medicine* **33**, 1698–701.

Parker, G. and Hadzli-Pavlovica, D. (1984) Modification of levels of depression in mother-bereaved women by parental and marital relationships. *Psychological Medicine* **14**, 125–35.

Parker, R.A. (1966) *Decision in Child Care: A Study of Prediction in Fostering*. London: George Allen and Unwin.

Parry-Jones, W.L. (1985) Adolescent disturbance. *In* Rutter, M. and Hersov, L. (Eds) *Child and Adolescent Psychiatry : Modern Approaches* pp 584–98. Oxford: Blackwell Scientific Publications.

Porteous, M.A. (1979) A survey of the problems of normal 15-year olds. *Journal of Adolescence* **2**, 307–23.

Prosser, H. (1978) *Perspectives on Foster Care*. Windsor: National Foundation for Educational Research.

Quinton, D. and Rutter, M. (1984) Parenting behaviour of mothers raised in care. *In* Nicol, A.R. (Ed), *Longitudinal Studies in Child Psychology and Psychiatry : Practical Lessons from Research Experience.* Chichester: John Wiley and Sons.

Robins, L.N., West, P.A. and Herjanic, B.L. (1975) Arrests and delinquency in two generations: a study of black urban families and their children. *Journal of Child Psychology and Psychiatry* **16**, 125–40.

Rose, M. (1986) The design of atmosphere: ego-nurture and psychic change in residential treatment. *Journal of Adolescence* **9**, 49–62.

Ruff, G.E. and Korchin, S.J. (1967) Adaptive stress behaviour. *In* Appley M.H. and Trumbull, R. (Eds), *Psychological Stress.* New York: Appleton-Century- Crofts.

Rutter, M. (1966) *Children of Sick Parents. Institute of Psychiatry Maudsley Monographs, No. 16.* London: Oxford University Press.

Rutter, M. (1979) *Changing Youth in a Changing Society.* London: Nuffield Provincial Hospitals Trust.

Rutter, M. (1982) Epidemiological- longitudinal approaches to the study of development. *In* Collins, W.A. (Ed), *The Concept of Development. Minnesota Symposia on Child Psychology* 15, pp 105–44. New Jersey: Lawrence Erlbaum.

Rutter, M. and Cox, A. (1985) Other family influences. *In* Rutter, M. and Hersov, L. (Eds), *Child and Adolescent Psychiatry: Modern Approaches*, pp 58–81. Oxford: Blackwell Scientific Publications.

Rutter, M. and Giller, H. (1983) *Juvenile Delinquency.* Harmondsworth: Penguin Books.

Rutter, M., Graham, P., Chadwick, O. and Yule, W. (1976) Adolescent Turmoil : Fact or Fiction? *Journal of Child Psychology and Psychiatry* **17**, 35–6.

Rutter, M. and Madge, N. (1976) *Cycles of Disadvantage : A Review of Research.* London: Heinemann Educational.

Rutter, M., Maughan, B., Mortimore, P., Ouston, J. and Smith, A. (1979) *Fifteen Thousand Hours : Secondary Schools and their Effects on Children.* London: Open Books.

Rutter, M. and Mittler, P. (1972) Environmental influences in language development. *In* Rutter, M. and Martin J.A.M. (Eds), *The Child with Delayed Speech. Clinics in Developmental Medicine No. 43*, pp 52–67. London: Heinemann.

Rutter, M. and Quinton, D. (1984) Long-term follow-up of women institutionalised in childhood: factors promoting good functioning in adult life. Quoted in Wolkind, S. and Rutter, M., Separation, Loss and Family Relationships. *In* Rutter, M., and Hersov, L. (1985) *Child and Adolescent Psychiatry : Modern Approaches*, pp 34–57. Oxford: Blackwell Scientific Publications.

Rutter, M. and Quinton, D. (1977). Psychiatric disorder – ecological factors and concepts of causation. *In* McGurk (Ed), *Ecological Factors in Human Development*, pp 173–87. Amsterdam: Holland.

Rutter, M. Tizard, J. and Whitmore, K. (1970) *Education, Health and Behaviour*. London: Longman.

Shaffer, D. (1985) Brain damage. *In* Rutter, M. and Hersov, L. (Eds) *Child and Adolescent Psychiatry : Modern Approaches*, pp 129–51. Oxford: Blackwell Scientific Publications.

Shields, J. (1980) Genetics and mental development. *In* Rutter, M. (Ed), *Scientific Foundations of Developmental Psychiatry*, pp 8–24. London: Heinemann Medical Books.

Steinberg, D. (1983) *The Clinical Psychiatry of Adolescence. Clinical Work from a Social and Developmental Perspective*. John Wiley and Sons, Chichester.

Steiner, J. (1986) Bridges over troubled waters. *Bulletin of the Royal College of Psychiatrists*. 10, 9, 246 (Correspondence).

Tizard, B. (1977) *Adoption : A Second Chance*. London: Open Books.

Triseliotis J. and Russell, J. (1984). *Hard to Place : The Outcome of Late Adoptions and Residential Care*. London: Heinemann.

Van Eerdewegh, M.M., Bieri, M.D., Parrilla, R.H. and Clayton, P.J. (1982) The bereaved child. *British Journal of Psychiatry* **140**, 23–29.

Von Bertalanffy, L. (1968). *General Systems Theory*. New York: George Brazillier.

West D.J. and Farrington, D.P. (1973) *Who Becomes Delinquent?* London: Heinemann Educational Books.

Williams, M. (1986). The Thatcher Generation. *New Society* **75**, 1208, 312–15.

Wolkind, S. (1974) The components of 'affectionless psychopathy' in institutionalised children. *Journal of Child Psychology and Psychiatry* **15**, 215–20.

Wolkind, S. and Rutter, M. (1985a) Separation, loss and family relationships. *In* Rutter, M. and Hersov, L. (Eds), *Child and Adolescent Psychiatry : Modern Approaches*, pp 34–57. Oxford: Blackwell Scientific Publications.

Wolkind, S. and Rutter, M. (1985b) Sociocultural factors. *In* Rutter, M. and Hersov, L. (Eds), *Child and Adolescent Psychiatry : Modern Approaches*, pp 82–100. Oxford: Blackwell Scientific Publications.

Chapter 4

Disorders: Classification and Prevalence

The broad categories of problems

The young people the adolescent psychiatrist sees include (a) a variable minority with a major mental illness or other seriously disabling disorder; (b) a proportion where individual problems are clearly directly related to social and family circumstances; and (c) a number with nothing psychiatrically wrong at all. How many there will be in each of these broad categories will depend on the type of service in which the psychiatrist works.

Within these categories the type of problem seen will be immensely variable; many will defy our clear-cut diagnoses. Nevertheless, the idea of classification should go hand-in-hand with recognition of the unique characteristics of each new adolescent and family seen. The skill which enables the psychiatrist to be a clinician and not simply a technologist depends on being able to recognize those aspects of the patient and situation which are unique, and for which a response is needed that is human, empathic and creative; and those aspects which are similar to other people's problems. These latter similarities enable us to make classification systems and from them informed predictions – for example, about the likely effects of different sorts of treatment.

Classification is complicated. There are two alternative systems at the moment, although they are likely to learn from each other and grow closer with successive revisions. One is the *International Classification of Diseases*, 9th Revision (ICD 9), which is widely used in the United Kingdom (see Rutter *et al.*, 1975a, 1975b). The other is the *Diagnostic and Statistical Manual*, 3rd edition (DSM III) which is used in the United States (see American Psychiatric Association, 1979). Their relative merits have been reviewed by Rutter and Shaffer (1980) and Rutter and Gould (1985).

There are a number of problems in trying to classify children's and adolescents' disorders. First, every individual is unique, and labelling the disorder can become confused with labelling the person.

Second, classification systems are imperfect and provisional; they should assist thinking about clinical issues, not replace it. Making a diagnosis should therefore be a start to how we think about the nature of each adolescent's problems, not a conclusion.

Third, many problems simply do not fit neatly into the available categories. Often an adolescent's set of difficulties will be unlike any other; we should then acknowledge that the disorder can *not* be clearly categorized, but is similar to one or two others. A moment's thought will show that this is far more in the scientific tradition than is forcing observations into pre-set categories. (There was a time when the whale was thought to be a fish; in psychiatry, no doubt, there are still many mis-identified and misunderstood denizens of the deep.)

Fourth, many problems in child and adolescent psychiatry require description in both individual terms and in terms of the family or social circumstances. Perhaps this is most apparent with conduct problems, but even when a disorder seems primarily determined by the adolescent's internal physio-chemical state (for example a manic-depressive illness, or brain damage), there remain family and social interactional problems needing attention.

Finally, it clarifies matters to differentiate between problems and disorder (Steinberg 1983). Thus delinquency, a legal term, is a problem but may not be due to a disorder. Self-poisoning or 'overdosing', school non-attendance and repeated absconding are all serious problems, but may or may not be the result of disorder.

The multi-axial approach to classification

The multi-axial classification system was introduced in both the ICD and DSM III schemes (see above) to bring some order into the confusion which can arise in the description of young people's problems, and in this respect both systems represent an important advance. ICD-9 uses the following dimensions or axes:

Axis I: Clinical psychiatric syndrome (e.g. anorexia nervosa, schizophrenia, depressive illness).
Axis II: Specific delays in development (e.g. specific reading retardation).
Axis III: Intellectual level (e.g. normal range, moderate retardation).

Axis IV: Medical conditions (e.g. epilepsy, diabetes, asthma).
Axis V: Abnormal psychosocial situations (e.g. familial over-involvement, inconsistent parental control, adverse discrimination).

The descriptive diagnosis is made up of a statement about each axis, including of course the possibility of 'no significant problem' (coded as zero) in any or indeed all of the categories. Thus a mentally handicapped child in an over-anxious family and attending an inappropriate school might have problems recorded under Axes III and V (and under IV too, if there were identifiable brain disorder) while Axes I and II could record no abnormality. Similarly, a child with specific reading retardation or 'dyslexia' would have the problem recorded under Axis II but there need be no significant abnormality under any other heading.

It is important to remember that the system was designed to be a reliable descriptive system, without aetiological implications.

Disorder in the community

The prevalence of adolescent disorder in the community varies from place to place and with age, and depends on the criteria used. The figures given vary between around 10 and 20 percent. The lower end of the range is associated with younger adolescents with recognized (i.e. known to adults) psychiatric problems in more rural or suburban areas, and the upper figures are associated with older adolescents, with industrial and inner city areas and with the inclusion of problems not so evident to parents and teachers. (For example, see studies by Krupinski *et al.*, 1967; Graham and Rutter, 1973; Leslie, 1974; Rutter *et al.*, 1976; Lavik 1977). A reasonable rough guide to the prevalence of significant psychiatric disorder (i.e. causing distress or disability) in an adolescent population is the figure 15 per cent. (This also happens to be the approximate proportion of adolescents in most general populations, but this too varies considerably, depending of course on what the birthrate happened to be 10-20 years earlier.)

The prevalence of different types of disorder is discussed in the appropriate chapters.

Disorders seen in clinical practice

Table 4.1 is a composite picture of the types of disorder likely to be seen in a general psychiatric service for adolescents, and is based on data drawn from several accounts. (Warren, 1965a, 1965b; Bruggen *et al.*,

Table 4.1 Presenting problems and clinical diagnostic categories in
adolescent psychiatry.

(a) Problems on referral

1. *Misbehaviour,* including disruption and quarrelling at home and/or
   school, stealing at home or outside, association with an antisocial
   or delinquent peer group. (20 per cent)

2. *More serious misbehaviour,* including violence, fire-setting, running
   away from home, or serious risk-taking behaviour, e.g. drug and
   alcohol abuse or sexual promiscuity. Delinquent behaviour,
   including requests for Court reports. (10 per cent)

3. *School non-attendance.* (10 per cent)

4. *Threatened or attempted self-injury,* e.g. drug overdose. (10–15 per cent)

5. *Concern,* usually presented by adults rather than the adolescent,
   about the boy's or girl's mood (anxiety, misery, withdrawal),
   symptomatic behaviour (oddness, repetitive habits) or things they
   seem unwilling or unable to do (eat, sleep, mix socially, talk). (40
   per cent)

6. *Further opinion or help requested for a problem* (as above) where attempts
   at diagnosis and treatment have already been made, sometimes
   over several years and with several agencies. (10–20 per cent)

(b) Clinical diagnostic categories (in approximate order of frequency)

Mood disorders: emotional or mixed emotional/conduct disorders, or
   adult-type anxiety or depressive disorders, including obsessive-
   compulsive and phobic states.
Conduct disorders.
Problems of personality development with mood and/or conduct problems,
   including 'borderline' and schizoid personality disorders, and
   problems of sexual identity.
Schizophrenic, schizoaffective and affective (manic-depressive) psychoses.
Anorexia nervosa and bulimia nervosa, enuresis, encopresis, tics.
Hysterical disorders e.g. with paralysis and serious self-neglect.
Autism.
Brain disorder, including epilepsy and neurodegenerative disorder.

1973; Framrose, 1975; Steinberg *et al.*, 1981; Place *et al.*, 1985a, b; Pyne *et al.*, 1985; Steinberg, 1986). The picture presented is of the range of problems to be expected in clinical practice rather than their precise proportions. As would be anticipated, studies from in-patient units report more young people with psychotic disorders, child psychiatric clinics seeing more adolescents with school, family and social problems.

Changes in prevalence with age and sex

The overall pattern seems to be a gradually increasing prevalence of psychiatric disorder from around 10 per cent in children through 10-15 per cent in mid-adolescence, to around 20 per cent in adulthood, although some studies report a peak of about 20 per cent being reached in adolescence (e.g. Leslie, 1974). This is especially so where, as mentioned earlier, systematic studies reveal symptoms not already evident to the adults in contact with the teenagers (Graham and Rutter, 1973).

In adolescence, enuresis and encopresis are less common than in earlier childhood. Hyperactivity presents less often, but children who have been hyperactive in earlier childhood sometimes present in adolescence with behavioural and other social problems. In general more clear-cut, adult-type symptoms are seen in adolescence, so that we begin to see the classical symptoms of depressive illness, and anxiety, phobic and obsessional states, as well as the less well differentiated mood disorders of younger children.

In earlier childhood, equal numbers of girls and boys are affected by emotional disorders. In adolescence, however, as in adult life, more girls than boys are affected. The reverse is the case with conduct disorders, which are more prevalent among boys than girls in childhood and adolescence.

Delinquency, which as already stated is a legal term, not a clinical one, increases markedly in adolescence, and declines from early adulthood onwards. Again, it is more common in the male than the female population, but recent data show that girls are catching up. In the twenty years from 1957 to 1977 the ratio of male:female delinquency among teenagers changed from around 11:1 to 5:1 (Rutter and Giller, 1983). In absolute terms, the number of offenders of both sexes in the age range 14-17 years is currently of the order of 10,000 per 100,000 of the total population (Rutter and Giller, 1983).

Concluding note

Classification complements the other clinical skills. It is true that there are disadvantages to people of any age group being 'labelled', but the stigma of labelling or stereotyping is likely to depend on many factors other than whether or not the psychiatrist makes a diagnosis. For example, the young people attending a psychiatric clinic or admitted to hospital, or resident in a Children's Home or special school are likely, unfortunately, to be labelled and stigmatized by virtue of that status alone, and not only because a psychiatrist has described their problems or symptoms in a particular way.

Care should be taken in the way such descriptions are used, whether one is talking to the adolescent, other members of the family, or writing a letter or report. I think one should avoid thinking or writing of a patient of any age as 'a schizophrenic' or 'an anorexic'. It is not only discourteous but untrue, because the cluster of symptoms and signs (i.e. the syndrome) referred to by such a term does not convey enough to justify referring to *anyone* in that way. If we refer however to 'a girl with anorexia nervosa' this is a reminder that we are talking about someone who may be a sister, daughter, cousin, friend, student, stamp collector, amateur disco dancer, keeper of a cat and a member of a youth club (among other classifications), as well as having the characteristics of a particular disturbed way of functioning.

References and further reading

American Psychiatric Association (1979) *Diagnostic and Statistical Manual* (DSM III). 3rd edition. Washington, D.C: American Psychiatric Association.

Bruggen, P., Byng-Hall, J. and Pitt-Aikens, T. (1973) The reason for admission as a focus of work in an adolescent unit. *British Journal of Psychiatry*, 122, 319–29.

Framrose, R. (1975) The first seventy admissions to an adolescent unit in Edinburgh : general characteristics and treatment outcome. *British Journal of Psychiatry*, 126, 380–89.

Graham, P. and Rutter, M. (1973) Psychiatric disorder in the young adolescent: a follow-up study. *Proceedings of the Royal Society of Medicine* 66, 1226–9.

Krupinski, J., Baikie, A.G., Stoller, A., Graves, J., O'Day, D.M. and Polke, P. (1967). A community mental health survey at Heyfield, Victoria. *Medical Journal of Australia* 1, 124–36.

Lavik, N.J. (1977). Urban-rural differences in rates of disorder. A comparative psychiatric population study of Norwegian adolescents.

In Graham, P.J. (Ed) *Epidemiological Approaches in Child Psychiatry*, pp 223–51. London: Academic Press.

Leslie, S.A. (1974) Psychiatric disorder in the young adolescents of an industrial town. *British Journal of Psychiatry* **125**, 113–24.

Place, M., Framrose, R. and Wilson, C. (1985a) The difficult adolescents who are referred to a psychiatric unit. I : Classification. *Journal of Adolescence* **8**, 4, 297–306.

Place, M., Framrose, R. and Wilson, C. (1985b) The difficult adolescents who are referred to a psychiatric unit. II : Clinical features and response to treatment. *Journal of Adolescence* **8**, 4, 307–20.

Pyne, N., Morrison R., and Ainsworth, P. (1985) A follow-up study of the first 70 admissions to a general purpose adolescent unit. *Journal of Adolescence* **8**, 4, 333–45.

Rutter, M. and Giller, H. (1983). *Juvenile Delinquency*. Harmondsworth: Penguin Books.

Rutter, M. and Gould, M. (1985) Classification. *In* Rutter, M. and Hersov, L. (Eds) *Child and Adolescent Psychiatry : Modern Approaches*, pp 304–21. Oxford: Blackwell Scientific Publications.

Rutter, M., Graham, P., Chadwick, O. and Yule, W. (1976) Adolescent turmoil : fact or fiction? *Journal of Child Psychology and Psychiatry* **17**, 35–6.

Rutter, M. and Shaffer, D. (1980) DSM III: a stepforward or back in terms of the classification of child psychiatric disorders? *Journal of the American Academy of Child Psychiatry* **19**, 371–94.

Rutter, M., Shaffer, D. and Shepherd, M. (1975a) *A Multi-axial Classification of Child Psychiatric Disorders*. Geneva : World Health Organization.

Rutter, M., Shaffer, D. and Sturge, C. (1975b) *Guide to a Multi-axial Classification for Psychiatric Disorders in Childhood and Adolescence*. London: Institute of Psychiatry.

Steinberg, D. (1983) *The Clinical Psychiatry of Adolescence*. Chichester: John Wiley and Sons.

Steinberg, D. (1986) Developments in a psychiatric service for adolescents. *In* Steinberg, D. (Ed), *The Adolescent Unit : Work and Teamwork in Adolescent Psychiatry*, pp 209–21. Chichester: John Wiley and Sons.

Steinberg, D., Galhenage, D.P.C., and Robinson, S.C. (1981) Two years' referrals to a regional adolescent unit : some implications for psychiatric services. *Social Science and Medicine* **15E**, 113–22.

Warren, W. (1965a) A study of adolescent psychiatric in-patients and the outcome six or more years later. I. Clinical histories and hospital findings. *Journal of Child Psychology and Psychiatry* **6**, 1–17.

Warren, W. (1965b) A study of adolescent psychiatric in-patients and the outcome six or more years later. II. The follow-up study. *Journal of Child Psychology and Psychiatry* **6**, 141–60.

Chapter 5

The Clinical Interview: Assessment and Diagnosis

Introduction

It will be clear from the earlier chapters that assessment and management in adolescent psychiatry cannot be a matter of simply diagnosing a clinical syndrome and prescribing a treatment. Too many other questions intrude: for example, is there a treatment? Is there, for that matter, a disorder? Might parental anxiety about a depressed child be contributing to the depression? And whatever the problem, how much help for it can be provided by people other than the psychiatrist – for example, by the adolescent's parents and teachers? Further, the psychiatrist may clarify the problem, but the help needed may be the skills of quite different professional workers, such as a remedial teacher or a probation officer or education welfare officer. Finally, suppose the adolescent disagrees with the parents about the need for help?

Assessment in adolescent psychiatry therefore requires a far wider appraisal of who is concerned about what, and who is in a position to help, than the traditional clinical diagnosis can possibly provide.

An outline of assessment

The process of assessment can be considered as follows:

(1) Sources of information.
(2) Authority to proceed.
(3) Whom to invite to the assessment interview.
(4) When to meet : urgency.
(5) Where to meet : on whose territory?

(6) Problem clarification : the family's point of view, and the beginning of family assessment.
(7) The history.
(8) Individual assessment.
(9) Diagnosis.

(1) Sources of information

The information the clinician needs will be found partly with the referred adolescent, partly with the rest of the family, and partly with the schools the boy or girl has attended. Important information will also be with the referring professional worker (e.g. the family doctor or a social worker), and with others who may have been involved – for example, educational welfare officers, probation officers or a clinical or educational psychologist.

In practice:

(i)   Assume to begin with that all the family living together at home can help in the assessment, and invite them to it.
(ii) Find out which workers other than the referring professional have been involved.
(iii) Seek the parents' permission (and the adolescent's, if aged 16 plus) to contact them. Younger adolescents should also be consulted about contacting other people, but their formal permission is not essential. Permission should be in writing; your clinic should have its own form.
(iv) My own advice and practice is always to seek the family doctor's agreement about seeing someone who is on his list.

(2) Authority to proceed

If the adolescent is 16 years old or more you need only his or her permission to go ahead with the assessment, although it usually remains important for practical purposes to involve the family. If the adolescent is under 16, you should obtain the parents' permission. For a child in care, parental authority rests with the social worker concerned.

Informal authority is also important. Those under 16, and the parents of those over 16, still need to be fully consulted even if there is no strict legal requirement to do so. This is courteous, but in any case may be crucial for work to be done.

(3) Whom to invite to the assessment interview

This issue generates strong and conflicting views. There are family therapists who will not see the referred adolescent unless the whole family attends, including brothers and sisters who are busy at work and school. Conversely, there are psychiatrists and individual psychotherapists who prefer to emphasize the importance of the boy or girl having the chance to be seen alone.

My own argument is for adaptability, and balancing how the professional team likes to work against what the clientele want. The prevailing approach, for example, in many centres, is for compulsory whole-family attendance with the assessment supplemented by one-way screens and banks of video-recording equipment, and there are indeed important arguments for these as aids to teaching and supervision. However, some patients and families prefer greater privacy. They should be listened to.

My practice is to invite the whole family unless the young person is leading an essentially independent life. If any single member of the family wants to attend alone to discuss a family problem, I point out that there may be little I can do if I see just one member, but I will occasionally agree to a single consultation in order to clarify the situation for myself and for whoever comes. Often, this leads to a second interview with the necessary people present. This 'pre-assessment' work should be seen not as an inconvenient diversion but as a focus for work in itself.

An important alternative to clinical assessment is a consultative meeting with the referring professional workers and any others who are involved. They may well have all the necessary information and skills but be temporarily stuck, and there may then be no real need for a second (it may be a third or fourth) full diagnostic assessment. (See Chapter 18, on consultative approaches).

As well as a full clinical assessment, and a consultative meeting with the professionals involved, there is a third approach which is often useful. This is to invite a key professional worker (e.g. a social worker who is already involved) to the assessment meeting, and involve him in the discussion with the family about how best to proceed.

Bear in mind two related matters: *confidentiality*, which is a legal and ethical requirement, and *privacy*, which is a necessary courtesy and may be crucial to therapeutic work. Doctors may share freely with each other information about the patient, but to discuss a patient's case with other professionals, permission is needed. Official legal guidance on this can be surprisingly restrictive; it is not crystal clear, legally, that a psychiatrist can freely discuss a patient's case even with his or her team, even though it may make nonsense of the work not to do so. It is therefore important for professionals meeting a new patient and family to explain who they are and with whom they need to work.

(4) When to meet: urgency

It may be important to arrange the assessment very urgently, for example when psychiatric disorder is endangering anybody or causing acute distress. However, it is a matter of fact that the referral process in adolescent psychiatry is often quite arbitrary, and sometimes determined by inappropriate anxiety, misunderstanding, or poor service organization (see Steinberg *et al.*, 1981; Steinberg, 1981, 1983, 1987) and not all urgently presented matters are truly urgent. Occasionally an 'emergency' referral is simply due to a pressing wish on the part of the referrer to transfer the young person's care to you, and the reasons may not justify an emergency appointment. The latter may lead to other people having to wait longer or have their appointments displaced, and to cutting corners in the assessment process. Treatment already in hand for other patients and families can be quite unnecessarily disrupted. Of course, the adolescent psychiatric team must be responsive and helpful; but there can be so much anxiety generated in adults by troubled adolescents that unless an adolescent psychiatric team keeps a tight and realistic grip on its referral and assessment procedures it will rapidly clog up and be little use to anybody, least of all to young people genuinely needing an urgent response.

(5) Where to meet

Giving specific advice here is less important than the simple reminder that the choice of where the clinician should meet the patient and family does have impact, and has implications for therapeutic work. In general I prefer to see patients at a clinic, with home visits when there are special reasons for this – for example, a domiciliary consultation requested by the family doctor. However, some of the meetings described above, sometimes with other professional workers, and sometimes with them plus the patient and family, may be more appropriately held on their own territory. For example, a problem which primarily affects family and school, and where the answer lies in what the family and teachers can do together, can usefully be held on school premises.

The foregoing preliminaries to the clinical assessment may be surprising to some clinical workers. After all, an approach which has stood the test of time is simply for patients to be 'booked in' to a clinic by a receptionist without preamble. There are some services and some clientele where this approach may work satisfactorily, but in a general adolescent service, for the reasons given in earlier pages, efficient work requires some prior matching of the type of response to the apparent problem. The reasons behind this are discussed more fully elsewhere (Steinberg, 1983).

(6) Problem clarification: the family's point of view, and the beginning of family assessment

The clinical tradition maintains that history-taking comes first and the examination second. (I remember a distinguished professor of psychiatry looking quite shaken when a fellow registrar, now an eminent consultant, explained in a case conference that it made more sense to him to get the routine physical examination done before getting to know properly the patient and his or her story.)

The way the family describes different perspectives of the adolescent's problem, however, is the beginning of the history-taking *and* the beginning of the family assessment, and says much about the adolescent as an individual too. I do not know any way of separating these functions of the interview, although what is learned should be placed under separate headings.

The family-oriented practitioner may want to conduct nearly all of the diagnostic assessment with the family group. The family therapist certainly would, and would usually have no place for Item 8 (individual assessment) on the above list.

At Bethlem Royal Hospital the approach I recommend is to have family and individual assessment on a sliding scale as follows.

(i)   As a routine, family and individual assessments take up roughly equal time.
(ii) For some family-based problems, however, (e.g. mutual complaints about behaviour), the family assessment may make up all or nearly all of the clinical interview.
(iii) For problems where the adolescent's personal difficulties seem primary, private or needing a more formal mental state examination (e.g. suspected psychosis) the individual assessment is allowed more time than average.

It is natural for the family to be more or less uncomfortable and embarrassed at first. Mutual introductions should be conducted in a way that shows respect for all concerned. Ace therapists should not be above the ordinary social exchanges that put people at their ease – the journey to the clinic, the state of the waiting room, or whatever helps establish as comfortably as possible the fact of a meeting which is essentially a peculiar event.

It is important to address all those who have been invited (younger children, for example) even if the discussion tends to shift towards adolescent and parents. A very young child may soon demonstrate either boredom or a wish to be the centre of attention and the parents can be invited to give them something appropriate to do with toys and materials available in the consulting room.

One way of starting is to explain that one has been asked by (for example, the family doctor) to help with the problem, and then to invite the referred adolescent to say how he or she sees the difficulty. The parents and then the other children can be asked how they see the problem, and by conversation with everyone, but with special attention paid to the referred adolescent and both parents equally, the problem list can be compiled. Observing the way the family responds to the interview and to each other will begin to show some of the ways they operate together; and they can be asked explicitly how they have tried to cope so far with the presenting problem. Drawing a family tree can be helpful, especially when there are complex family relationships following remarriage.

While noting the adolescent's various difficulties, it is important to remember the difficulties and other events in the family as a whole. Younger and older siblings may be changing schools, starting jobs, leaving home and so on, and the parents may sometimes be having mid-life personal or marital difficulties of their own. Their own parents may be elderly, too close or too distant, and will be in various states of health. Remember that the focus for work at this stage is the adolescent. Permission and explanation are needed for a shift of emphasis. Both family and parental capacity for having fun together and leading a satisfying social life should be discussed.

Many parents feel guilty about their children's problems, and assume that the family assessment is about what they have done wrong. Since they may well not be doing the right thing, one should avoid fulsome reassurance; but it is important to draw attention to the more important part of the issue, namely that the referred child's problem is of course of concern to the whole family, that every member's view of the problem is useful, and that, with some outside assistance, everyone can be helped to deal with the problems they have identified.

The large amount of information that will be coming from this part of the assessment can be put together under the following headings:

Who is present (names, occupations, ages)?
Who is absent (names, occupations, ages)?

Sociocultural and socioeconomic state
Formal relationships (father, daughter, etc.)
Informal relationships (hierarchy, authority, alliances, etc.)
Main current, recent and anticipated events (e.g. arrivals and departures)
Important past experiences (events, perhaps similar to the presenting problem, in the parents' own childhoods; past similar experiences in the adolescent's earlier childhood: e.g. consultation with a paediatrician).
How the presenting problem is handled: Is it confronted, faced equably, avoided? Is it reinforced? What works and what doesn't work in their attempts to help with it? Do different family members respond differently? What is the effect of the presenting problem on the family? How have the family responded to the family assessment?

In the approach described here the parents are then seen by themselves while the adolescent is being interviewed. Some clinics and teams do not take this approach. You then need to decide how to respond when one or both parents take you aside 'for a private word, doctor'. I think it is reasonable, usually but not always, to agree to a 'private word', but in my view it is best, first, to see if there is some way the parents can talk in front of the adolescent; and if they can't, or can't do so yet, to ask if the request (and the agreement) can be made in the family meeting, not for example in the corridor. Remember to comment on those many things the family will be doing right, since they are likely to be more conscious of their deficiencies.

(7) The history
The overlap between obtaining two different sorts of information – what happened, and observations about people's personalities and relationships – has already been noted.

The historical information should be organized under the headings given below. Try to be alert to chronological connections and co-incidental events, although premature assumptions about one thing causing another should not be made. For example, it could be important if the following sequence occurred in the adolescent's infancy:

(a) parental anxiety about a grandparent's admission to hospital;
(b) dissatisfaction with obstetric care when the mother was pregnant with the referred adolescent;
(c) post-natal depression;
(d) the father's promotion, just in time to save the family's finances, but involving him in a lot of travelling;
(e) difficulty in managing the new-born baby who had screaming

attacks and seemed to have tummy-aches which no-one could diagnose or help.

Such a sequence, in which mother and child are left feeling helpless with a problem for which the experts cannot be trusted with an answer, can reverberate over the years and be amplified at adolescence. Such apparent connections can be of the greatest importance, but may be red herrings.

(i) Problems

Describe precisely and in plain language – as used by your informants – who is concerned about what. *The referring doctor* may be concerned about persistent 'hypochondria' in the adolescent; his problem is a diagnosis that hasn't led to any of his interventions (e.g. counselling, antidepressants) being helpful. *The adolescent's* problem may be about being brought to see a psychiatrist ('It's nothing really – they're just all making a fuss.') *The mother's* problems are (a) the adolescent's complaints about not feeling well, and (b) increasing pressure from the school about the reason for so many school days being missed. *The father's* complaints might be (a) the family doctor's failure to treat the condition satisfactorily, (b) his wife's constant worrying, (c) his own lack of time to get involved.

(ii) Developmental milestones

Pregnancy and delivery, including family attitudes to the pregnancy, health in pregnancy, maternal health and mood and the experience of obstetric care.

Behaviour and responsiveness as a baby.

Eating, sleeping and elimination habits and progress.

Growth – weight, height and general physical development over the years.

Learning to walk and talk; sight, hearing, speech, reading.

Attention and concentration; ability to play – to become happily absorbed in solitary play and to share in play with others; ability to generate and pursue interests.

(iii) Social and personality development

Academic and social progress throughout school career (note schools, dates, key teachers).

Confidence, friendships, ability to separate from parents, be alone, make new relationships, function in groups.

Ability to play, relax, enjoy himself or herself.

Sexual development, education, relationships.

Misbehaviour, response to discipline, (and what type of discipline), delinquency. Court record, if any.

Use of alcohol, drugs, other toxic substances.

Bizarre or unusual ideas, speech, experiences, habits, behaviour.

Mood – anxiety, phobias, compulsions, rituals, sadness.

Suicidal or other self-destructive or self-neglectful ideas, threats or behaviour.

(iv) Physical health

Major or minor illnesses, accidents, allergies (note any adverse drug reactions).

Major or minor medical, surgical or other specialist attention.

Fits, faints, headaches, dizziness, weakness.

Diarrhoea, vomiting, abdominal pains; disturbance of bowel or bladder function.

Appetite; sleep; personality changes, especially in relation to physical disorder.

Physical development; weight, height, and sudden changes in these.

Onset and progress of adolescent development.

(v) Family history

Draw a family tree, with mental and physical illnesses and other problems noted. Note also miscarriages and the deaths of children, parents and others. Note the adolescent experience of other family members: how was leaving home coped with? Have there been problems similar to those of the referred adolescent? How managed?

Is there a family view (or views) of emotional disorder, doctors, clinics, etc?

What do they think the cause might be?

What changes have the presenting problems brought about in the family?

(vi) Development of the presenting problems

This story will be obtained partly in the family assessment and partly in the individual clinical interview, and supplemented by reports from other sources.

Putting together a coherent story is difficult and can be frustrating. The accounts from different people will vary and they will emphasize different things, and the information will come at different times. Something crucial to understanding the problem may not emerge until a second or third individual or family interview, or even later. For such reasons the clinician should accept that a neatly buttoned up history taken on the first occasion may look nice for the notes but is likely to be misleading.

Rather, regard the first account as a working document which is essentially a provisional and unedited guide to further exploration.

In outline, ask about these areas:

What has actually been happening? (Obtain factual, descriptive information, with times, places and people.)

What seemed to be the causes (i.e. antecedents) of problematic feelings and behaviour? And the consequences?

Who tried to help, and how? What were the results? (Look for modest changes for better or worse as well as great achievements and disasters.)

What sort of feelings have been generated by all this? What was the effect on memories, relationships, attitudes, hopes and plans?

What good things have been happening too? Look for strengths and successes as well as difficulties.

Note what else you need to find out on future occasions, and possible sources of information.

(8) The individual assessment

To recapitulate, the basic though adaptable sequence we follow at the Adolescent Unit at Bethlem Royal Hospital is as follows:

(i)   Psychiatrist and family worker introduce themselves to the adolescent and family and confirm with them the key problems. (a nurse joins in if admission is a possibility.)

  The developmental history is taken and the family assessment begun.

(ii) The psychiatrist then sees the adolescent individually while the family worker talks further to the parents. If psychological or physical assessment is needed, this takes place now.

(iii) The clinical team then discuss the adolescent's case while the family has coffee.

(iv) Finally, two or three key people (who may include a 'visiting' worker involved in the referral) meet the family to discuss the team's advice, answer any questions, and discuss how to proceed.

Individual assessment involves:

(i)   Engagement : establishing rapport and eliciting feelings.
(ii)   Clarifying the adolescent's personal concerns.
(iii) Formal examination of the boy's or girl's mental state (supplemented by psychological testing then or on a later occasion).
(iv)   Physical assessment or examination when appropriate.
(v)   Psychological testing, sometimes.
(vi)   Physical investigation, sometimes.

(i) Engagement

By the time you see the referred adolescent other people will no doubt have been pressing the boy or girl to say 'what is the matter'.

Engagement in this context (as opposed to engagement in psychotherapy, which is a larger matter) means that sufficient friendliness and trust is established for the adolescent to feel it is worthwhile talking to this new stranger about how he feels and what he thinks.

One way of beginning is to explain to the adolescent who you are, if you have not done so before, and why you are seeing him; for example, that his teachers and school doctor thought he seemed so upset about something that his work was suffering, and that his parents wanted your advice. What follows depends on the confidence and maturity of the boy or girl; but note that a chatty, forthcoming and self-revealing style on the adolescent's part might be due to anxiety rather than tranquillity, and you may be misled into thinking the young person is relaxed. He or she is likely to be anxious and unsure how to talk to you, and it will often help if you adopt a conversational style, and begin by talking about the facts of the referral, and what difficulties and what help (if any) the adolescent would like to talk about. In other words, you can begin by establishing the agenda rather than homing straight in on what you think is the central problem. For you the problem may be suicide or incest or the diagnosis of psychosis; for the adolescent it is likely to be how to talk to the stranger the adults have called in to help.

Do not contrive a hearty, jokey, matey, Dutch Uncle, pseudo-youthful or other artificial approach unless this is what you are like naturally. In manner, try to 'be yourself' and if this is difficult, perhaps because you find talking to this age group does not come easily, discuss this with your supervisor.

Try not to be prejudiced, which is difficult when of necessity (as in this book) one refers again and again to 'the adolescent'. Young people, like old people, are all different.

Finally, the traditional medical advice is *listen* to the patient, he is telling you the diagnosis.

(ii) Clarification of problems, and completion of the history

List what everyone is concerned about. In the initial meeting with the family this exercise can be shared, so that we hear what the father is worried about, what the mother is worried about, what concerns teachers, and so on, and the boy or girl may have joined in. In the separate interview, however, check that you are aware of the adolescent's main concerns. You may hear 'I'm not bothered about anything. It's only Mum who's fussing', or something similar. Well, that is an observation to be noted. Or, you may receive only a shrug, a disappearance behind a curtain of hair or deep into an anorak, or no apparent response at all.

(iii) Formal mental state examination

Avoid, if you can, working steadily down a check-list of things to ask. (If you are just beginning, and have to have an *aide-mémoire* by you, then tell the adolescent that you are using it because you don't want to leave anything out. You will always find that such honesty will help break the ice, while squinting at a secret crib will make both of you lose confidence.)

Instead, have a conversation about:

- past and recent happenings and experiences;
- worries and disappointments;
- things the adolescent finds difficult, and things he or she likes to do;
- things liked and disliked about himself or herself;
- interests and hobbies; how the day and the week is spent at school, at home and with friends;
- things done with the family (outings, holidays);
- friendships with both sexes;
- interests or worries about sex (behaviour, experiments, experience, identity as a boy or girl, sexual interference or assaults);
- plans, hopes and ambitions (training, career, social).

While doing this, have in mind for your notes:

(a) General appearance and behaviour:
   Dress, (whose influence?), posture, demeanour, spontaneity, alertness or withdrawal; aggressive, assertive or compliant; preference for being seen with or without family; self-care.

(b) Conception of problem:
   Attitude to referral, to the interview, to the idea of being helped; feelings about confidentiality and privacy; what is the problem? Whose problem is it? (His? The parents'?) Is anyone to blame for it? What will it take to put things right again?

(c) Mood:
   Distress, anxiety, sadness, hopelessness, despair; excitement, euphoria, hypomania, mania; shame, embarrassment; range and appropriateness of emotional expression. Suicidal or other self-destructive ideas, thoughts or plans.

(d) Thought form and content:
   Perplexity, muddle, mixed feelings, avoidance of central issues; worries and preoccupations; preconceptions, misunderstandings, misinformation, misinterpretations, overvalued ideas, delusions; hallucinations and illusions; depersonalisation, derealisation, *déjà vu*; obsessive-compulsive thinking; thought disorder; balance between introspection and attention to external reality; assumptions about

self and relationships e.g. self-esteem and esteem of others. Feelings about other people.

(e) Language:
Speech (clarity, vocabulary, syntax), comprehension. Expression, posture and gesture accompanying speech. Writing and spelling. Comprehension.

(f) Cognitive functions:
General knowledge and information. Orientation, short and long-term memory. Attention span and concentration. Capacity for reflection. Perceptiveness, imagination and curiosity. General impression of intellectual level.

(iv) Physical assessment
The psychiatrist should always form an impression of the adolescent's general state of physical health, growth and nutritional state, and should find out (by questioning about menstruation, ejaculation and pubic hair) if puberty has been reached. History-taking will have included questions about general health and symptoms and these will alert the doctor to the possibility of physical illness.

A fuller neurodevelopmental examination (cranial nerves; head circumference; right- or left-handedness; speech production (dysphasia, dysarthria, stutter); involuntary movements; stiffness of movements; incoordination; tone, power, muscle wasting; reflexes; plantar responses) is possible with the removal of very little clothing. The pulse and thyroid function can be similarly examined.

(v) psychological testing
Formal testing by a psychologist has sometimes been conducted as a routine. I think it is better for the information to be made available to the psychologist on the team, for his or her advice about the sort of questions to ask, the further information to be sought, and the tests, if any, that are indicated. The adolescent clinic's psychologists will usually undertake a whole range of individual, family and group work, and formal assessments will only be part of their contribution. They include:

Intelligence testing (overall intelligence quotient (IQ) and performance on sub-tests). Well-established tests are the Wechsler Intelligence Scale for Children (WISC) and the Wechsler Adult Intelligence Scale (WAIS).
Behavioural assessment – e.g. systematic study of precisely what happens in precisely which circumstances. This may be done as a preliminary to working out a behavioural training strategy.
More specific testing – e.g. of reading problems, co-ordination, or of areas of mental functioning that may indicate general or local brain dysfunction.
Projective techniques, in which a stimulus such as an ambiguous drawing

(Thematic Apperception Test) or abstract 'ink blots' (Rorschach Test) are used to provoke ideas and fantasies which might give insight into unconscious or disguised thought and feeling. There is controversy about their usefulness.

(vi) Physical investigation

There are no routine physical investigations, but a full blood count with erythrocyte sedimentation rate (ESR) and blood urea and electrolyte analysis should be performed for a young person whose general physical health or weight seems poor or in decline.

The suspicion of neurological disorder should be discussed with a neurologist or developmental paediatrician, who will usually appreciate the availability of an electro-encephalogram (EEG) and computer tomography (CT scanning) of the skull. These and other investigations are outlined in Chapter 17.

(9) Diagnosis

The diagnosis should be in two parts.

(1) First, one of the multi-axial diagnostic systems (ICD-9 in the UK) should be used to categorize the identified problems (or their absence) under the headings:

- Clinical psychiatric syndrome
- Developmental delay
- Intellectual level
- Physical disorder
- Abnormal psychosocial situation

Although an adolescent's case should not be forced into an unsatisfactory category for clinical purposes, it is a useful exercise for learning and for communication with others if a provisional diagnosis is selected from those available.

(2) Second, a diagnostic formulation should be made. This should include all potentially useful information or ideas. It should consist of:

(i) A brief description putting together basic information about the patient, e.g. 'a sixteen-year-old schoolgirl of normal intelligence, living at home, and referred by her family doctor because of a recent recurrence of anxiety symptoms'. Briefly list the main problems.

(ii) A short paragraph on possible aetiological factors. As a guide, select from:

- genetic
- early environmental
- developmental (skills, behaviour)
- intellectual
- physical
- psychological
- developing personality and
- family/social factors

and think in terms of

- predisposing factors
- precipitating factors
- perpetuating factors
- protective factors

to put together a hypothesis about why this young person in this family at this time is presenting the problems described.

(iii) A brief note on the prognosis. This is not a guessing game for which the safest answer is 'guarded'; rather, put down what might happen, e.g. that suicidal attempts or threats may be anticipated, dangerous behaviour may be repeated, or a restless, excited state may turn into acute mania.

(iv) Outline the broad lines along which management will proceed, for example:

- further enquiries or tests needed
- how and with whom treatment will begin
- how progress will be monitored
- any special precautions.

Outline : how an adolescent's case can be presented

(1) Basic information: name, age, address, school and domestic situation; by whom referred. The day's date.
Factors affecting authority to proceed : e.g. if in care, or custody of child unclear.
Who came to the assessment?
(2) Main problems for key people (patient, family, referrers).
(3) Details of the problems and their development.
(4) Developmental history from pregnancy to the present.
(5) Social and personality development.

(6) Physical health and medical attention.
(7) Family history, and family disorders and problems.
(8) Family assessment.
(9) Individual assessment   mental
                             physical
(10) Psychological assessment, performed or indicated.
(11) Physical investigations, performed or indicated.
(12) Diagnostic statement:
     (i)   Multi-axial categories;
     (ii) Diagnostic formulation.
(13) Note action taken: appointments made, explanations given, letters
      sent, etc.

References and further reading

Barker, P. (1984) *Basic Child Psychiatry*. Fourth edition. London: Collins.
Barker, P. (1986) *Basic Family Therapy*. Second edition. London: Collins.
Cox, A. and Rutter, M. (1985) Diagnostic appraisal and interviewing. *In*
    Rutter, M. and Hersov L. (Eds), *Child and Adolescent Psychiatry : Modern
    Approaches*, pp 233–48. Oxford: Blackwell Scientific Publications.
Steinberg, D. (1981) *Using Child Psychiatry*. Sevenoaks: Hodder and
    Stoughton.
Steinberg, D. (1983) *The Clinical Psychiatry of Adolescence*. Chichester: John
    Wiley and Sons.
Steinberg,. D. (1987) Management of crises and emergencies. *In* Hsu,
    L.K.G. and Hersen, M. (Eds), *Recent Developments in Adolescent Psychiatry*.
    New York: John Wiley and Sons.
Steinberg, D., Galhenage, D.P.C., and Robinson, S.C. (1981) Two years'
    referrals to a regional adolescent unit.*Social Science and Medicine* **15**,
    113–22.

Chapter 6

Educational and Developmental Problems and Mental Handicap

Mental Retardation and Handicap

Mental retardation is the most recent term in a series which has included mental subnormality and mental handicap. The term mental impairment has now been introduced in the Mental Health Act 1983. These terms are defined below.

Understanding mental retardation makes most sense if seen in the light of multi-axial diagnosis, as described in Chapter 5. Mental retardation is not a psychiatric disorder, although a mentally retarded adolescent may also develop a major or minor psychiatric disorder. Nor is it in the same category as specific developmental delay : thus, by definition, specific reading retardation refers to a reading problem out of proportion to the young person's general level of intelligence. Similarly, a mentally retarded child may or may not have physical brain damage or a brain disorder.

Example 1
The patient is Terry, a young man of 17 who is mildly mentally retarded. His IQ score is 58. He is a senior pupil in a special residential school and training centre for mentally handicapped young people. The visiting psychiatrist has been asked to see him because of a series of uncharacteristic violent outbursts. He is seen with his parents and, separately, with a member of staff whom he knows and trusts.

He has brought to the interview a piece of carpentry of which he is proud: a model boat, carefully painted. He is anxious and puzzled, but looks relieved when asked some straightforward questions about what he has done that day, whom he works with, and about his boat. Questions about what might upset him or worry him are evaded with an anxious smile and he then concentrates on his boat or looks hopefully at the door and asks 'Can I go now?' Asked what he wants to go and do he says 'Play with Jimmy', but he doesn't want to say any more than that. After that he begins to wander round the room, picking up things. When asked to come and sit down again he starts crying noisily and wants to go to the lavatory.

His parents, who are in their fifties, are deeply distressed and talk for an hour. They are sure there is something wrong with Terry's brain and point to an electroencephalogram report that referred to 'non-specific abnormalities', but which they say no-one takes seriously. They like some aspects of the school, but don't feel the place has the resources, medical or educational, for someone like Terry; on the other hand there's nowhere else that they prefer. They acknowledge that a change now, with him coming up to the last year, could be unsettling. They've worried for years about whether this is the right place, but there has always been one reason or another against a move.

Once they had some family meetings with a social worker attached to the school, and felt much calmer about things, but she left. They could never get on with her successor and they stopped attending. They are concerned about the possibility of Terry being given medication, and have brought along a cutting from a newspaper, an article about tardive dyskinesia.

A big worry for them is: 'Why is Terry getting so violent? He was such a gentle boy'. As big a worry is: 'Suppose they can't keep him here? Where will he go?' A third worry, the biggest one of all, is: 'What will he do when he leaves here, especially if he's violent?' Eventually they say 'We're not getting any younger. What will happen to him when we've gone?'

The staff are very kind, very matter-of-fact. They have carried out a behaviour training programme which 'didn't work'. Someone sees Terry for counselling. There's an art therapist. The visiting general practitioner, whom Terry likes (he has a lot of minor and transient health problems) once gave him some imipramine for a time but it didn't help. Most of the staff can handle his outbursts, as long as they don't get worse. So far he's all right at night or they really would be in difficulties. But his behaviour is now too disruptive for their senior training group, and without this opportunity in his last year they fear his chance of achieving a little independence in a supervised flat or a hostel will be jeopardized. 'If the only way of controlling him is medication he may end up in a long-stay hospital.'

Terry's case illustrates a number of common features of psychiatric problems with mentally handicapped young people. In no special order of priority (which will of course vary with each person's case) they include:

(i)   Parental distress about what they cannot do for their child, and uncertainty about entrusting care and upbringing to others.

(ii)   Two special anxieties as adolescence proceeds : first, will he become still more difficult? Often, when there is a primary concern about assertiveness and physical aggression there is anxiety about sexually disinhibited behaviour, minor or major, not far behind. Second, fear for the young man who, although physically full grown in a year to two, may not be able to lead anything like an independent life.

(iii)   There is sometimes persisting disappointment, sadness or grief about the ideal child they never had, and painful mixed feelings of anger as well as affection for the problematic child they do have. Such natural feelings may be long coped with in a mature way; or, at the other extreme, may be the source of major distress and bitterness, sometimes expressed towards those who try to help. Feelings about death may be prominent; for example that the child might have died, but perhaps is believed to have been saved by the doctors; or nearly died because of medical misdiagnosis and mishandling that might have made the mental handicap worse; or that there will be no-one to look after the child properly when they themselves die. It is possible to understand this as a half-conscious wish to give up an intolerable life-long burden, but it also has some basis in reality.

(iv)   Is Terry mentally handicapped or mentally disturbed? There can be confusion about the distinction even in otherwise well-informed circles. In fact it may not be clear whether the young man is (a) going through essentially normal emotional crises but expressing them badly because of his social and intellectual limitations, or (b) whether he has developed a real psychiatric disorder.

(v)   Both the formal mental state assessment, and the finer aspects of personal and therapeutic engagement, can be more difficult because of problems with comprehension and expression. (Note, however, that some mentally handicapped young people can also be refreshingly straightforward and clear about their problems too.)

(vi)   Is there 'something wrong' with Terry's brain? There may be, but it may be hard to establish what it is; and if a diagnosis can be made, there may not be any useful treatment. (Sometimes potentially manageable social, family, psychological and educational problems will have been set on one side while the diagnosis and the 'cure' are pursued, perhaps from clinic to clinic and specialist to specialist over a number of years.)

(vii)   Is he in the best possible place? Young people with mental handicap can have multiple problems. Ideal care could include highly skilled psychological assessment (behavioural as well as cognitive) and management, psychotherapy and family therapy as well as the right qualities in the staff and environment. A residential setting may be excellent in some crucial respects but deficient in others, with little likelihood of change.

(viii) Medication with neuroleptic drugs can produce its own problems (see Chapter 18) and can interfere with new learning (Eisenberg and Connors, 1971; McAndrew *et al.*, 1972) Tardive dyskinesia may result from long-term medication started in childhood. Drugs given for the epilepsy which may accompany the more severe forms of mental retardation may themselves cause behavioural problems (Stores 1975, 1978). On the other hand it can be necessary to use medication to keep a child manageable in a setting that is proving helpful.

In the case described the key issue was Terry's rising anxiety as people began to point out to him the next step, i.e. participating in the senior educational programme as a preliminary to leaving the school and moving to a more independent role. He was unable fully to conceptualise this fear, still less express it. His parents' similar anxieties fed into his, not only during school holidays but in every contact with him. The key move which made a significant difference was to re-introduce supervised family work, with fear about dependence and independence as an important focus for work.

Some Definitions

Mental retardation, or better still *intellectual retardation*, is the term to be preferred for an uncomplicated deficit in intelligence. *Mental handicap* is best used for intellectually retarded people in whom there are additional social, psychiatric or physical handicaps (Corbett, 1985).

The revised Mental Health Act for England and Wales 1983 uses the terms *mental impairment* and *severe mental impairment* for mental handicap associated with 'abnormally aggressive or seriously irresponsible conduct' (Department of Health and Social Security, 1983). These terms replace subnormality and severe subnormality respectively, as used in the 1959 Act.

The classification system ICD-9 (Chapter 4) uses the following categories of mental retardation:

Normal variation: any intellectual level over 70
Mild mental retardation: IQ 50–70
Moderate mental retardation: IQ 35–49
Severe mental retardation: IQ 20–34

Profound mental retardation: IQ under 20

These categories refer to IQ levels based on tests with a mean of 100 and a standard deviation of 15, such as the WISC and the WAIS (Chapter 5).

It is important to note that mental retardation refers to two different concepts of normality. One is the normality of *how most people happen to function*. Intelligence tests are devised on the basis that most people will score in an arbitrarily chosen average range, i.e. 70–130. Any spectrum of naturally occurring phenomena will show the normal distribution curve (see Fig. 6.1). A curve describing the range of height, weight or visual acuity in the community would be similar.

However, the lower down this normal distribution curve the individual is placed, the more likely is the intellectual deficit to be caused by a disorder of the brain, which brings in a different notion of abnormality, namely the presence of actual pathology. People with severe mental handicap usually have gross brain abnormalities. Brain abnormality may also be found, though less frequently, in those who are only mildly retarded. Kirman (1985) gives a helpful account of mental retardation and those major disorders that cause it.

Mental retardation and psychiatric disorder

An adolescent with mental retardation may have no mental disturbance at all. Most do not. Adolescents with mental retardation may, however, experience the same normal turbulent emotions as any other boy or girl, although they may be expressed differently.

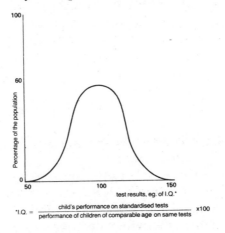

Figure 6.1.

Mental disturbance in the sense of psychiatric disorder, however, does have a higher prevalence among mentally retarded young people compared with those of normal intelligence. Thus in the Isle of Wight study of 10 to 11 year old children, psychiatric disorder was regarded as present in 7 per cent of the general child population, in about a third of mentally retarded children, and in half of the severely retarded group. (Rutter *et al.*, 1970)

Among mildly mentally retarded children and adolescents, the psychiatric disorders seen are similar to those occurring in young people of normal intelligence, and are treated in much the same way, although allowing for the additional factors outlined in the case example.

The psychiatric disorders seen among severely retarded children, however, include a greater preponderance of such conditions as autism, disintegrative psychosis, stereotyped behaviour including severe, repetitive self-injury, and, in younger children rather than in adolescence, hyperactivity (Corbett, 1985). Pica, the ingestion of inedible substances (Bicknell, 1975) occurs throughout the range of mental retardation, and occasionally in children of normal intelligence too.

Mentally retarded adolescents in severe emotional crises sometimes present with extreme distress, chaotic or withdrawn behaviour and bizarre fears and fantasies which appear descriptively like psychotic states, and which may be acute or persistent. It may be very difficult to confirm or exclude the presence of schizophrenic or depressive delusions, and these disorders can be hard to diagnose with precision.

In his excellent review of the relationships between mental retardation and psychiatric disorder Corbett (1985) mentions the association between low IQ in early childhood and emotional symptoms and delinquency in adolescence; the increased susceptibility of children with organic brain dysfunction to psychiatric disorder; the likelihood that such characteristics as overactivity and poor concentration may increase the possibility of poor parent-child relationships and conduct problems; the effect of problems in language development; the effect of educational failure; and the effects of social rejection and poor self-esteem.

Mental retardation and active brain disorder

In principle the differences between mental retardation, psychiatric disturbance and organic brain dysfunction are clear-cut. In clinical practice the distinction is not always easy, and a recurring question in adolescent psychiatry is whether deteriorating mental function in a mentally retarded adolescent is due to (a) emotional problems anomalously expressed; (b) the onset of a major mental illness; or (c) the appearance of a neurological disorder. The neurological disorders that may present in this way are discussed in Chapter 17. For the present, it can be said that the early diagnosis of physical brain disorder in a mentally retarded adolescent may be very difficult, and the guidelines for diagnosis and management are:

(i) Repeating clinical examination, EEG and psychometry at intervals appropriate to the apparent rate of change so far.
(ii) Specific biochemical investigations in collaboration with a specialist in the field (see Chapter 17).
(iii) Dealing with the other problems of the adolescent and family, which include the fact of the diagnostic and prognostic uncertainty; and attention to the young person's handicaps. These are likely to persist whatever the final outcome of investigation.

Developmental disorders

The term 'developmental' appears in a number of quite different diagnostic contexts, and this causes confusion. The classification system ICD-9, Axis 2, refers to Specific Delays in Development. These are delays in the development of reading, arithmetical, speech and language or motor co-ordination skills, and they are described separately from any other condition (such as psychiatric disorder, or intellectual retardation) that may be present. Thus specific reading retardation refers to a degree of reading retardation not explained by the young person's age and general level of intelligence.

There is controversy about the relationship between specific reading retardation and 'dyslexia' or 'developmental dyslexia'. All these terms refer to severe reading and spelling difficulties, usually persisting through adolescence and into adult life, and occurring in three times as many boys as girls. Yule and Rutter (1985) in a comprehensive review of these and related conditions, argue against the concept of dyslexia on the grounds that its proponents seem to imply that (a) it is a distinct condition (rather than one within the spectrum of specific reading problems) and (b) that the environmental influences on this biological condition are relatively unimportant.

Disorders of language development have a close and complex relationship with learning in general, and with the capacity to play and acquire social skills. While this can be severe if associated with mental retardation on the one hand or autism on the other, it may also be seen as a problem in its own right in some emotional and conduct disorders and problems of personality development. In such persisting problems in adolescence, enquiry into the development of play and language forms an important part of the history and examination.

A number of other disorders are also commonly referred to as 'developmental' in that delays in biological maturation are central to the problem. Thus enuresis and encopresis (Chapter 9) and hyperactivity (Chapter 8) are included in this category.

Autism, (Chapter 14), once confused with both mental handicap and with schizophrenia, and more recently classified as a psychosis, is now better categorized as a pervasive developmental disorder: i.e. a disorder of psychological development with multiple effects on the child's cognitive, language, emotional and social development.

Descriptive diagnostic systems attempt to operate without the assumptions of theories of aetiology. Thus the term 'developmental' is used descriptively in the ICD-9 classification of specific reading retardation. Sometimes, however, it is used to refer to the developmental concept of disorder used in child and adolescent psychiatry, namely the idea of the emerging interaction of different levels and aspects of functioning as the child grows up. These varied uses of the term and the concept contribute to the confusion.

Elective mutism

Elective mutism is generally defined as a condition in which a child or adolescent, without a handicap in language comprehension or speech production ceases to talk, except, usually, to a small group with whom he or she may whisper, sometimes in secret. It is variously classified with language disorders, emotional disorders and adjustment reactions. It usually develops in middle childhood after several years of normal language development. In a study by Kolvin and Fundudis (1981) most cases had developed insidiously from very early in life and in only very few cases had it appeared for the first time in later childhood. One quarter were shy, and half showed anger at home and sulkiness with people outside the home. Nearly half were enuretic, and one sixth were encopretic. Most were in the lower range of average intelligence. This group were followed up for five to ten years, during which time just under half improved.

Elective mutism: management issues
(i) Confirmation is needed that there is no language disorder or sensory condition that could account for the lack of speech.

(ii) Elective mutism should also be distinguished from mutism due, for example, to a schizophrenic or depressive illness.
(iii) Shyness and social awkwardness should be helped by social skills training and, where appropriate, desensitization.
(iv) The relationship with minor speech defects is unclear. Some children have a speech handicap which is insufficient to account for the mutism alone, and there may be a history of abandoned speech therapy. For these and others the opinion of a speech therapist should be obtained. (Smayling, 1959; Wright, 1968).
(v) Behaviour modification using operant training can be helpful (Straughan *et al.*, 1965; Reid *et al.*, 1967).

Educational issues

The school is complementary to the family in the life of most children. An adolescent's problems may present as problems at school, and these may be behavioural, emotional or in terms of academic performance. The problems listed earlier in this chapter are those that can profoundly affect a child's educational development. By the time a boy or girl is seen in adolescence decisions will have already been taken about his or her need for special education, in a particular school or unit or through special tuition. However, this is by no means always the case, and from time to time the clinical team will come across general or specific handicaps that were either unrecognised, or to which insufficient attention had been paid. Such problems may become apparent for the first time when an adolescent is referred because of disturbed conduct.

The adolescent's past and present performance in school is important in understanding the emergence of disorder (Chapter 3), history taking (Chapter 5) and in many aspects of planning management (Chapter 18). Administrative terms that are on the decline include 'educational subnormality', i.e. intellectual unfitness for the range of normal education provided, and 'maladjustment' for behavioural problems that interfere with schooling. There are still a range of very different schools for different degrees of handicap and problems of behaviour, but the thinking behind the Education Act of 1981 is for as full as possible an integration of children with handicaps into the normal schools system.

Concluding note

Often it is quite difficult to know whether a problem in the field of mental handicap and educational achievement is going to require quite complex handling (e.g. neuropsychiatric investigation or behavioural analysis) or a relatively straightforward approach (e.g. a modification of parents' and teachers' expectations of the child – not that this is always easy). The key to understanding the presenting situation is a careful teasing out of the precise problems and handicaps, as described in Chapter 5, and the use of a multi-axial approach to diagnosis.

The use of family or individual psychotherapeutic or counselling techniques is perfectly appropriate for mentally handicapped young people. As in all forms of psychotherapy, it is necessary to meet the patient at least halfway, and sometimes on his or her own ground, to ensure that relevant difficulties are explored together in a way that feels right and makes sense (see Chapter 18). It is also important to do as much as one can through those most in contact with the adolescent – for example, teachers and residential workers, – using collaborative and consultative techniques (Chapter 18). This is because for the most part the difficulties are to do with learning and development rather than the treatment of disorder.

Whatever approach is taken, it is important to remember the adolescent's sense of self-esteem, whether the problem is one of major retardation or a problem in school. A poor self-image will result from and also compound poor achievement. Conversely, encouragement for even a little progress can lead to further achievement.

We do not know enough about the development of self-esteem, but its deficiency is evident in many psychiatric problems of adolescence, a time of life when self- concept, positive or otherwise, is changing and consolidating (Coleman, 1980). The mentally handicapped adolescent, or the boy or girl suffering from a specific difficulty in a cognitive skill, is likely to have major problems in confidence and self-concept, and the clinician should be conscious of this in understanding the handicapped young person's problem, in planning management, and in the way he or she is handled.

References and further reading,

Bicknell, J. (1975) *Pica : A Childhood Symptom*. London: Butterworth.

Coleman, J. (1980) *The Nature of Adolescence*. London: Methuen.

Corbett, J. (1985) Mental retardation : psychiatric aspects. *In* Rutter, M. and Hersov, L. (Eds) *Child and Adolescent Psychiatry : Modern Approaches*, pp 661–78. Oxford : Blackwell Scientific Publications.

Eisenberg, L. and Connors, C.K. (1971) Psychopharmacology in childhood. *In* Kagan, S. and Eisenberg, L. (Eds) *Behaviour Science in Pediatric Medicine*. Philadelphia: W.B. Saunders

Kirman, B. (1985) Mental retardation : medical aspects. *In* Rutter, M. and Hersov, L. (Eds), *Child and Adolescent Psychiatry : Modern Approaches,* pp 650–60. Oxford: Blackwell Scientific Publications.

Kolvin, I. and Fundudis, T. (1981) Elective mute children : psychological development and background factors. *Journal of Child Psychology and Psychiatry* 22, 219–32.

McAndrew, J.B., Case, Q. and Treffert, D.A. (1972) Effects of prolonged phenothiazine intake on psychotic and other hospitalised children. *Journal of Autism and Childhood Schizophrenia* 2, 75–91.

Reid, J.B., Hawkins, N., Keutzer, C., McNeal, S., Phelps, R., Reid, K. and Mees, H. (1967) A marathon behaviour modification of a selectively mute child. *Journal of Child Psychology and Psychiatry* 8, 27–30.

Rutter, M., Tizard, J. and Whitmore, K. (1970) *Education, Health and Behaviour.* London: Longman.

Smayling, L. (1959) Analysis of six cases of voluntary mutism. *Journal of Speech and Hearing Disorders* 24, 55–8.

Stores, G. (1978) Anticonvulsants. *In* Werry, J. (Ed), *Paediatric Psychopharmacology.* New York: Brunner-Mazel.

Stores, G. (1975) Behavioural effects of anti-epileptic drugs. *Developmental Medicine and Child Neurology* 17, 647–58.

Straughan, J., Potter, W. and Hamilton, S. (1965) The behavioural treatment of an elective mute. *Journal of Child Psychology and Psychiatry* 6, 125–30.

Wright, H. (1968) A clinical study of children who refuse to talk in school. *Journal of the American Academy of Child Psychiatry* 7, 603–17.

Yule, W. and Rutter, M. (1985) Reading and other learning difficulties. *In* Rutter, M. and Hersov, L. (Eds), *Child and Adolescent Psychiatry : Modern Approaches.* pp 444–64. Oxford: Blackwell Scientific Publications.

Chapter 7

Emotional Disorders and Depression

Emotional Disorders of Childhood and Adolescence

The relationship between syndromes of unhappiness and anxiety in childhood and the psychoneurotic disorders of adults is not clear, either in theoretical terms or in terms of the continuities in time between childhood and adult conditions. What is clear is that they are different in their presentation; thus young children generally do not show, and may be too young to describe, the classical 'textbook' symptoms of anxiety and phobic states and depression. In adolescent psychiatry we see young people who in years or in maturity may be more like young children or more like adults, and so we see both the childhood conditions and adult-type conditions. Often, the adolescent's problems include features of both.

Example 2
Lorraine, aged 17, is referred to the psychiatric clinic from the Casualty Department. She was seen there for a third overdose of aspirin tablets. After each admission for physical treatment and psychiatric assessment she appears brighter, and denies that the problems with school or boyfriends which led to each overdose were all that important to her. On the third occasion she is seen by a social worker who concludes that she is still depressed 'behind' a smiling front.

Lorraine has no wish to see a psychiatrist. She and her mother (her parents are separated) stress that she is anxious to get back to her job and find it difficult to agree a time for an appointment. When seen, Lorraine's mother seems far more sad than does her daughter. Her mother is often near to tears; Lorraine's role seems to be to persist with saying 'cheer up, Mum'. It emerges that Lorraine's maternal grandmother spent many years in and out of psychiatric hospitals with 'depression', had several courses of ECT which 'helped for a time', and killed herself when Lorraine was small. Lorraine's mother has also been depressed on and off for years, worsening considerably in the year that Lorraine left school and started going out with boys. Her husband left home soon after.

Lorraine denies feeling sad. She says she was angry and fed up, not depressed, when she took the drug overdoses. About the dangers she says she 'doesn't care'. She denies suicidal intentions but imagines it could happen again. She doesn't have very definite hopes or plans for the future, but 'lives from day to day'. Her mother says 'she only cares about boys'. It does seem that when she goes out with friends she has a lively time and enjoys herself. 'You should see her when she's all dressed up.' Her mother fears she is promiscuous. The overdoses have all been within the last few months, during which time her appetite and sleep have been poor. About attending the clinic again she comments: 'It's a waste of time really'.

Figure 7.1 The range of emotional and mood disorders seen in adolescence.

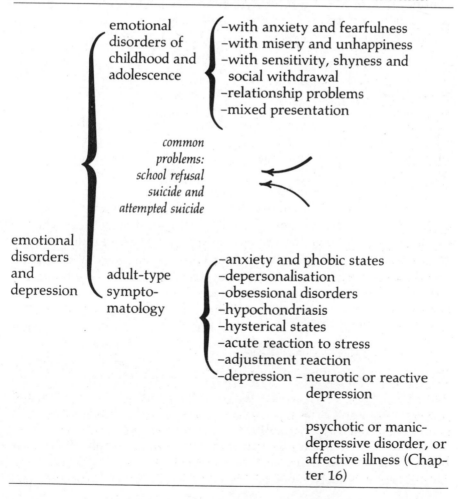

emotional disorders of childhood and adolescence
- –with anxiety and fearfulness
- –with misery and unhappiness
- –with sensitivity, shyness and social withdrawal
- –relationship problems
- –mixed presentation

common problems: school refusal suicide and attempted suicide

emotional disorders and depression

adult-type sympto-matology
- –anxiety and phobic states
- –depersonalisation
- –obsessional disorders
- –hypochondriasis
- –hysterical states
- –acute reaction to stress
- –adjustment reaction
- –depression – neurotic or reactive depression

psychotic or manic-depressive disorder, or affective illness (Chapter 16)

Lorraine's case illustrates some common diagnostic difficulties for the psychiatrist. Different clinicians could each make a case that her problems are psychoneurotic, (or neurotic, emotional or reactive) in type; that the problems clearly have their origin (and possibly their resolution) in family functioning; or that her family history and symptoms indicate a depressive illness. Many adolescents with psychiatric problems present with this heterogeneous picture.

In this chapter the range of emotional and depressive disorders in adolescence will be considered according to the schema in Fig. 7.1.

Emotional disorders

Emotional disorders are those which are less well differentiated than the adult-type syndromes they resemble. The adolescent may present with anxiety and fearfulness, or may be unhappy, with disturbance of sleep and appetite. There may be disturbed relationships, e.g. sibling jealously, or the child may be abnormally shy, with marked sensitivity and social withdrawal. Emotional disturbance associated with disturbance of social behaviour is classified as mixed disturbance of emotions and conduct. As mentioned earlier, the *symptoms* in these categories are worth distinguishing from the *problems* they cause; a number of quite different clinical syndromes may be behind school refusal, for example, or attempted suicide.

Descriptively, these conditions contain the seeds of the adult-type neurotic disorders shown in the above list. This does not mean that one precedes the other, however. The relationships between the emotional disorders of childhood and the neurotic disorders of adult life are not straightforward. The following continuities and discontinuities may be noted : (i) the sex ratio for emotional disorders is equal in childhood, but changes during adolescence so that in adult life females predominate for psychoneurotic disorder; (ii) most children with emotional disorder appear to become normal adults (Robins, 1972), and where emotional disturbance persists it is as the neurotic and depressive disorders described; (iii) there is some evidence that obsessional disorders in adolescence are preceded in some cases by related, anxiety-laden habits and preoccupations (see Hersov's review, 1985); and (iv) fears and phobias are quite common in young children, and are related to such things as animals, the dark, death, noise and school; most respond to being handled sensibly by parents. Many fears fall off during adolescence, although fears of illness, death, injury, separation and crowds are more likely to persist (Hersov, 1985). Agoraphobia and social phobias and anxieties tend to appear in adolescence or early adult life (Marks and Gelder, 1966).

School non-attendance

School refusal is the term preferred by Hersov (1985) to encompass both actual phobias of an aspect of school on the one hand, and fear of separation from home and parents on the other. Hersov stresses that although there are common themes in each case, diversity of aetiology, psychopathology, prognosis and treatment is more usual. School refusal is a common reason for referral in adolescence, with a gradual onset of problems contrasting with the more acute onset seen in younger children.

The various patterns of non-attendance at school may be broadly classified in Fig 7.2.

Truancy has many of the associations of conduct disorder rather than emotional disorder – for example, large families with poor or inconsistent supervision and discipline, and school problems such as frequent changes of school and poor academic performance. Both the school (Reynolds *et al.*, 1980) and the peer group seem influential in the incidence of truancy. Among truants, the presentation is misbehaviour, defiance, taking illicit jobs or going about with a gang, rather than anxiety.

In contrast, school refusal is associated with anxiety-laden and depressive affect (mood) in the child, and with higher family incidence of psychoneurosis. The children tend to be passive, dependent and overprotected and usually work and behave well (Hersov, 1960a, b, 1985). However, within the family it is common to find the school-refusing youngster dominating by tears, anger and sometimes violence, and

Figure 7.2   Patterns of non-attendance at school.

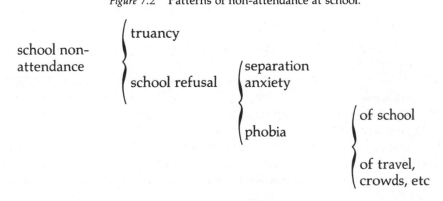

thereby preventing the parents bringing about any effective change in the situation.

Major mental disorder such as a schizophrenic or depressive illness may lead to school refusal, but this is relatively rare. School refusal may present with psychosomatic symptoms such as nausea, vomiting, abdominal pain or syncope, or a fear that these and other symptoms might happen (Schmitt, 1971).

The overall prevalence of school refusal has proved hard to determine. Hersov suggests a clinic incidence of around 5 per cent of all children referred with a higher rate in early adolescence than in earlier childhood. It occurs equally in both sexes.

There have been very many suggestions about the aetiology and psychopathology of school refusal (see review by Hersov, 1985). The best-supported notion is that separation anxiety plays an important part in its genesis. From this psychodynamic and family dynamic model for the generation of anxiety, it is a small step to the anxiety becoming firmly school-related through maladaptive learning, reinforced by persisting parental anxiety about placing the child in school firmly and with confidence. My own impression is that in many cases of school refusal the psychodynamic model explains how the symptom has been generated and the behavioural model explains its persistence. This is consistent with the approach taken by many family workers.

School refusal : management plan

(i) Remember that general practitioners, paediatricians and the better organized school welfare and psychological services manage many, perhaps most, cases of incipient school refusal effectively (this may account for the uncertainty in the psychiatric statistics) and the first step is to make sure that whatever useful efforts are made are encouraged. Psychiatric help should be used to supplement rather than replace efforts already in hand. By the same token it will be helpful for the anxious child to see that parents and the involved professionals are co-operating in his or her care, rather than operating at cross purposes. Assessment therefore includes a review of what is being done so far, and its successes as well as failures.

(ii) A detailed clinical assessment should attempt to show (a) the broad type of school non-attendance (see Fig. 7.2); (b) how far the problem seems to be 'in' the adolescent, e.g. as a true phobia, and how far maintained largely by family dynamics or by the way the family and education authorities are managing the situation; (c) the child's individual state, including phobic, depressive and other psychiatric syndromes, but also his or her intellectual and academic ability and specific learning problems.

(iii) Establish the goal of treatment, e.g. a return to school or, if appropriate, a change of schools. Some adolescents display extremes of emotional distress on separation from the parents, yet once separated rapidly settle down quite happily – at least until the next contact and separation. This may be shown by a period of admission to a psychiatric unit, but only for those with intractable problems.

If this picture should emerge, and the point of separation remain a major problem, a new focus for family work is : can the adolescent return home, and to day school, or does it seem that a residential school is the more sensible choice? If a change of schools seems indicated, it is essential to liaise closely with the educational authority (with parental permission) from the early stages of intervention, because the administrative procedures can take a long time. The schools psychological service will be an important source of advice and help in this and other respects.

(iv) Clarify who is going to work on what, with whom. Some family therapists will work entirely with the family, regarding the re-assertion of parental authority as a key goal (e.g. Skynner, 1974). In many cases a combination of family work and individual work is valuable : family work to provide the necessary parental authority for the treatment programme as well as its aim, and individual work (e.g. psychotherapy or systematic desensitization) for the adolescent. All work should be sharply focussed on the urgency of helping the boy or girl with what is a serious handicap that is not only undermining his or her education, but also seriously interfering with peer relationships and therefore normal social and emotional development.

Medication has only a very limited place in this individual work. In a careful study Gittelman-Klein and Klein (1971) reported significantly better results with children on imipramine plus psychosocial treatment, compared with imipramine plus placebo. However, a similar study with clomipramine found no improvement with medication (Berney *et al.*, 1981). On clinical principles, it may be supposed that a highly motivated but highly anxious adolescent may be assisted in a return to school by a small dose of a benzodiazepine drug for a limited period to supplement other forms of anxiety management.

What happens to school refusers? Hersov's very thorough review of the subject (Hersov, 1985) suggests that the outcome of any treatment is usually good, with a success rate of two-thirds or more, but with a poorer outcome with older children. There is a tendency for psychiatric problems such as agoraphobia and work problems of a neurotic type to persist into adult life (see, for example, Warren, 1965a, b; Hodgman and Brayman, 1965; Pittman et al., 1968; Tyrer and Tyrer, 1974).

Suicide, attempted suicide and self-injury

As with school refusal, this cluster of problems represents a wide range of possible disorders, and in some cases no real psychiatric disorder at all.

The suicide and attempted suicide rates for young children appear to be extremely low, although doubt has been cast on this on two grounds: first, reluctance of adults to attribute suicidal intent to young children, and second, the difficulty of disentangling suicidal intent from despairing self- negligence resulting in death. Among older children and young adolescents, Shafffer (1974) found that only one child in 800 000 committed suicide in England and Wales during the seven year period under study. It has long been recognized that both suicide and attempted suicide rates rise from puberty onwards (Morgan et al., 1975; Holding et al., 1977; Wexler et al., 1978; Lumsden Walker, 1980) and there is evidence of a rising rate of suicide for older adolescents throughout the world (Brooke, 1974; Sainsbury et al., 1980; Shaffer and Fisher, 1981; Holinger, 1978, 1979; Holinger et al., 1986) including England and Wales (McClure, 1986).

Attempted suicide, in which self-poisoning predominates, is also increasing, among younger adolescents too. Most of those who attempt suicide are girls; boys predominate in actual suicide. In Hawton's study of 13 to 18 year old adolescents who attempted suicide in England, 90 per cent were girls, and one-third had physical problems such as juvenile arthritis or asthma. Family, school and peer-related problems were common, and in most cases the type of problem precipitating the overdose was in itself a transient one. The outlook in terms of further overdoses was worse where self-poisoning was part of a range of behaviour that included habitual drunkenness, stealing and fighting. (Hawton et al., 1982 a, b). The study supported some of the impressions reported by Leese (1969) and Lumsden Walker (1980) in which self-injury was associated with a cluster of problems such as absent parents or poor communication with them. In the series reported by Hawton and his colleagues 14 per cent of the children had been in care of the local authority. This compares with only 4 per cent of sixteen-year-olds in general. One-third of the young people in Hawton's account (Hawton 1982b) said they had wanted to die. Despite this range of family and personal problems, the presence of a specific psychiatric illness is the exception rather than the rule.

Suicide and attempted suicide: management plan

(i) All threats or hints of suicide should be taken seriously. A recent attempt constitutes, in effect, a threat. Having said this, it does not follow that every risk of suicide requires maximum supervision. Not only is this impracticable, but absolute security (which would require personal surveillance round the clock) could in many cases be anti-therapeutic and in the long run raise the risk of repeated suicide attempts. Taking the attempt seriously means taking the adolescent seriously, and in particular paying careful attention to the distress or circumstances which, by the attempt, the adolescent was trying to influence. The parents should be expected to take part in this effort to listen to the boy or girl. There are two intentions here: first, to attempt to make self-injurious acts redundant by opening up alternative paths of communication; second, to make the suicidal attempt serve its purpose by generating appropriate concern. This too can help make further attempts superfluous.

(ii) A careful individual assessment is necessary to look for the following high risk factors: (a) hallucinatory instructions to carry out dangerous acts; (b) the firmly held belief (sometimes a delusional conviction) that the adolescent is worthless and better off dead, or not worth helping; (c) feelings of despair and hopelessness; (d) unassuaged anger; (e) the expressed intention of making a further attempt. Background high-risk factors include : previous attempts; alcoholism or drug abuse; and social isolation.

My own experience is that once a relationship is established with an adolescent he or she is very often straightforward about his or her intentions. An undertaking not to attempt further self-harm between, say, now and the next appointment can, in the context of a therapeutic relationship, usually be relied upon. Correspondingly, a threat to do so is likely to be carried out. However, it is most important that such undertakings are based on a reasonable degree of engagement and a full conversation; a hastily extracted 'agreement' whose purpose is primarily to reassure the enquirer is not the same thing, and is unsafe.

(iii) Beyond the above, the management of suicide threats or attempts is as for emotional, conduct and depressive disorder in general. If actual poisoning has occurred, the greatest care must be taken. If there is the slightest doubt that the adolescent may have taken a larger or more serious overdose than he or she will admit to, emergency referral to a general medical department or poisons unit is necessary, sending with the patient an appropriate escort, a note about his or her mental state, and (in safe hands) any leftover tablets. Note that both aspirin and paracetamol overdoses can have very serious and sometimes fatal delayed effects, despite the patient, when seen, being quite alert. Make a note of your local centre of the National Poisons Information service. (The London and National Centre number is 01 407 7600).

Anxiety and phobic states

Anxiety accompanies most psychiatric conditions but can occur as the main distressing symptom, either as a general, 'free-floating' sense of fear or worry; or as a specific fear of an object or situation, which is avoided (phobic anxiety). Anxiety states sometimes present in adolescence as a continuation of fearfulness in earlier childhood, now made more disabling and distressing by the increasing expectations and responsibilities of adolescence. Some adolescents appear to be frightened of their peers, and seek the company of older or younger companions. Anxiety states also arise in relation to frightening events (illness, death or mental illness in a parent) or may appear determined by intrapsychic problems without a clear external cause.

Anxiety as a reason for referral in its own right is unusual among adolescents, although it was found to be a common problem in a psychiatric survey of the general adolescent population (Rutter *et al.*, 1976). It seems likely that anxiety among young people is referred for professional help when it becomes disabling or alarms others, for example as hypochondriasis, obsessional behaviour, school refusal or as a phobia, rather than as a distressing symptom in its own right. Possibly it is insufficiently recognized as a primary symptom, and other mood states like depression or anger attributed as a primary problem instead. Generalized anxiety may also be hard for a young person to put into words; well-meaning adults may propose the description that they are feeling 'depressed' and this be accepted by an adolescent who does not know how better to put it. In the clinical interview it can be helpful to explain that troubled feelings are often a mixture of worry and sadness, and to explore whether the predominant feelings are about something lost, missed or regretted, a feeling of being 'low' and miserable; or about worries or scared feelings that something might go wrong or something unpleasant happen.

There are many accounts of the sources of anxiety, including anxiety as something learned from anxious parents (Eisenberg, 1958); as an expression of long-standing environmental stresses, temperamental vulnerability or both (Thomas *et al.*, 1968; Chess, 1973); or as the outcome of attempts to cope with intrapsychic conflict, for example those summed up by Poznanski (1973) as representing fears of abandonment, fears of mutilation and sexualized fears.

Phobias involve a dread of objects and situations which are therefore avoided by the affected individual. Handicapping phobias such as social phobias and agoraphobia tend to make their first appearance in adolescence, although as already mentioned, school refusal in younger children *may* be accompanied by degrees of true phobic avoidance (see above). As with anxiety states in general, phobias can be attributed to the learning of maladaptive responses, reinforced by the 'reward' of further avoidance; by the externalization and displacement of inner, unconscious sources of anxiety onto outside situations and objects; by the persistence into one developmental phase of a fear appropriate for an earlier one; or by the maintenance of phobias by interpersonal relationships, e.g. in the family (Miller *et al.*, 1974). A point made several times in this book in relation to other conditions is that these conceptual models are not necessarily incompatible with each other (see also Tyrer and Steinberg, 1987)

Phobias of one sort or another are common in the population as a whole. One figure suggested is 77 in 1000 of the general population, of which 22 in 1000 were actually disabling (Agras *et al.*, 1969). Agras *et al.*, (1972) found that untreated phobics tended to improve gradually, and this was particularly true of the small number of cases in which the onset of the phobic symptoms was in adolescence. (See reviews by Marks (1969) Marks and Gelder (1966))

Anxiety and phobic states : management plan

(i)   Three aspects of assessment require particular attention. First, as precise a clinical impression as possible about whether the anxiety is primary or secondary to a depressive or other abnormal mental state; second, as objective an account as possible of phobic symptoms : what precisely is feared (object, time, place, circumstances) and how the patient deals with the fear; third, confirmation that there is no physical cause (e.g. anaemia, hyperthyroidism, hypoglycaemia, medication) or effect (e.g. hyperventilation) of the anxiety.

(ii) Look for those ways in which the adolescent alone or with the family has been able to overcome some of the anxiety. Loss of confidence and lowered self-esteem may be seen in the boy or girl, or the family may be actively though unconsciously undermining the adolescent. See if there are strengths and partial solutions that may be reinforced and shaped up by straightforward encouragement and advice. In this context, note that some anxiety states appear to represent a general, ill-defined disquiet in the adolescent. Once the step has been taken to identify a problem and bring it to the attention of a trusted person outside the family, a sense of relief and the beginning of the resolution of other problems may follow. During the process of history taking, perhaps over more than one session, look for positive features in the story, and positive results from the therapeutic effect of paying attention to the adolescent's and family's fears, and from helping them reflect about them.

(iii) If systematic treatment is embarked upon, set up the means of monitoring results – for example, a simple self-rating chart. Different clinicians will have different views about the treatment of first choice. My own is to use the following sequence: (a) family work to deal with any obvious ways in which family or parental behaviour is contributing to the problem. Small things may make a big difference; one may occasionally see children show visible and lasting relief when a parent confesses that he or she had similar problems in adolescence; (b) individual psychotherapy (see Chapter 18) accompanied by a behavioural approach such as relaxation training or desensitization; (c) if necessary, low dose anxiolytic medication (see Chapter 18) to supplement, not replace, these approaches.

Depersonalization

Depersonalization refers to a feeling of unreality; derealization refers to the surroundings seeming unreal. Either may occur in normal people of any age as a transient experience when tired, when under stress or when something out of the ordinary happens suddenly. It has been reported as an experience related to sleep and sensory deprivation, and a symptom in anxiety, depressive and phobic states, in epilepsy, and in schizophrenia. In a classic account, Ackner (1954 a, b) attributed some of his cases to schizoid personality or hysterical syndromes. It has also been reported as an effect of hallucinogenic and benzodiazepine drugs.

Depersonalization has also been described as a syndrome in its own right, beginning in adolescence or early adult life and persisting for years with occasional variation and remission. This puzzling disorder has received surprisingly little attention in recent years. Useful accounts have been given by Shorvon *et al.* (1946), Ackner (1954 a, b,) and Sedman (1970). There are many theories about its nature and cause (Sedman, 1970).

Depersonalization : management plan

(i)   Make certain of the diagnosis. The experience seems hard for most people to describe and must be differentiated from reports of anxiety, depression, confusion, or delusional thinking. It is important to be alert to the possibility of physical disorder.
(ii) The symptom is often secondary to other conditions, including transient stressful phenomena. These should be identified and treated.
(iii) No treatment has been demonstrably effective. Stress management techniques and anxiolytic medication may be helpful. The disorder sometimes seems closer to being a perceptual rather than affective anomaly, and cognitive psychotherapeutic methods might in principle be useful.

Obsessional disorders

Although ICD-9 describes the obsessive-compulsive symptom as one which the individual tries to resist, resistance is not an essential feature of obsessional feelings and behaviour (Stern and Cobb, 1978) and this is particularly true of adolescents. Rather, obsessive symptoms in childhood and adolescence tend to be characterized by the experience of their being a distressing and unwelcome but *necessary* chore.

Example 3
An intelligent 16 year-old is referred because of increasingly furious arguments at home, mostly between his mother and himself. He perceives dirt and germs being brought into the home as people come and go, and insists on having his own plates and cutlery, which must also be washed in a special way. So must the things the family shares, for example tablecloths. No-one else may sit on the chairs he uses; and he will not sit on those of other people. His parents have gone along with his wishes 'for the sake of a quiet life' but he is becoming increasingly demanding: more 'decontamination' chores are being added to his mother's duties, and he increasingly requires them to be repeated if not perfectly carried out. Moreover, repetitions must be in threes – thus, if a third rewashing of a plate fails to satisfy him, they must proceed to six, or he will

have a violent tantrum. The whole household now revolves around these rituals.

Mental state examination shows that the patient is not deluded. His rationale for his behaviour boils down to this : he does not think that he will be harmed by germs, but only that he could be; it is only a possibility, but the possibility nags at his mind, preoccupies and seriously distresses him. He feels fine when the cleaning rituals have been properly conducted. Note that interviews with obsessional adolescents can get pulled towards fascinating but time-wasting intellectual discourse. The psychiatrist asks whether the domestic chaos and upheaval is justified, bearing in mind the negligible risk of being harmed by germs. His answer is a definite yes. The remote possibility, however minute, causes him too much anguish. The psychiatrist might feel comfortable about the risk, but he doesn't.

In adolescence it is common to find some or all of the family drawn into 'helping' with rituals (Bolton et al., 1983). One family who were required by their intensely obsessional son to retrace every step taken on a trip, long or small, balked only at his demand to go anticlockwise around roundabouts on the way home. One common reason for referral is the young person's violent rage when his demands are not met. Another is the length of time a boy or girl may indulge in washing themselves in the morning, so that they cannot get to school before the early afternoon, unless they rise in the early hours. Patients may damage their hands and perineal areas with cleaning and re-cleaning, sometimes with disinfectants.

Obsessional behaviour was found to be uncommon in the Isle of Wight study, (Rutter et al., 1970), although Adams (1973) found that the 39 boys and 10 girls he studied had developed their symptoms in middle childhood. Studies by Kringlen (1965) and Pollitt (1969) found that most adult cases began in adolescence. Family tendencies to obsessional behaviour are common but there is no clear evidence for a genetic influence. Adams considered that there was a relationship between middle- class strictness about being orderly and well-behaved and obsessional symptoms. The classical psychoanalytic view is that obsessional behaviour represents 'doing and undoing', a quasi- magical ritual that attempts to deal with unconscious conflict about death, aggression and guilt. Whatever the cause, a factor in its persistence may be the spurious and short-lived reward of tension relief when the obsessive thought or compulsive act is undertaken, rather like the similar effect of taking illicit drugs.

Obsessional disorders: management plan

(i)   Confirm that it is obsessive-compulsive thinking and behaviour, rather than delusional thinking, that is behind the problem. It is extremely rare for true obsessional disorder to present later as a schizophrenic illness (4 per cent in Pollitt's series, 1969); but obsessional preoccupations sometimes occur as an early symptom in adolescent schizophrenia.

(ii) Look for depressive features, especially when obsessive symptoms are more marked during depressive periods. This clinical picture may be improved with use of the tricyclic antidepressant clomipramine (Marks *et al.*, 1980).

(iii) Look also for maintenance of symptoms by family participation in rituals and see if this can be avoided through family work. Seriously handicapped obsessional young people have been helped successfully by combined behaviour therapy and family work (Bolton *et al.*, 1983). However, some young people seem to make progress only away from the family, and this may be revealed by admission to hospital. If strategies for a return home aren't successful, a move away (e.g. to a residential school) is helpful for some.

(iv) Behavioural methods like self-monitoring, thought-stopping, modelling and response-prevention may help adolescents who have relatively mild symptoms or who are relatively mature and highly motivated for treatment. Many adolescents, however, will be found to be ambivalent or openly resistive about treatment and a firm approach e.g. using response prevention on a residential basis, may be needed.

(v)   Obsessional patients are often angry, and generate anger. Take care to avoid an unthinking fight over symptoms and treatment. An improvement in those symptoms that are most handicapping should be the goal, not an over-zealous struggle for a 'cure'.

Hypochondriasis

Hypochondriasis is a state of worried preoccupation on the part of the patient that something is wrong with his or her physical (or occasionally mental) health. Like obsessional thinking, it is an intense anxiety about 'what if' rather than a delusional conviction that something is definitely abnormal. Sometimes it is felt that something 'looks wrong' or 'smells wrong' in which case the disorder is closer to *dysmorphophobia*, which is an overvalued idea or sometimes a delusion that a part of the body is deformed. Dysmorphophobia (which by definition is not really a phobia) may occur in schizophrenic or depressive disorders.

Hypochondriasis in children sometimes represents the somatization of anxiety or depressive states – i.e. their expression in physical terms. Physical symptoms may also be adopted half-consciously as an acceptable reason for avoiding school or other challenging situations; or be a misinterpretation of the physiological expression of anxiety. The symptoms may be copied from an earlier time of life, or from another child in the family. An adolescent who is depressed or under stress may reproduce the tummy-aches that, in infancy, elicited a degree of parental concern that he or she finds hard to get now. Fears about growing up physically may also be represented by fears that something is going wrong with physical development.

Hypochondriasis : management

(i)   Do not jump to the conclusion that because the adolescent has been referred by a physician or surgeon to a psychiatric clinic nothing physical is likely to be wrong. Nor does a classical psychopathological picture in the individual or in the family mean that there isn't physical disorder. (Corbett *et al.*, 1977) Physical ill-health can produce worries that the individual and family then present in their own way, which may be in a 'neurotic' style. The physical symptoms require very careful exploration, examination and, if appropriate, investigation. My own experience is that physical disorder among adolescents in psychiatric units is common (Steinberg, in preparation).

(ii) The confident assertion that 'nothing physical is wrong' may be appropriate for some clinicians and some patients. For others, a helpful approach is to explain that the history, examination and tests show no evidence of physical disease; that the body can express tension and depression as physical feelings; and moreover, the psychiatrist can see that there are a number of emotional problems that do need help. If there is real doubt it is better to face it, with child and family, than to treat non-existent physical disease on the one hand, or prematurely to rule it out on the other. I have seen children prescribed anticonvulsants for no reason beyond conduct problems, a mildly anomalous EEG and parental certainty that 'something is wrong with the brain'. On the other hand it is a feature of psychiatric practice that physical disorder capable of explaining the presenting symptoms does regulary emerge, sometimes after a long delay, even after thorough examination and repeated examination by the appropriate specialists. (Caplan, 1970; Rivinus *et al.*, 1975; Corbett *et al.*, 1977)

(iii) For clues about what feelings or conflicts lie behind a hypochondriacal symptom, look carefully at what it achieves or helps to avoid. See if these needs can be met in other ways, or if they are needs that can be rendered redundant, e.g. by help towards emotional maturity. See also the discussion, below, on the management of hysteria.

Hysterical states

Hysteria (conversion hysteria) refers to a physical or mental disturbance or disability, including abnormalities of consciousness or arousal, which appear to be due to a motive on the part of the patient.

There are three main problems with the concept of hysteria. First, the classical definition required unconscious motivation, i.e. an explanation in psychodynamic terms, something which not all clinicians can accept. Second, motivation does seem to operate on a spectrum of awareness with (in my view) truly unconscious motivation at one end and deliberate behaviour at the other, so that it is not always possible to differentiate clearly between hysteria on the one hand and deliberate deception on the other. This is particularly true in immature people of any age where deception and self-deception can operate together. Third, a number of studies have demonstrated that conditions that appeared psychogenic, including hysterical disorders, can turn out in due course to have an organic basis (e.g. Slater, 1965; Caplan, 1970; Rivinus *et al.*, 1975).

The adolescent psychiatrist will see a number of young people with physical disability and sometimes mental abnormalities (e.g. atypical psychotic states with floridly bizarre behaviour and reported experiences) where there is evidence of neither physical disease nor a characteristically schizophrenic or affective clinical picture. Commonly it is not difficult to find in the history or circumstances a major stress or conflict which could explain the symptoms in terms of avoidance, e.g. by becoming unwell. Such 'illness behaviour' can achieve the following:

(a) Attention is drawn to the adolescent's distress, but without the child or family having to make clear the nature of the problem. It may be something which cannot be talked about, e.g. real or imagined incest, marital discord or a fear of illness and death, e.g. in a parent.

(b) Individual or family dynamics may make an adolescent feel inappropriately responsible. For example, an eldest child 'escapes' from a troubled household, leaving the most competent child behind feeling responsible for holding a distraught family together. The adoption of 'illness behaviour' is one way of abandoning responsibility without loss of respect and self-esteem. Indeed, it may hold the family together.

(c) It provides a focus which is comprehensible to the family if not the doctor. Instead of the patient and family being anxious, confused, guilty and helpless about a psychological or social conflict they cannot begin to grasp, the picture suddenly clears : the child is ill, and the doctors, who are after all responsible for illness, can be anxious, confused, guilty and helpless instead.

Epidemic hysteria refers to outbreaks of distressing and alarming behaviour such as collapsing and overbreathing in groups of adolescents – for example, in schools, communities or large meetings such as pop concerts. What characteristically happens is that symptoms affect one young person (who may be psychiatrically disturbed) and in the atmosphere of heightened tension that follows, the symptoms spread. Most such outbreaks last a few days and may affect up to a third of the community concerned, involving both normal and mildly disturbed young people (see accounts by Moss and McEvedy, 1966; McEvedy *et al.*, 1966; Benaim *at al.*, 1973; Levine *et al.*, 1974; Levine, 1977; Mohr and Bond, 1982). One outbreak in a large comprehensive school lasted for two years (Mohr and Bond, 1982).

Conversion hysteria : management plan

(i) See hypochondriasis, above. Here, too, it is important to complete and if necessary repeat physical investigations, be straightforward about diagnostic doubts, and look for what the symptom is achieving.

(ii) There can be physical consequences of prolonged psychogenic symptoms, e.g. muscle weakness in paralysis, or loss of stomach volume in anorexia. Account must be taken of this.

(iii) Even when the motives behind the symptoms are not 'close to consciousness' there is usually a degree of doubt and ambiguity about the genuineness of the disorder among staff and indeed in the patient and fellow patients. Treatment strategies which allow for this ambiguity are helpful; thus physiotherapy gives confidence, helps restore lost function and lost confidence, and provides an acceptable reason for recovery.

(iv) Conversion disorders may follow mild organic illness. Whether or not they do so, physiotherapy, a behaviour modification programme and family work aimed at helping the disability is appropriate even when there is no evidence of an active disease process. This approach has been shown to help with both psychological and secondary physical problems, and enables progress without loss of face (Dubowitz and Hersov, 1976; Delamater *et al.*, 1983.)

(v) In individual or psychodynamic work the clinical team should begin by taking at face value the patient's or family's overt concerns (e.g. the child's mysterious paralysis) and explore its consequences (that the child may not be able to live an independent life; that the parents have no time for anything beyond caring for the patient; that the other children are being neglected; that parental ambitions have had to be postponed; and so on). In my own experience, just as the symptoms act by proxy for an unspoken problem, so psychotherapeutic work with the consequences of the symptoms can begin to deal by proxy with that problem. In due course, as trust is established, the work moves from the proxy problem to the real one (Steinberg *et al.*, 1988).

Example 4
An adolescent girl is referred for admission having been in two previous treatment programmes. She is unable to move, swallow, or see; her parents, and now the nursing staff, have to help her with every basic function (feeding via a nasogastric tube, toileting). For family meetings she is carried, lying horizontally, into the treatment room. There is no detectable physical abnormality on examination, and although she cannot swallow food or drink she manages saliva. She is losing weight and muscle bulk and strength, and previous attempts at family and individual psychotherapy and behaviour programmes have not been successful. The clinical team assess her and point out to the family that the previous, highly experienced teams have tried everything; 'we have nothing else to offer in the way of active diagnosis or treatment. We will offer to admit her as a seriously disabled young person and at least will be able to care for her physically; moreover, she will be among other young people even though she cannot join in with what they do. We will not set a time limit for her admission; but, at her age, we would be able to keep her for a few years'. The question is raised whether she would not be better looked after at home. First, home nursing would be possible but she would not be among her peers; second, not only do her parents need to live their own lives, but the patient needs them as mother and father, not as nurses.

We therefore make no claims to be able to bring about improvement – i.e. we do not challenge the girl's problems or symptoms – but nor are we completely pessimistic. We point out that these disorders do wax and wane, 'things' (deliberately put impersonally) may change for the better, and if they do, she is in the right place for education and rehabilitation. Family work with the focus on sadness and despair begins, and the girl receives basic physical care, physiotherapy and the general support and counselling appropriate for a seriously disabled and perhaps incurable teenager.

One of the most difficult tasks for the key workers and senior staff is to allay anxiety among staff who fear she will deteriorate and even die if 'nothing' is done. Another is that staff should show no great excitement or astonishment when she begins to improve, but accept her slow and steady improvement. This approach avoids the confronting implication that 'you could do it if you wanted to', which is likely to make the patient's symptoms more entrenched. This is easier said than done, especially with successive changes of staff. A few months later she is one of the most active, talkative and physically and mentally normal girls in the unit and is discharged to continue family therapy, which has meanwhile developed some new themes. (This is discussed more fully in Steinberg *et al.*, 1988.)

Epidemic hysteria : management plan

(i)　Make sure that the clinicians involved are working together on the same principles.

(ii)　There may well be public anxiety that the 'cause' is some unidentified infective or toxic agent. The reasons why the clinicians think this is not the case should be fully explained.

(iii)　The 'trigger' adolescents should be identified, isolated from the others and given whatever help is needed.

(iv)　Attention is needed to group tension and anxieties which may involve parents, teachers and others.

Acute reactions to stress, and adjustment reactions

Acute reactions to stress are identified in ICD-9 as very transient disorders, settling within hours or days, occurring in normal people in response to severe stress such as bereavement, extreme danger, an accident or a natural catastrophe. Anxiety or hysterical symptoms may be seen. When such reactions last longer, e.g. weeks or months, they are termed adjustment reactions in ICD-9.

Stress and adjustment reactions : management plan

(i)   Basic attention to physical care, safety and practical management, especially when the stressor is continuing.

(ii) Encouragement of natural coping methods, particularly helping those with automatic responsibilities to the patient (the family, obviously, and civil agencies such as the police or rescue organizations if they are involved). In so far as they want help or advice, it should be consultative help which enables them to do their own work effectively.

(iii) Carry out whatever supportive or psychotherapeutic work seems appropriate, and give short-term sedation for extremes of distress which are not responsive to other forms of help. The aim should be to minimize clinical intervention, and expect the most of ordinary healing, coping and helping methods within the patient and among his or her family and other involved people. However, in a proportion of cases longer-term clinical problems may supervene, e.g. natural grief may become a prolonged depressive reaction, and need one of the treatments for depression.

Neurotic or reactive depression

These terms are generally taken to mean rather different things. 'Neurotic' depression implies that the depression expressed is disproportionate to the problem, so that the patient is thought to be already psychologically vulnerable in temperament or personality, even though there has been an external cause such as a significant loss. 'Reactive' depression has been used to distinguish depression due to external circumstances (whether neurotically determined or otherwise) from depressive illness due to neurophysiological disorder 'within'.

In practice the terms are often used synonymously, to distinguish these two 'understandable' depressive states from those due to a postulated physiological disorder, i.e. 'endogenous' or psychotic depression.

The advent of depressive states in adolescence raises a number of complex questions. First, it is not easy to say where 'normal' sadness ends and depression as a disorder starts. In studies of the normal adolescent population quite large numbers report feelings which in adults would be regarded as depressive (e.g. Rutter *et al.*, 1970; Albert and Beck, 1975; Rutter *et al.*, 1976).

Second, children and adolescents sometimes show disturbances (e.g. conduct problems or psychosomatic problems) in circumstances where one may think they 'ought' to be depressed. For example, a boy becomes delinquent and indulges in solvent abuse, or a girl becomes promiscuous, after a parent's death, but both deny feeling sad. In adolescents and younger children this common clinical finding has led to the concept of 'atypical' depression or 'depressive equivalents' (e.g. see Toolan, 1962; Glaser, 1967; Weiner, 1970). One way of understanding this is that adult-type depressive symptoms require sufficient maturation for their expression. This is a reasonable notion, but could apply to cognitive, expressive, intellectual, biochemical, emotional or social aspects of maturation, or to interactions between these components of functioning; hence the matter is a complicated one.

Third, adolescents are seen who do indeed show the adult-type pictures of 'reactive' or 'neurotic' depressive states or of major affective disorders such as manic-depressive illness. The latter are discussed further in Chapter 16.

The assessment of depressive states in adolescence is therefore complicated. The clinician should treat what he finds, and look for:

(a) the possibility that the adolescent's sadness is an entirely appropriate response to circumstances (e.g. being not academically skilled enough for a highly academic school, but under pressure from parents and teachers to do well). Whether one calls this 'reactive depression' or not depends on whether the adolescent's mood is an appropriate unhappiness about educational expectations, or a sadness that is interfering with other aspects of life, e.g. appetite, sleep, leisure activities.

(b) the possibility that the adolescent's developing personality (attitudes to self and others, expectations and belief systems, confidence, motivation, social competence) shows a tendency to react in an excessively depressed way to difficulties. He or she is 'thrown' easily by circumstances, assumes too readily that it will be difficult or impossible to manage, or that a distressing experience can never be overcome.

(c) the possibility that the depressive state is strongly or primarily determined by psychophysiological processes by definition beyond the reach of the patient's psyche, and beyond the reach of a conversation with the clinician for that matter. The sadness is not readily explained by the adolescent's family or other circumstances; it is not readily understood in psychosocial, or psychodynamic terms; it isn't possible to construct a convincing reactive hypothesis; there may be the more physiological symptoms of depression, e.g. lack of energy, withdrawal, poor appetite and weight loss, poor concentration and sleep disturbance, and there may have been periods of elation or excitability and a family history of depressive disorders.

(d) Finally, and most commonly, the adolescent is neither neurotic, nor the circumstances grossly traumatic, and yet the young person's still-developing emotional and social skills are not coping with various external pressures. The parents' marriage may be under strain at a time when that particular boy or girl (for intrapsychic developmental reasons) most needs security and stability; or a parent or school may be emphasizing academic success during a period when the adolescent's self-esteem is particularly precarious and he needs encouragement of an unconditional sort.

Conversely, parents may be indulgent and permissive with a youngster who knows he is 'getting away with it' and recognizes that his parents' support is thereby on a shaky foundation. There are endless permutations of possible demands versus capacities, and many examples of adolescent depression seeming to result from a period of disequilibrium rather than true pathology in the individual or the family. Indeed such 'decompensation' is part of the vicissitudes of ordinary life: it may put itself right, or drag on for years, sometimes leading to further problems, and may or may not come the way of psychiatrists and other professional workers.

Management plan : depression

'Depression' has become something of a shorthand term, along with anxiety, euphoria and anger, as if half a dozen such words could serve as the compartments for the range of human emotions. An adolescent in mental pain and those trying to help him may well grasp the word 'depression' as something to hold on to without it being clear that a depressive state of mind is at the core of the problem. One should try to understand what type of predicament the adolescent is in, or feels that he is in. If there is a strong sense of loss, of something or someone gone (or given up by the adolescent in anger or by misjudgement), of having been abandoned or let down, of something fouled up on which self-esteem depends, or of an ambition (even an unrealistic one) which is not going to come about, then in psychodynamic terms one is describing depression. One must then make a clinical judgement about how this understanding of the patient's inner life matches with external circumstances past and present, and with the clinical signs and symptoms, and whether it all adds up to a depressive state. Recommended reading: Bowlby (1969, 1973 and especially 1980) and Pedder (1982).

(i)   Clarify whether the adolescent's problem is best described in terms of depression. He or she may have learned to describe the feeling as 'depression' when it is something else. If the state is depressive, what are its components in reactive (usually family), personality and physiological terms? How much weight can you give to each?

(ii)   Assess and decide about the risks of depression, which include self-devaluation and self-neglect as well as self-injury and suicide.

(iii) Decide whether the formulation in these terms points to a primarily 'external' (e.g. family, school) or individual approach, and consider the sequence of approaches if more than one might be needed. The management of depressive states is discussed further in Chapter 16, pp. 199–200.

References and further reading

Ackner, B. (1954a) Depersonalisation I : aetiology and phenomenology. *Journal of Mental Science* **100**, 939–53.

Ackner, B. (1954b) Depersonalisation II : the clinical syndromes. *Journal of Mental Science* **100**, 954–72.

Adams, P.L. (1973). *Obsessive Children : A Sociopsychiatric Study*. London: Butterworth.

Agras, W., Sylvester, D. and Oliveau, D. (1969) The epidemiology of common fears and phobias. *Comprehensive Psychiatry* **10**, 151–6.

Agras, W., Chapin, H., Jackson, M. and Oliveau, D. (1972). The natural history of phobia. *Archives of General Psychiatry* **26**, 315–17.

Albert, N. and Beck, A. (1975) Incidence of depression in early adolescence : a preliminary study. *Journal of Youth and Adolescence* **4**, 301–7.

Benaim, S., Horder, J., and Anderson, J., (1973) Hysterical epidemic in a classroom. *Psychological Medicine* **3**, 366–73.

Berney, T., Kolvin, I., Bhate, S., Garside, R., Jeans, J., Kay, B. and Scarth, L. (1981) School phobia: a therapeutic trial with clomipramine and short-term outcome. *British Journal of Psychiatry* **138**, 110–18.

Bolton, D., Collins, S. and Steinberg, D. (1983). The treatment of obsessive-compulsive disorder in adolescence : a report of 15 cases *British Journal of Psychiatry* **142**, 456–64.

Bowlby, J. (1969) *Attachment and Loss. Volume I : Attachment*. London: Hogarth Press.

Bowlby, J. (1973) *Attachment and Loss. Volume II : Separation : anxiety and anger.* London: Hogarth Press.

Bowlby, J. (1980) *Attachment and Loss. Volume III : Loss : sadness and depression.* London: Hogarth Press.

Brooke, E.M. (1974) *Suicide and attempted suicide. Public Health Paper no. 58.* Geneva: World Health Organization.

Caplan, H. (1970) *Hysterical 'Conversion' Symptoms in Childhood.* University of London: M. Phil dissertation.

Chess. S. (1973) Marked anxiety in children. *American Journal of Psychotherapy* **17**, 390–5.

Corbett, J., Harris, R., Taylor, E. and Trimble, M. (1977) Progressive distintegrative psychosis of childhood. *Journal of Child Psychology and Psychiatry* **18**, 211–19.

Delamater, A.M., Rosenbloom, N., Conners, C.K., and Hertweck, L. (1983) The behavioural treatment of hysterical paralyses in a 10 year-old boy : a case study. *Journal of the American Academy of Child Psychiatry* **22**, 73–9.

Dubowitz, V. and Hersov, L. (1976) Management of children with non-organic (hysterical) disorders of motor function. *Developmental Medicine and Child Neurology* **18**, 358–68.

Eisenberg, L. 1958) School phobia : a study in the communication of anxiety. *American Journal of Psychiatry* **1141**, 712–18.

Gittelman-Klein R. and Klein, D., (1971) Controlled imipramine treatment of school phobia. *Archives of General Psychiatry* **25**, 204–7.

Glaser, K. (1967) Masked depression in children and adolescents. *American Journal of Psychotherapy* **21**, 565–74.

Hawton, K., Cole, D., O'Grady, J. and Osborn, M. (1982a) Motivational aspects of deliberate self-poisoning in adolescents. *British Journal of Psychiatry* **141**, 286–91.

Hawton, K., O'Grady, J., Osborn, M. and Cole, D. (1982b) Adolescents who take overdoses : their characteristics, problems and contacts with helping agencies. *British Journal of Psychiatry* **140**, 118–23.

Hersov, L. (1960a) Persistent non-attendance at school. *Journal of Child Psychology and Psychiatry* **1**, 130–6.

Hersov, L. (1960b) Refusal to go to school. *Journal of Child Psychology and Psychiatry* **1**, 137–45.

Hersov, L. (1985) Emotional Disorders. *In* Rutter M. and Hersov L. (Eds) *Child and Adolescent Psychiatry : Modern Approaches*, pp 368–81. Oxford: Blackwell Scientific Publications.

Hodgman, C. and Brayman, A. (1965) College phobia : school refusal in university students. *American Journal of Psychiatry* **12**, 801–5.

Holding, T., Buglass, D., Duff, J. and Kreitman, N. (1977) Parasuicide in Edinburgh : a seven year review 1968–1974. *British Journal of Psychiatry* **130**, 534–43.

Holinger, P. (1978) Adolescent suicide : an epidemiological study of recent trends. *American Journal of Psychiatry* **135**, 754–6.

Holinger, P. (1979) Violent deaths among the young : recent trends in suicide, homicide and accidents. *American Journal of Psychiatry* **136**, 1144-7.

Holinger, P. and Offer, D. (1986) Suicide, homicide and accidents among adolescents : trends and potential for prediction. *In* Feldman, R. and Stiffman A. (Eds). *Advances in Adolescent Mental Health, Volume 1, B*, pp 119-45. Greenwich, Connecticut: JAI Press.

Kringlen, E. (1965) Obsessional neurotics: a long term follow up. *British Journal of Psychiatry*, **111**, 709-22.

Leese, S., (1969) Suicide behaviour in 20 adolescents. *British Journal of Psychiatry* **115**, 479-80.

Levine, R., Sexton, D. Romm, F., Wood, B. and Kaiser, J. (1974). Outbreak of psychosomatic illness at a rural elementary school. *Lancet* **2**, 1500-3.

Levine, R. (1977) Epidemic faintness and syncope in a school marching band. *Journal of the American Medical Association* **238**, 2373-6.

Lumsden-Walker, W. (1980) Intentional self-injury in school-age children. A study of 50 cases. *Journal of Adolescence* **3**, 217-28.

Marks, I., (1979) *Fears and Phobias*. London: Heinemann.

Marks, I. and Gelder, M. (1966) Different ages of onset in varieties of phobia. *American Journal of Psychiatry* **123**, 218-21.

Marks, I., Stern, R., Mawson, D., Cobb, J. and McDonald, R. (1980) Clomipramine and exposure for obsessive-compulsive rituals. *British Journal of Psychiatry* **136**, 1-25.

McClure, G. (1986) Recent changes in suicide among adolescents in England and Wales. *Journal of Adolescence* **9**, 135-43.

McEvedy, C., Griffith, A. and Hall, T., (1966) Two school epidemics. *British Medical Journal* **2**, 1300-2.

Miller, L., Barrett, C. and Hampe, E. (1974) Phobias of childhood in a prescientific era. *In* Davids, A. (Ed), *Child Personality and Psychopathology : Current Topics*. Chichester: John Wiley and Sons.

Mohr, P. and Bond, M. (1982) A chronic epidemic of hysterical blackouts in a comprehensive school. *British Medical Journal* **284**, 961-2.

Morgan, H., Burns-Cox, J., Pocock, H. and Pottle, S. (1975) Deliberate self-harm: clinical and socio-economic characteristics of 368 patients. *British Journal of Psychiatry* **127**, 564-74.

Moss. P. and McEvedy, C. (1966) An epidemic of overbreathing among schoolgirls. *British Medical Journal* **2**, 1295-300.

Pedder, J. (1982) Failure to mourn, and melancholia. *British Journal of Psychiatry* **141**, 329-37.

Pittman, F., Donald, L. and Deyoung, C. (1968). Work and school phobia : a family approach to treatment. *American Journal of Psychiatry* **124**, 1535-41.

Pollitt, J. (1969) Obsessional states. *British Journal of Hospital Medicine* **2**, 1146–50.

Poznanski, E. (1973) Children with excessive fears. *American Journal of Orthopsychiatry* **43**, 428–38.

Reynolds D., Jones, D., St Leger, S. and Murgatroyd, S. (1980) School factors and truancy. *In* Hersov, L. (Ed), *Out of School – Modern Perspectives in School Refusal and Truancy*, pp 85–110. Chichester: John Wiley and Sons.

Rivinus, T., Jamison, D. and Graham, P. (1975) Childhood organic neurological disease presenting as psychiatric disorder. *Archives of Diseases of Childhood* **50**, 115–19.

Robins, L. (1972) Follow-up studies of behaviour disorders in childhood. *In* Quay, H. and Werry, J. (Eds), *Psychopathological Disorders of Childhood*. New York: John Wiley and Sons.

Rutter, M., Graham, P., Chadwick, O. and Yule, W. (1976) Adolescent turmoil : fact or fiction? *Journal of Child Psychology and Psychiatry* **17**, 35–56.

Rutter, M., Tizard, J. and Whitmore, K. (1970) *Education, Health and Behaviour*. London: Longman.

Sainsbury, P., Jenkins, J. and Levey, Q. (1980). The social correlates of suicide in Europe. *In* Farmer, R. and Hirsch, S. (Eds), *The Suicide Syndrome*. London: Croom Helm.

Schmitt, B. (1971) School phobia – the great imitator : a paediatrician's viewpoint.*Paediatrics* **48**, 433–442.

Sedman, G. (1970) Theories of depersonalization : a reappraisal. *British Journal of Psychiatry* **117**, 1–14.

Shaffer, D. (1974) Suicide in childhood and early adolescence. *Journal of Child Psychology and Psychiatry* **15**, 275–91.

Shaffer, D. and Fisher, P. (1981) The epidemiology of suicide in children and young adolescents. *Journal of the American Academy of Child Psychiatry* **20**, 545–65.

Shorvon, H., Hill, J., Burkitt, E. and Hastead, H. (1946) The depersonalisation syndrome. *Proceedings of the Royal Society of Medicine* **39**, 779–92.

Skynner, A. (1974) School phobia : a reappraisal. *British Journal of Medical Psychology* **47**, 1–16.

Slater, E. (1965) Diagnosis of hysteria. *British Medical Journal* 1395–9.

Steinberg, D., Bolton, D., Savoury, G., Kean, W. and Fortune, B. (1988) Hysterical disorders in adolescence : treatment by family and milieu approaches. In preparation.

Stern, R. and Cobb, J. (1978) Phenomenology of obsessive-compulsive neurosis. *British Journal of Psychiatry* **132**, 233–9.

Thomas, A., Chess, S., and Birch, H. (1968) *Temperament and Behaviour Disorders in Childhood*. New York: Universities Press.

Toolan, J.M. (1962) Depression in children and adolescents. *American Journal of Orthopsychiatry* **32**, 404–15.

Tyrer, P. and Steinberg, D. (1987) *Models for Mental Disorder : Conceptual Models in Psychiatry.* Chichester : John Wiley and Sons.

Tyrer, P. and Tyrer, S. (1974) School refusal, truancy and neurotic illness. *Psychological Medicine* **4**, 416–21.

Warren, W. (1965a) A study of adolescent psychiatric in-patients and the outcome six or more years later. I. Clinical histories and hospital findings. *Journal of Child Psychology and Psychiatry* **6**, 1–17.

Warren, W. (1965b) A study of adolescent psychiatric in-patients and the outcome six or more years later. II. The follow-up study. *Journal of Child Psychology and Psychiatry* **6**, 141–60.

Weiner, I. (1970) Psychological disturbance in adolescence. New York: John Wiley and Sons.

Wexler, L., Weissmann, M., and Kasl, S. (1978) Suicide attempts 1970–1975: updating on US study and comparisons with international trends. *British Journal of Psychiatry* **132**, 180–5.

Chapter 8

Conduct Disorders and Delinquency

Misbehaviour in adolescence

Problem behaviour, which may or may not also break the law, may result from a psychiatric disorder or it may occur in a young person who is psychologically normal. Some young people appear to be psychologically disturbed primarily in terms of their patterns of social behaviour, and the term conduct disorder is then applied to them. However, the family and social influences closely associated with conduct disorder make it difficult, clinically and theoretically to make an absolutely clear distinction between disorder 'in' the adolescent, and misbehaviour caused and maintained by external circumstances – e.g. poor upbringing.

Example 5
Wayne is a fourteen-year-old boy who is referred to the child psychiatric clinic by his family doctor because his mother thinks he is being treated unfairly by the education authority. Wayne has always been difficult and disruptive but has now broken a teacher's nose, and his mother thinks the school's reaction, to exclude him, and press assault charges, is disgraceful. The psychiatrist is quite surprised at the mother's attitude which seems almost to encourage Wayne's defiance. She says he isn't a bad boy, that particular teacher always 'had it in for Wayne', and she has been complaining for a long time about the poor standard of the teaching and behaviour there. 'Wayne isn't the worst, but he gets picked on, and that's what winds him up. And he still can't read properly'. When asked what Wayne's father has to say, his mother says, with an anxious glance at Wayne, 'That's why I wanted to see you by myself, Doctor'.

She is scared of Wayne, and for him. If she doesn't take his side he attacks her verbally and sometimes physically. Her husband (it is her second marriage) is fed up with Wayne and now wants nothing to do with him. When she has tried to involve Wayne's stepfather in his care there have been two quite different outcomes : occasionally, Wayne's stepfather will take him off on one of his fishing outings from which both return in good spirits 'like a pair of kids – they have a great time'. More often, when stepfather is called in to help it ends with Wayne getting hit by him.

It had been agreed initially that his stepfather would be asked to attend. But Wayne's mother hasn't passed the message on. She says that her husband has already had enough of Wayne, and fears that he could walk out if asked to get involved in his problems. He doesn't even know about the appointment.

Many young people with conduct disorders have some such background to their difficulties, and these are described in this chapter. Also characteristic is the fact that the problems tend to be multiple.

Some definitions

Conduct disorders are characterized by aggressive, destructive and disruptive behaviour in the absence of another psychiatric condition that might account for it (e.g. autism or a schizophrenic illness). Conduct disorders can be sub-categorized into unsocialized and socialized conduct disorder.

Socialized conduct disorder refers to misbehaviour carried out in a peer group; the identified patient might be a leader or follower in a group, or simply liable to be drawn into the behaviour of other groups. Fighting, stealing, avoiding school and delinquency may be among the repertoire of undesirable behaviour.

Unsocialized conduct disorder refers to misbehaviour confined to a narrower field of relationships. There may be defiance and disobedience, aggressive and destructive behaviour within the home, lying, stealing and bullying, largely initiated by the adolescent. The boy or girl might sometimes generate attention from peers e.g. as the class clown, but the child is essentially solitary in his or her misbehaviour.

Where emotional disturbance such as anxiety or sadness is marked, the term *mixed disorder of conduct and emotions* is used. However, most if not all young people with conduct disorders are unhappy or anxious about their behaviour, though this may not be obvious at first.

Delinquency refers to behaviour which breaks the law. Most adolescent delinquents do not have conduct disorders. Correspondingly, many young people with conduct disorders do not break the law, and hence are not delinquents.

The term behaviour disorder is sometimes used synonymously with conduct disorder. The latter is the better term, since it refers in a more general way to the overall social conduct of the boy or girl.

Is it a disorder?

The essence of the notion of conduct disorder is that it is behaviour that gives rise to social disapproval (Rutter, 1975). An alternative term is antisocial disorder (Rutter *et al.*, 1970). It can be argued that we are defining this disorder primarily in terms of what society happens to disapprove of, and it should therefore not be regarded as a clinical disorder at all.

However, the adolescents the psychiatrist diagnoses as having conduct disorders are not nonconformists who have taken a thought-out dissenting position on some aspect of the community's demands, but young people who have several or all of the following individual characteristics: they are often socially unskilled, mismanaging relation-ships and activities in which they are motivated to succeed, as well as those (e.g. keeping appointments) they want to subvert; they are often male, the male:female preponderance for conduct disorder being about 3 or 4 to 1; the boys, but not the girls, may be slightly below average intellectually (Rutter *et al.*, 1970); educational difficulties, lack of academic success and, in particular, reading retardation is common in both boys and girls with conduct disorder.

In addition, they often come from large families which are socially disadvantaged, live in disadvantaged neighbourhoods and may be at a disadvantaged school; there is often discord between the parents, which may include violence and broken marriages.

In earlier childhood they are likely to have been aggressive, impulsive and non-compliant, while long-term follow-up studies reveal problems in many areas of their lives, including problems with relationships, jobs and health (physical as well as emotional) including a tendency to abuse alcohol (Robins, 1966, 1970). Of course these factors alone do not cause conduct disorder; a male in a large family is not at risk by virtue of these two characteristics alone. But this range of personal and environmental characteristics is associated very strongly with conduct disorders in children and adolescents, and justifies their recognition in terms of individual dysfunction. However, the social and family influences are clearly very important (see also Rutter and Madge, 1976).

The psychiatrist will also see two groups of adolescents who present conduct *problems* but not necessarily conduct *disorders*. First, psychiatric help is sometimes sought to help with older adolescents who are going their own way against their parents' wishes but are neither psychiatri-cally disturbed nor breaking the law. There may sometimes be a case for family or parental counselling, if that is wanted by all concerned, but this should not be confused with diagnosing the adolescent as 'disturbed'.

Second, some young people are naughty because they manage to get away with behaviour that their parents or teachers ought not to tolerate; they are being handled and brought up inexpertly, and work with the family or advice to the parents and school may help. Although this should not be confused with conduct disorder, it is reasonable to suppose that a spectrum could be constructed with inept upbringing at one end and a cluster of social disadvantages at the other. Adolescents in family therapy or attending psychiatrists and counsellors are likely to be found at all points on this spectrum.

Hyperactivity

Hyperactivity, which means excessive activity, is another term which is a source of much confusion. It is associated with two other terms : the hyperkinetic syndrome, and attention deficit disorder. There is considerable disagreement and even confusion in the literature, and Taylor (1985), with admirable frankness, urges caution about accepting any account, even his own, of hyperactivity.

The following definitions, based on Taylor's thorough review, are recommended:

(a) *Overactivity*: excessive movement, not necessarily due to any abnormality.

(b) *Hyperactivity* (= *hyperkinesis*): a behavioural style which includes overactivity, impulsive restlessness and inattention, and which varies depending on the situation the child is in.

(c) *Hyperkinetic syndrome*: an uncommon condition, if it exists at all, in which hyperactivity (as described above) is pervasive, i.e. occurs in a wide range of situations or in all situations the child is in.

Descriptively, overactive (or hyperactive, or hyperkinetic) children show disturbed conduct.

Example 6

Kevin, aged 10, shows extreme hyperactivity. He brings into the counsulting room an armful of toys and models which he begins to show the psychiatrist before diving onto the floor and under the desk to set out one of his games. He swiftly abandons it in order to argue noisily with his mother about something she had promised him as a reward for seeing the doctor. While she is explaining he goes out into the waiting room; he is brought back and starts another game, then abandons it to make a series of demands of the psychiatrist. His questions are turned into a discussion of how he feels, which he attends to for some ten to fifteen seconds before turning to the bookcase in the room and trying to get at the contents. A toy car from the bookcase is given to him and he agrees to sit down at the desk to look at it, but by the time he has done so the car is abandoned and he begins a struggle with his mother about something in her bag.

Given the uncertainty about the condition, it is not surprising that its prevalence is unclear. In the United States of America it is widely regarded as a common condition, with up to 40 per cent of the children attending some child psychiatric clinics receiving this diagnosis (Safer and Allen 1976). In England a clinic population prevalence of 1.5 per cent (Taylor, 1985) and a child population prevalence of only 2 in 2199 (Isle of Wight study of 10 and 11 year-olds, Rutter *et al.*, 1976) shows rates of a quite different order. The likely reason for the difference is the inclusion in the American reports of a wide range of children with conduct disturbance who are judged to be overactive.

The diagnosis *attention deficit disorder* ('ADD') has now been introduced in the United States, and picks out distractability and short attention span as a psychological problem and clinical disorder in its own right. As Taylor (1985) points out, the relationship between the neuropsychological problem on the one hand and the overactivity on the other is not clear (e.g. which causes which), and 'attention' is not a single cognitive function but the end result of a number of quite different psychological and behavioural operations.

Children with brain disorder (including 'minimal brain dysfunction' or 'minimal brain damage', sometimes elevated and abbreviated to 'm.b.d.') show a higher incidence of hyperactivity (Seidel *et al.*, 1975), as do children with intellectual retardation and autistic children. However, children with these conditions often do not show hyperactivity.

The term hyperactivity, like conduct disorder, should be used with caution, because it is sometimes used to describe a symptom, sometimes a syndrome, and sometimes as if referring to a specific disorder.

Hyperactivity through childhood and adolescence

Overactivity among three-year-olds is a strong predictor of conduct disorder in later childhood (Richman *et al.*, 1982). 'Hyperactivity' as a problem in the clinic is seen largely in middle childhood, when any propensity to impulsiveness and non- compliance is likely to cause more problems. By the age of puberty the incidence is reducing. However, hyperkinetic children followed up into adolescence continue to be impulsive, distractible and poorly organized, with relatively poor social skills (Weiss *et al.*, 1979; Minde *et al.*, 1972), while Strachan (1981) showed that in a conduct-disordered group those with pervasive overactivity did worst. In adult life there is no striking incidence of problems in adjustment in work or socially (Hechtman, 1976), nor mental illness, although their personalities are sometimes described as impulsive or immature (Weiss *et al.*, 1979) and they do seem to be impulsive, accident-prone people.

The causes of conduct disorder and hyperactivity

Aetiological factors in conduct disorders and delinquency were discussed in Chapter 3. In brief, conduct-disordered children are often aggressive and hard to manage from an early age, with the probability that either temperamental or early upbringing factors are operating, or an interaction between the two. Socially, family discord with extremes of handling (e.g. punitive, permissive or inconsistent) is common, as is membership of a large, poor family in a deprived neighbourhood and with poor schooling. The common association of reading retardation with conduct disorder has been mentioned.

There does seem to be a genetic component to the aetiology of hyperactivity (Willermann, 1973) and the families of hyperkinetic children contain a higher prevalence of antisocial conduct, alcoholism and hysterical disorders (Cantwell, 1972). There has been much excitement about food additives as a cause of hyperactivity (as with other disorders); Taylor (1979, 1985) and Connors (1980) conclude that evidence for this is very scanty but there may be 'islands of justification', and that families experimenting in this direction should be helped and advised, which includes making sure that other aspects of help and care are not neglected.

Some research has focussed on the details of family life of conduct-disordered children. The families of aggressive and delinquent children may be particularly punitive, provide unclear rules, do not persist consistently with such rules as there are, and do not provide positive guidance on how to behave reasonably. Nor is there much encouragement or experience of normal conversation (Patterson, 1982).

For many years research into conduct disorders, delinquency and psychopathy has produced intriguing evidence of abnormal neuropsychological functioning in some individuals (e.g. low autonomic reactivity) but its relationship with other (e.g. social) influences and disturbed behaviour remains unclear. These and other possible neurophysiological influences are reviewed in Lewis (1981), Rutter and Giller (1983) and

West (1985). There have also been indications that lead, as an environmental intoxicant of the central nervous system affecting cognitive function, could affect behaviour (Rutter, 1980). Although the evidence remains uncertain it is strong enough for active steps to be required to reduce this form of pollution.

Overall, biological impairments great and small, from major and minor brain disorder to lowered self esteem from minor handicaps and anomalies could contribute to persistent misbehaviour, just as in other children they could contribute to unhappiness. Whatever these primary causes, if such they are, it would be surprising if subsequent family and social shaping of behaviour by various processes did not play a major part.

Conduct disorder, with and without hyperactivity, is a most complicated social and biological phenomenon, and neither its social management nor psychiatric treatment is in any way satisfactory. In a thoughtful paper, Wolff (1987) urges psychiatrists and their colleagues not to abandon their attempts to study and help with the problem of antisocial conduct. She sees this as a greater risk in adult than in child psychiatry; certainly it is during later adolescence that adults may begin to lose patience, interest or hope with misbehaving young people.

Delinquency

Delinquency is universal. Many quite respectable people break the law as motorists, often regularly. However, the motorist is not the stereotype image of the delinquent. When we turn to the more widely accepted image of delinquency, largely stealing, violence, vandalism and disruption of public order, we find that the number of offenders in England and Wales in the 14 -17 age group was just under 8000 per 100,000 in 1977 among males, and around 1500 for females – a male:female ratio of about 5 : 1 (Home Office figures quoted in Rutter and Giller, 1983).

Three things should be said about these figures. First, the offences are for the most part criminal damage and taking cars, i.e. not violence against the person, and across the range of offences tend to be less serious than the equivalent offences in adults (West, 1985). Second, there has been a real increase in recorded delinquency in the last 25 years in many areas of Western society. Third, while the increase in male delinquency in this age group was about 150 per cent between 1959 and 1977, it was almost 380 per cent for females (Rutter and Giller, 1983). Thus the rate for boys rose during that period (though has changed little since) while the rate for girls rose much faster.

The backgrounds of delinquent young people show similarities to those with conduct disorders. Both delinquents and those who self-report offences in surveys tend to come from large, poor families in which other members have been delinquent, to have experienced problems in their upbringing and to be of lower than average intelligence (West and Farrington, 1973). The same study suggested that being of higher intelligence and coming from a good home could be protective factors against being convicted even when, according to self-report, offences had been carried out.

Acts of delinquency are common, but do not usually lead on to a delinquent career. Much repeated delinquency is due to a relatively smaller group of persistent offenders; in the study by West and Farrington (1977) less than one quarter of the convicted youths were responsible for over half of the offences that led to conviction. West (1985) suggests that the worse the behaviour at school and the worse the school background, the more likely are offenders to become persistent offenders. However, for most acts of delinquency the picture is of only one or two offences against property and no further convictions.

For the persistent offender, several studies demonstrate some continuity between childhood conduct problems and later antisocial behaviour, including adult delinquency (Jessor and Jessor, 1977; Robins, 1978). There have been a number of studies showing correlations between persistent antisocial behaviour, neurological impairment causing attention deficit (Orris, 1969), low frustration tolerance, aggressiveness, poor educational attainment and low or below average intelligence. As with conduct disorder and hyperactivity, it is difficult to draw firm conclusions about the relationships between these correlating factors.

Vandalism

Vandalism, the more or less casual damage and defacement of public and private property, deserves mention as a delinquent phenomenon influenced by as well as affecting the physical environment. There is some evidence that designing housing estates so that people's own property was readily identified, and other people's homes and public places were readily overlooked by neighbours, may reduce vandalism (Newman, 1973) although Rutter and Giller (1983) suggest that it would be optimistic to expect too much from this alone.

It is also likely that delapidated, neglected areas encourage further disfigurement; one could suppose that badly maintained areas devalue themselves and their inhabitants, prompt bored groups into ideas about how to spend a few minutes, and demonstrate the evidence that others have 'successfully' created a mess. One could also speculate that the type of village or close community where quite modest disturbance from youngsters resulted in adults coming out of their houses to see what was happening and remonstrate with them, would have a different vandalism rate from areas where adults were inhibited about intervening.

Fire-setting

Young people who start fires, even quite modest blazes in wastebins, cause serious concern. Not only can very serious danger arise for large numbers of people, but the death and damage caused can be far beyond whatever intentions the child had, and rapidly grow quite beyond his control. The adolescent who acquires the reputation of being a possible fire-setter may in due course find few places prepared to look after him other than specialized high-security establishments. Fire-setting children tend to come from disrupted families and to have other conduct problems. A small number are diagnosed as impulsive, hyperactive or psychotic (Kaufman *et al.*, 1961). In general, younger children tend to start fires alone and at home; older children, and adolescents, away from home and in groups. Of those who are referred to psychiatrists, about three-quarters stop setting fires (Stewart and Culver 1982) and about a quarter carry on; but there is no clear evidence on which to base predictions of further fire-setting. The only reasonably safe course is to treat whatever disturbance is present and give high priority to supervision and safety. (see Lewis and Yarnall, 1951; Strachan, 1981; Stewart and Culver, 1982).

Conduct disorder and delinquency : management issues

(i)   The mental state of the adolescent referred because of unacceptable social behaviour may be entirely normal at one end of the spectrum, or reveal evidence of major mental illness at the other. Psychiatrically normal delinquents may be seen in psychiatric clinics and grossly disturbed offenders are found in young people's prisons.

(ii) Distinguish individual or family problems which may be helped in due course by psychiatric or psychological therapy, from unacceptable or possible dangerous behaviour which must simply be stopped by any means, regardless of the efficacy of treatment. It is not uncaring or unsympathetic to point out that parental firmness, supervision (e.g. by a probation officer) or even physical containment (e.g. in a secure centre) may be necessary to limit misconduct; quite the reverse. Appearance in Court, accompanied by a helpful report (see Chapter 18), should not be regarded as anti-therapeutic except for the most unwell patient. Clarifying that control and treatment are different, but that both are components of proper care, can be helpful for parents and child, all of whom may have come to associate limit- setting with hostility, perhaps with good reason.

(iii)   Even where a formal behaviour programme (Chapter 18) is not being used, agreement and precision are important between all concerned (parents, adolescent, helpers) about precisely what behaviour is unacceptable, and what are the goals of treatment.

(iv)   By the same token try to organize good communication and consistency between the people involved in helping. Problematic teenagers can accumulate large numbers of different workers, and mutually agreed pruning and division of labour can help focus help and avoid confusion.

(v)   The going is often difficult and all concerned can get dispirited. Monitoring actual progress towards agreed goals will help demonstrate objectively what is or is not being achieved over time.

(vi)   There can be a tendency to focus only on misbehaviour and what the adolescent cannot do. Attention should be paid to strengths, achievements and attainable goals in aspects of life outside the targeted misbehaviour.

(vii)   Many conduct disordered and delinquent adolescents have poor educational attainment, reading skills and social skills, and should be helped in these areas. Some aggressive youngsters do not know how to explain or assert themselves without getting confused, enraged and aggressive, and imaginative help here can boost self-esteem and reduce some aspects of misconduct.

(viii)   Stimulant (amphetamine-like) drugs may help some patients with hyperkinetic disorder, if there is also marked attention deficit which is not due to anxiety (Chapter 18).

(ix)   Tranquillizing medication is not usually useful, but I consider it reasonable to use it as a chemical restraint if there is no other way of keeping a violent young person safely in a therapeutic setting. Tranquillizing medication such as the phenothiazines and similar drugs, and carbemazepine and lithium are occasionally useful, and are discussed in Chapter 18.

(x)   Individual counselling or support should be considered (from either within the clinic or a social agency) particularly if there is no other, natural, source (e.g. in the family or school) to help with discussion and advice.

(xi) Individual psychotherapy does not have an encouraging record in the management of conduct disorder or delinquency. However, some young people in these two categories may be suitable for psychotherapy according to wider criteria, and this should be considered as a possible treatment as for any other patient.

(xii) Conduct problems can be intractable. On the one hand, persist- ence on the part of the clinician is to be encouraged, and quite often will be worth while. On the other, it is also proper to know when to stop.

References and further reading

Cantwell, D. (1972) Psychiatric illness in the families of hyperactive children. *Archives of General Psychiatry* **27**, 414–17.

Connors, C.K. (1980) *Food Additives and Hyperactive Children*. New York: Plenum.

Hechtman, L. (1976) Hyperactives as young adults. *Canadian Medical Association Journal* **115**, 625–30.

Jessor, R. and Jessor, S. (1977) *Problem Behaviour and Psychosocial Development : A Longitudinal Study of Youth*. New York: Academic Press.

Kaufman, I., Heims, L. W. and Reiser D. (1961) A re-evaluation of the psychodynamics of fire-setting. *American Journal of Orthopsychiatry* **22**, 63–72.

Lewis, D.O. (Ed) (1981) *Vulnerabilities to delinquency*. Lancaster: MTP Press Ltd.

Lewis, N.D. and Yarnell, H. (1951) *Pathological firesetting. Nervous and Mental Disease Monographs, No. 82*. New York: The Coolidge Foundation.

Minde, K., Weiss, G. and Mendelson, N. (1972) A five year follow-up study of 91 hyperactive schoolchildren. *Journal of the American Academy of Child Psychiatry* **11**, 595–610.

Newman, O. (1973) *Defensible Space*. London: Architectural Press.

Orris, J.B. (1969) Visual monitoring performance in three subgroups of male delinquents. *Journal of Abnormal Psychology* **74**, 227–9.

Patterson, G.R. (1982) *Coercive Family Processes*. Eugene, Oregon: Castalia Publishing Company.

Richman, N., Stevenson, J. and Graham, P.J. (1982) *Pre-School to School : A Behavioural Study*. London: Academic Press.

Robins, L. (1966) *Deviant Children Grown up*. Baltimore: Williams and Williams.

Robins, L. (1970) Follow-up studies investigating childhood disorders. *In* Hare E.H. and Wing J.K. (Eds), *Psychiatric Epidemiology*, pp 29–68. London: Oxford University Press.

Robins, L. (1978) Sturdy childhood predictors of adult antisocial behaviour : replications from longitudinal studies. *Psychological Medicine* **8**, 611–22.

Rutter, M. (1975) *Helping Troubled Children*. Harmondsworth: Penguin Books.

Rutter, M. (1980) Raised lead levels and impaired cognitive/behavioural functioning : a review of the evidence.*Developmental Medicine and Child Neurology*, (Supplement) **22**, 1–26.

Rutter, M. and Giller, H. (1983) *Juvenile Delinquency*. Harmondsworth: Penguin Books.

Rutter, M. and Madge, N. (1977) *Cycles of Disadvantage : A Review of Research*. London: Heinemann.

Rutter, M., Tizard, J. and Whitmore, W. (1970) *Education, Health and Behaviour*. London: Longman.

Rutter, M., Tizard, J., Yule, W., Graham, P. and Whitmore, K. (1976) Research Report : Isle of Wight studies 1964-1974. *Psychological Medicine* **6**, 313–32.

Safer, D.J. and Allen, R.P. (1976) *Hyperactive Children : Diagnosis and Management*. Baltimore: University Park Press.

Seidel, U.P., Chadwick, O. and Rutter, M. (1975) Psychological disorders in crippled children : a comparative study of children with and without brain damage. *Developmental Medicine and Child Neurology* **17**, 563–73.

Stewart M.A. and Culver K.W. (1982) Children who set fires : the clinical picture and a follow-up. *British Journal of Psychiatry* **140**, 357–63.

Strachan, J. G. (1981) Conspicuous firesetting in children. *British Journal of Psychiatry* **138**, 26–9.

Taylor, E. (1979) Food additives, allergy and hyperkinesis. *Journal of Child Psychology and Psychiatry* **20**, 357–63.

Taylor, E. (1985) Syndromes of overactivity and attention deficit. *In* Rutter M. and Hersov, L. (Eds), *Child and Adolescent Psychiatry : Modern Approaches*, pp 424–43. Oxford: Blackwell Scientific Publications.

Taylor, E. (Ed) (1986) *The Overactive Child*. Oxford : Spastic International.

Weiss, G, Hechtman, L., Perlman, T., Hopkins, J. and Wener, A. (1979) Hyperactives as young adults. A controlled prospective 10 year follow-up of 75 children. *Archives of General Psychiatry* **36**, 675–81.

West, D. (1985) Delinquency. *In* Rutter, M. and Hersov, L. (eds), *Child and Adolescent Psychiatry : Modern Approaches*, pp 414–23. Oxford: Blackwell Scientific Publications.

West, D. and Farrington, D. (1977) *The Delinquent Way of Life*. London: Heinemann.

West, D. and Farrington, D. (1973) *Who becomes delinquent?* London: Heinemann.

Willerman, L. (1973) Activity level and hyperactivity in twins. *Child Development* **44**, 288–93.

Wolff, S. (1987) Antisocial conduct : whose concern? *Journal of Adolescence* **10**, 105–18.

Chapter 9

Enuresis and Encopresis

Enuresis (bedwetting)

Acquiring bladder control is part of normal development and is achieved at different times by different children. By the age of seven about 15 per cent of boys and 12 per cent of girls are still occasionally wet at night; by fourteen 2 per cent and 1 percent respectively. For more frequent bedwetting of once a week or more, the prevalence is 1 per cent and 0.5 per cent respectively (Rutter *et al.*, 1973) Bedwetting is usually divided into primary enuresis (never been dry) and secondary enuresis (wet after a period of continence). Shaffer (1985) concludes from several longitudinal studies that secondary enuresis is more likely to appear in boys and in the age range 5 to 11 years.

Associated with bedwetting are (a) a strong genetic component – a higher incidence in relatives and a stronger concordance in monozygotic than dizygotic twins); (b) upbringing in an institution or large family; (c) being in a lower socio-economic class; (d) being male; (e) a tendency for below average intelligence; (f) a history of stress in early childhood; (g) a relatively small bladder capacity; and (h) urinary tract infection, especially in girls. Psychiatric disorder is not strongly associated with enuresis; but there is more of an association between psychiatric disorder and enuresis in girls than in boys. There does not seem to be the association between bedwetting and sleeping deeply that enuretics' parents sometimes report, and indeed no association with any particular stage of sleep (Mikkelsen *et al.*, 1980). Bedwetting has been reported as an apparent side-effect of neuroleptic drugs in children and adults (discussed in Shaffer's review, 1985).

Enuresis is particularly embarrassing in adolescence for obvious reasons. It seems a childish problem, and the boy or girl whose younger sibling does not have such a handicap will feel particularly ashamed. It can also cause anxiety about trips away from home, and similarly is a challenge to any ambitions the adolescent has for being more independent.

A common clinical impression is that a period of stress or emotional disturbance causes the habit of bladder control to be lost, and that the enuresis, potentially a transient problem, becomes maintained by continuing anxiety and preoccupation in the adolescent and in the family.

Example 7

Susan, 16, is referred because of persistent secondary enuresis. She has been prescribed a bell- and-pad which is proving ineffective. Enquiry about how it is used shows that not only is it being used competently, but the whole of a large, warm, turbulent and rather intrusive family is collaborating intensively in checking that it is used according to instructions and asking about the results. Her father keeps a chart. The wider problem is Susan's unhappiness and thoughts of taking overdoses because of repeated arguments with her parents about her boyfriends, her school, her future career, etc. Characteristically her parents 'take over' friends they like, and reject those they dislike.

At the first appointment, her father takes the lead in describing Susan's bedwetting problems; she doesn't seem to mind this, nor be surprised. The psychiatrist, however, does express surprise. He suggests that they meet as a family to discuss only the wider worries, and they are instructed to stop talking to Susan about her bedwetting. Having checked with her in an individual session that she is using the equipment properly, and provided a self-monitoring chart, the psychiatrist does not discuss it again until the last session when Susan reports that she is now dry at night.

She is advised to stop using the bell-and-pad for the time being, but to use it again for four days if enuresis occurs again. A year later however the enuresis had not apparently recurred.

Enuresis: management issues

(i)   The above girl's case was unusual in that a potentially effective treatment was in fact being persisted with, and the family's over-preoccupation with her problems was symptomatic of a general inappropriate intrusiveness, which responded to straightforward advice. Usually a counselling or psychotherapeutic approach is unnecessary, except where individual or family feelings are clearly getting in the way of applying a simpler (e.g. behavioural) treatment.

(ii) Urinary infection or another physical condition is an occasional cause of enuresis, and the clinician should ensure that this has been considered before embarking on psychological treatment.

(iii) Often one of the following approaches will have been tried before the patient comes to the psychiatric clinic:

(a) Restriction of fluids 2 hours before sleep.

(b) Waking the child in the night to empty the bladder.

(c) Use of a tricyclic antidepressant at night (Blackwell and Currah, 1973) e.g. 50 mg imipramine in the evening for older children and adolescents. It is not clear how it works; perhaps by affecting sleep, perhaps by affecting the bladder and its innervation, perhaps by affecting mood (see review by Shaffer, 1985).

(d) Sometimes behaviour therapy will already have been tried and abandoned, but quite often will be found not to have been applied properly or persistently.

(iv) The bell-and-pad, or night alarm, is an effective treatment in 60–100 per cent of cases (Kolvin *et al.*, 1972). There has been much discussion among psychologists about how it works; the simplest explanation is that the passage of urine, completing a battery-operated circuit and sounding an alarm, so that waking (the conditioned, i.e. learned, response) becomes associated with the indifferent stimulus of bladder contraction. It may become effective in four to six weeks, but in mentally handicapped children may take several months (Smith, 1981). Relapses should be treated by using the equipment for three or four consecutive nights.

(v) Some recommend an overlearning technique by giving the child extra fluid to drink in the evening once the bell-and-pad approach has worked, and then continuing with this conditioning method.

(vi) The adolescent should keep a progress chart. Explaining to the boy or girl that seeing a psychiatrist or psychologist does not mean they are 'neurotic', but that their bladder needs training, will help.

(vii) It is worth looking for the impact of the bedwetting on the adolescent's life in general, and family life in particular, in case an emotional need is being met or a family behavioural system operating to encourage continuation of the problem.

Encopresis

Encopresis, or faecal soiling, is defined as a disorder of bowel control in the absence of physical disease, and occurring after the age of 4 years, the time by which almost 100 per cent of children have achieved proper control (Bellman, 1966; Quay and Werry, 1979). The prevalence at age 10–12 years seems to be of the order 1.3 per cent in boys and 0.3 per cent in girls (Rutter *et al.*, 1970).

There is more than one sort of soiling. Some young people appear to have normal bowel control but leave their faeces in inappropriate places around the house, e.g. amongst clothes in chests of drawers. Others seem unable to control their bowels so that they soil their clothes, sometimes en route to the lavatory. The former child is likely to be producing stools of normal consistency; the latter may produce very fluid faeces, and if this is not due to physical illness may be due to diarrhoea caused by anxiety, or to retention with overflow. The anxiety may be due to fear of using the lavatory.

The retentive type of encopresis may arise from a battle over defaecation between parent and child, or a period of painful defaecation (e.g. due to constipation or an anal fissure). The lower bowel then becomes distended and packed with hard faeces around which watery faeces escape uncontrolled.

Bellman (1966) in a controlled study in a paediatric clinic concluded that the encopretic children she saw had a greater incidence of personality difficulties of a passive-aggressive type, their peer contact was less well established, and their family background more disrupted and more marked by a punitive, coercive approach by the parents. Other studies have shown that encopretic children are more likely to be aggressive, have educational problems, suffer from enuresis too, and come from socially disadvantaged families (Anthony, 1957; Rutter, 1975). Some encopretic adolescents will be found to be of low normal intelligence or just below the average range, and under increased emotional stress from other people's expectations of them, e.g. to show more independence.

Encopresis: management issues

(i)   It is always important to consider a physical cause and enquire carefully into physical investigations done so far. The disorder may be one that causes constipation, diarrhoea or impairment of neural control of the lower bowel and the perineal musculature.

(ii) A blocked bowel can overflow whatever the cause. A microenema containing sodium alkylsulphoacetate, followed by bowel training with rewards if necessary and the prescription of mild laxatives (e.g. Senokot) and a stool softener (e.g. lactulose) may all be sufficiently helpful to re-establish bowel control, autonomy and self- esteem.

(iii) Although parents should be involved with retraining methods for younger children, with older children and adolescents it may be more appropriate for the work to be done on an individual basis.

(iv) Biofeedback aimed at greater sphincter control has been tried with some success, and recommended for consideration in older children when all else has failed (Olness *et al.*, 1980).

(v) As with all problem behaviour, there is the prospect of the unpleasant symptom becoming an absorbing preoccupation for all concerned. It is important to attend to those wider social and educational or training matters that will help build confidence and self-esteem, and make it worth while and feasible for the adolescent to aim at a life free of soiling.

References

Anthony, E.J. (1957) An experimental approach to the psychopathology of childhood encopresis. *British Journal of Medical Psychology* **30**, 146–175.

Bellman, M. (1966) Studies on encopresis. *Acta Paediatrica Scandinavica Suppl.* 170.

Blackwell, B. and Currah, J. (1973) The psychopharmacology of nocturnal enuresis. In Kolvin, I., MacKeith, R. and Meadow, S. (Eds), Bladder Control and Enuresis, *Clinics in Developmental Medicine* **48 49** pp 231–57. London: Spastics International Medical Publications and Heinemann.

Kolvin, I., Taunch, J., Currah, J., Garside, M., Nolan, J. and Shaw, W. (1972) Enuresis: a descriptive analysis and a controlled trial. *Developmental Medicine and Child Neurology* **14**, 715–26.

Mikkelsen, E., Rapoport, J., Nee, L., Gruenau, C., Mendelson, W. and Gillin, J. (1980) Childhood Enuresis I: Sleep patterns and psychopathology. *Archives of General Psychiatry* **37**, 1139–45.

Olness, K., McParland, F. and Piper, J. (1980) Biofeedback : a new modality in the management of children with faecal soiling. *Journal of Pediatrics* **96**, 505–9.

Quay, H. and Werry, J. (Eds) (1979) *Psychopathological Disorders of Childhood*, pp 165–7. New York: John Wiley.

Rutter, M. (1975) *Helping Troubled Children*. Harmondsworth: Penguin.

Rutter, M., Tizard, J. and Whitmore, K. (1970) *Education, Health and Behaviour*. London: Longman.

Rutter, M., Yule, W. and Graham, P. (1973) Enuresis and behavioural deviance: some epidemiological considerations. In Kolvin, I., MacKeith, R. and Meadow, S. (Eds), Bladder Control and Enuresis. *Clinics in*

Developmental Medicine, **48, 49**, pp 137–47. London: Spastics International Medical Publications and Heinemann.

Shaffer, D. (1985) Enuresis. In Rutter, M. and Hersov, L. (Eds), *Child and Adolescent Psychiatry : Modern Approaches*, pp 465–81. Oxford: Blackwell Scientific Pulblications.

Smith, L. (1981) Training severely and profoundly mentally handicapped nocturnal enuretics. *Behaviour Research and Therapy* **19**, 67–74.

Chapter 10

Problems of Sexual Identity, Experience and Behaviour

Problems of sexual identity

There are many levels to sexual identity and behaviour : genetic sex; physique (i.e. primary and secondary sex characteristics); gender identity, i.e. the sex in which the young person has been brought up and which is partly assigned and partly adopted; sexual self-presentation (i.e. the physical appearance adopted, particularly in dress); and sexual (erotic) behaviour.

It is therefore important to be clear about the patient's problem and this is not always absolutely clear to the adolescent concerned. For example, (a) an adolescent may be genuinely homosexual and feel distressed and alienated as a result; (b) another adolescent may be experimenting with homosexual behaviour and causing his parents or teachers concern; (c) another adolescent may fear he is a homosexual and wish not to be; (d) another may believe he is 'really' a girl (transexualism) and be unhappy and frustrated in his attempts to complete that role; while (e) another adolescent may cross-dress (transvestism) for fun, or because of some complex identification with his mother or sister, or for erotic reasons which may be homosexual or heterosexual, but without doubting his gender identity.

Parental anxiety about sexual development

It is unusual for parents to worry about their daughters being 'tomboys' i.e. showing stereotypical boyish behaviour. But anxiety may be expressed about young boys who prefer to play with girls, dress in girls' clothes and play with dolls. In a major study of 4 to 11-year-old boys who showed this behaviour, two-thirds became bisexual or homosexual in young adulthood, while a control group of 'masculine' boys showed, in young adulthood, no bisexuality or homosexuality. In another part of the same study, about two-thirds of adult transexual men recalled preferring girl playmates and girls' toys in childhood, and half preferred girls' clothes (Green, 1976, 1985a). Green discusses the ethics of intervention in this behaviour (Green, 1985b) and suggests the strategy not of trying to force these boys into the male stereotype, but rather to help them to feel comfortable and positive about being physically male, about performing some culturally age-appropriate male behaviours, and about anticipating becoming an adult male. Green noted how fathers in particular tended to be alienated from feminine sons, and suggested strategies for helping to minimize this. Green's review (1985b) deserves reading, particularly for its discussion of the pros and cons of attempting treatment; for example, the need to bear in mind the unhappy experiences of adult transexuals whether or not they are physically 'reassigned' by surgical or hormonal procedures. His approach would help the developing child into the position where there is the prospect of making a real choice, and as far as possible reducing family and individual distress.

Do 'tomboy' girls grow up to be homosexual women? Studies by Bell *et al.*, (1981) and Saghir and Robins (1973) demonstrated an association between tomboy behaviour in childhood and adult lesbianism. Green *et al.* (1982) has begun a prospective study, and so far the most significant discriminator between tomboy and non-tomboy girls has been for the former group's greater participation in sports. By adolescence, both groups prefer to be female (Green, 1985b).

Transexualism

Transexual men and women have a powerful wish to be of the opposite sex, usually accompanied by the conviction that whatever their anatomical appearance their biological and therefore true sex is the opposite to what it appears to be. Christie Brown (1983) has explored the complexity of the phenomenology involved, and suggests that the feeling of 'really' being of the opposite sex is an intense wish rather than an obsession or delusion. He also describes transexuals' distaste for their own sexual anatomy, and a sexual preference for others of the same sex, while insisting that they are not homosexual.

Example 8
Eileen, aged 15, is referred because of depression and suicidal attempts

resulting from her frustration with her anatomical sex. The frustration has been compounded by the reminder from various sources that she cannot be seriously considered for the sex change operation she wants for some two or three years, and even then there can be no certainty about the decision. Meanwhile, Eileen tightly straps her breasts, and wears a 'codpiece' of screwed-up cloth under her jeans. She is experimenting with alcohol and drugs to relieve her distress and rejects practitioners who urge patience about her wish for a surgical operation.

The following things emerge, all with a bearing on the help and advice she is given. First, her denial of homosexual feelings is ambiguous. She actually has homosexual feelings, of which she is ashamed because of her parents' attitudes. However, she is enraged at the idea that she might be better off as a well-adjusted homosexual young woman than as someone converted surgically into a male. Second, she is so confused and depressed about herself and what her parents feel for her that she appears to have major problems of identity well beyond the limits of sexual identity alone. Quite apart from needing help with this wider problem, it seems unlikely that she is in a position to make any choice that will 'hold up' satisfactorily over the years, and even more unlikely that a competent surgeon would agree to operate on her unless her personality was more stable. Third, she has little idea about what a sex-change operation would involve, nor the outcome. This notion seems to have occupied a blind spot; she has only a vague idea that a surgeon could magically turn her into a man.

Working on these therapeutic and educational needs with her and her family (prolonged and stormy work) results in her moving towards being a more independent, happier young woman with ambivalent rather than negative feelings about becoming homosexual, and the willingness to postpone the issue of a physical sex-change until she is surer of what she wants.

Her case demonstrates a characteristic adolescent uncertainty of what is really wanted, based on real identity confusion, and accompanied by both depression and ignorance of the facts. It is crucial for the practitioners involved not to jump to premature conclusions about what is best for the boy or girl. Sexual identity problems are muddling for everyone involved, generate anxiety, and raise moral and ethical dilemmas for which individual workers and the team may be unprepared. (For example : is the patient to be referred to as Eileen or, as she wishes, Peter? And referred to as 'he' or 'she'? This was a subject for dispute in the family too.)

The approach taken was (a) to regard her firmly as the girl she in fact was, although respecting her choice of a male name; (b) to aim explicitly at working with her individual and family confusion and her distress, in order to be in the best possible position to make real choices when the time came; and (c) to find out, with her, what a sexual reassignment clinic would expect, which was (i) emotional stability, (ii) to be at least 18, and (iii) to be living successfully as if a member of the opposite sex for at least two years.

Transexualism raises complex issues in adolescence and adults (see Stoller, 1968; Christie Brown, 1983) and the results of physical intervention are variable in terms of anatomical outcome and the patient's satisfaction and future adjustment (see Noe, 1978; Lothstein, 1980, 1982, 1983). The recommended course for an adolescent is to adopt the general aims suggested above, which include sharing information as well as providing counselling and psychotherapy; and, if the patient is determined to have an operation or hormonal treatment in his or her late teens, to liaise with the family doctor to try to encourage the seeking of only competent, ethical, advice.

Homosexuality

Homosexuality is distinct from transexualism, but aspects of the studies outlined above, and the approach to management described, is relevant. When homosexuality is a cause of distress, the general strategy should be psychotherapeutic, to help the adolescent develop in a way that maximizes the chance of knowing his or her own mind and feelings, and enables mature decisions to be made. Advice and guidance may be needed to help an adolescent experimenting with homosexuality, or who is homosexual, to manage his or her affairs in a way that doesn't provoke unnecessary distress in the patient nor alarm in, for example, parents or teachers.

Although the attitude that homosexuality is a disorder appears to be passing, it may be the presented problem behind which lies personality or family difficulties, and as a secret or as a style of life it can lead to personal distress. Some young people are helped by being put in touch with responsible self-help and mutually supportive homosexual organizations.

Exhibitionism

Genital display is a common sexual offence, and the great majority of exhibitionists are males. They are characteristically young, rather passive and inhibited men responding to excitement and a powerful urge to expose their genitals to passing strangers, usually female and sometimes children. They tend not to attempt to take the incident beyond exposure, but there is a group with antisocial personality disorder, and it cannot be assumed that there is never a further danger of sexual assault or rape, although this is rare (see Rooth, 1973, 1980; Rosen, 1979; Snaith, 1983.)

A wide range of psychological formulations may be made, with the conclusion that the adolescent is angry, unhappy, seeking attention or contemptuous of women; sometimes this diagnostic exercise is undertaken without much participation by the adolescent concerned, who adopts an incredulous or bemused (if not denying) attitude to the event. It can be useful then to shift the focus from the exposed penis to the issue of the adolescent being inexplicably vulnerable to bizarre behaviour which may get him into repeated trouble. One should then explore the sort of difficulties often found in adolescent exhibitionists: shyness; few friends, particularly girlfriends; problems in social skills and assertiveness, often explicable in terms of family dynamics; occasionally sexual immaturity e.g. misgivings about masturbation. A wide range of treatments have been tried, and although there can be a good outcome there is a lack of systematic studies to help predict this (Snaith 1983).

Promiscuity

Most adolescents are not promiscuous in the sense of having large numbers of sexual partners (see Chapter 1). It is unusual for psychiatrists to see boys referred for promiscuous behaviour, presumably because of social attitudes to male and female sexuality being different. The promiscuous girls seen in psychiatric clinics and children's homes tend often to be unhappy young people in whom indiscriminate sexual activity seems determined by a mixture of impulsiveness, a need for comforting and affection, lack of interest and supervision by adults, and contact with groups of males willing to take advantage of them.

Apart from this stereotype of the promiscuous girl, whose first need very often is for adequate care and control (preferably by the family) promiscuity may also be a presenting symptom of mania or hypomania.

Preganancy and marriage in adolescence

Rutter (1979) and Rutter and Madge (1976) have reviewed the potential disadvantages for children of the rising divorce rate and the increasing number of one parent families, while pointing out that warring parents 'remaining together for the sake of the children' is not a solution either.

Too early (i.e. teenage) marriage is one contribution to marital discord and breakdown and subsequent divorce (Rutter and Madge, 1976).

Young people who marry early tend also to have children early and to be particularly vulnerable socio-economically (Gibson, 1974).

Pregnancy in adolescence is associated also with obstetric and psychiatric complications (Gabrielson *et al.*, 1970; Sugar, 1976; Lambert, 1976), and often the pregnancy is a result of psychological problems as well as a cause (Hatcher, 1973; Jense, 1976; Zongker, 1977; and a brief review in Parry-Jones, 1985). Cheetham (1977) provides a helpful account of the problems of unwanted pregnancy in adolescence.

There has been much recent controversy over the issue of whether or not doctors should give contraceptive advice and prescriptions to girls under the age of 16 in confidence, i.e. without their parents' knowledge. The issue was first raised by a member of the public, Mrs Victoria Gillick, in a failed claim against the West Norfolk Area Health Authority, and became subsequently widely known as the Gillick case. After much huffing and puffing from all sides the outcome was that a doctor may give a girl of fifteen or under confidential contraceptive advice or contraceptives, if that doctor considers she is mature enough and intelligent enough to understand the implications of the treatment she is receiving. The judgment contains 'grey areas', e.g. Mr Justice Woolf considered it unlikely that a girl under fifteen could legitimately give consent to being sterilized, but thought that her consent would be acceptable for most methods of contraception. The judgment was hailed as a triumph by organizations claiming to speak for children's rights. There has been to date (two years later) a noticeable lack of public debate in adolescent psychiatric circles, perhaps because of the conflict between concern for individual children's rights on the one hand, and recognition, on the other, of the primary importance of involving parents or competent people *in loco parentis* in the affairs of younger adolescents.

My own impression of the girls of fifteen and under I have seen over the years in a variety of psychiatric units and clinics, children's homes and assessment centres is that it is difficult to think of a single one for whom a confidential decision about contraception taken between the girl and a doctor would have seemed appropriate. However, these settings are selective, and those who value the recent ruling presumably see advantages in it for their own practice, which is presumably with young girls for whom any hope of being involved in a caring family or its equivalent has for some reason been abandoned, and for whom the most urgent priority is that they should not reproduce. This strikes me as a grimly pessimistic view of children and child care.

Sexual abuse

The sexual abuse of children and adolescents is being increasingly reported, and is part of the wider spectrum of child maltreatment (see review by Mrazek and Mrazek, 1985.) It may take the form of physical interference with the child's genitals, their exploitation e.g. in pornography or prostitution, or involvement in the adult's sexual activity. The abuse may involve persuasion, seduction or violence. It may or may not amount to rape.

Incest refers to sexual relationships between people closely related (most commonly between father or stepfather and daughter). Studies suggest that those who perpetrate incest tend to have personality problems, with paranoid personality disorder being prominent, and there is often the abuse of alcohol and marital discord (Burton, 1968; Herman, 1981). Mrazek and Mrazek (1985) describe the possible role of the mother as passively colluding, although occasionally the mother may be perpetrator too. Although mental retardation has been reported as a factor in the perpetrators of incest, recent studies have not confirmed this. Mrazek and Bentovim (1981) have pointed out that sexual abuse can be seen as one among several manifestations of role, boundary and parenting problems in the family.

Perhaps surprisingly, there is relatively little good evidence of the subsequent effects of child sexual abuse in general and incest in particular. Quite a lot of what information there is has come from the retrospective reports of adults in psychotherapy. Among the problems in this area of research are difficulties of defining different categories of abuse, uncertainty about how far abuse causes psychological problems and *vice versa*, and the effects of background (e.g. family) on both. In a review by Mrazek and Mrazek (1981) of the short term and long term effects the authors found problems and preoccupations with sexual matters frequently reported as an outcome in young people, with the suggestion that sexually abused boys may themselves become, during adolescence, sexual abusers. In adolescence and adulthood, sexual problems may be manifested as prostitution or the passive or active involvement in the sexual abuse of children. The disclosure of sexual abuse may be followed by suicide attempts in some girls (Goodwin, 1981). Overall, Mrazek and Mrazek (1985) conclude that research on the effects of child sexual abuse remains inadequate. It is commonly said that 'the response of the authorities causes more distress than the incident itself'. No doubt this can happen, but it is not clear how generally true this observation is.

Sexual problems : notes on management issues

(i)   Sexual problems may have any or all of the following effects : they may cause social offence, break the law, be related to psychiatric problems (as a cause or effect), or simply cause distress. They are also likely to provoke different emotional and moral reactions among those trying to help. These very different aspects of attitudes to sexuality can profoundly affect management.

(ii)   At the time of writing there appears to be, in many areas of child psychiatry, muddle and blurring over the issue of gathering of information for diagnostic and therapeutic purposes on the one hand, and on the other the gathering of information to see if a crime has been committed – 'disclosure' as it is known. It would seem sensible clearly to separate these two functions, so that the people trying to help a child and family are not the same people as those trying to establish the facts for legal purposes.

(iii)   In complex cases arousing strong and conflicting feelings, especially in residential settings, it can be helpful for the key workers to have additional meetings chaired by an uninvolved person so that emotion-laden attitudes do not cause inconsistency and confusion.

(iv)   The basic strategy of assessment (who is anxious or distresed about precisely what, and why? (Chapter 5)) is of particular importance in cases involving sexual behaviour, because of the extremes of personal reaction and legal response that can be triggered by quite finely graded differences in perceptions of the incident. Cool heads will be needed to sort out what is pathological, what is merely 'deviant', what is unacceptable, what is illegal, and what is unwise.

     To take just one example, e.g. homosexual activity, work may be needed to make sure that the patient pays attention to the concerns of family, school and the community. Correspondingly, work is needed with family and school to ensure that the problem is kept in perspective, and that anxiety and heated feelings do not get in the way of constructive help.

(v)   Management is likely to need general attention to social, family and personal developmental issues before help is focussed on the specifically sexual problem by, for example, sexual or behaviour therapy. This is because success with the latter will require the collaboration of a patient able to reflect about his problem, and capable of making some reasonably mature and responsible choices.

References and further reading

Bell, D., Weinberg, M. and Hammersmith, S. (1981) *Sexual Preference : Its Development in Men and Women*. Bloomington: Indiana University Press.

Burton, L. (1968) *Vulnerable Children*. London: Routledge and Kegan Paul.

Cheetham, J. (1977) *Unwanted Pregnancy and Counselling*. London: Routledge and Kegan Paul.

Christie Brown, J. (1983) Paraphilias : Sadomasochism, fetishism, trasvestism and transexuality. *British Journal of Psychiatry* **143**, 227–31.

Gabrielson, I., Klerman, L., Currie, J., Tyler, N. and Jekel, J. (1970) Suicide attempts in a population pregnant as teenagers. *American Journal of Public Health* **60**, 2289–301.

Gibson, C. (1974) The association between divorce and social class in England and Wales. *British Journal of Sociology* **25**, 79–93.

Goodwin, J. (1981) Suicide attempts in sexual abuse victims and their mothers. *Child Abuse and Neglect* **5**, 217–21.

Green, R. (1976) One hundred and ten feminine and masculine boys. Behavioural contrasts and demographic similarities. *Archives of Sexual Behaviour* **5**, 425–46.

Green, R. (1985a) *Sissy Boys to Gay Men. A Fifteen Year Prospective Study*. Connecticut: Yale University Press.

Green, R. (1985b) Atypical psychosexual behaviour. *In* Rutter M. and Hersov L. (Eds), *Child and Adolescent Psychiatry : Modern Approaches*, pp 638–49. Oxford: Blackwell Scientific Publications.

Green, R., Williams, K. and Goodman, M., (1982) Ninety-nine 'tomboys' and 'non-tomboys' : behavioural contrasts and demographic similarities. *Archives of Sexual Behaviour* **11**, 247–66.

Hatcher, S. (1973) The adolescent experience of pregnancy and abortion : a devolopmental analysis. *Journal of Youth and Adolescence* **2**, 53–102.

Herman, J. (1981) *Father-Daughter incest*. Cambridge, Massachusetts: Harvard University Press.

Jense, G.P. (1976) Adolescent sexuality. *In* Sadock, B., Kaplan, H. and Freedman, A. (Eds), *The Sexual Experience*. Baltimore: Williams and Wilkins.

Lambert, P. (1976) Perinatal mortality : social and environmental factor. *Population Trends* 4. London: Her Majesty's Stationery Office.

Lothstein, L. (1980) The post-surgical transexual : empirical and theoretical considerations. *Archives of Sexual Behaviour* **9**, 547–64.

Lothstein, L. (1982) Sex reassignment surgery – historical, bioethical and theoretical issues. *American Journal of Psychiatry* **139**, 417–26.

Lothstein, L. (1983) *Female to Male Transexualism. Historical, Clinical and Theoretical Issues*. London: Routledge and Kegan Paul.

Mrazek, P. (1981) Sexual abuse of children (Annotation). *Journal of Child Psychology and Psychiatry* **21**, 91–5.

Mrazek, P. and Bentovim, A. (1981) Incest and the dysfunctional family system. *In* Mrazek, P. and Kempe, C. (Eds), *Sexually Abused Children and their Families*, pp 167–78. Oxford: Pergamon Press.

Mrazek, D. and Mrazek, P. (1985) Child maltreatment. *In* Rutter, M. and Hersov, L. (Eds) *Child and Adolescent Psychiatry : Modern Approaches*, pp 679–97. Oxford: Blackwell Scientific Publications.

Mrazek, P. and Mrazek, D. (1981) The effects of child sexual abuse : methodological considerations. In Mrazek, P. and Kempe, C., (Eds), *Sexually Abused Children and their Families*, pp 235–45.

Noe, J., Sato, R., Coleman, C. and Laub, D. (1978) Construction of male genitalia; the Stanford experience. *Archives of Sexual Behaviour* **8** 523–7.

Parry-Jones, W.L. (1985) Adolescent disturbance. *In* Rutter, M. and Hersov, L. (Eds), *Child and Adolescent Psychiatry : Modern Approaches*, pp 584–98. Oxford: Blackwell Scientific Publications.

Rooth, F. (1973) Exhibitionism, sexual violence and paedophilia. *British Journal of Psychiatry* **122**, 705–10.

Rooth, F. (1980) Exhibitionism : an eclectic approach. *British Journal of Hospital Medicine* **23**, 366–70.

Rosen, I. (1979) Exhibitionism, scopophilia and voyeurism. *In* Rosen, I. (Ed), *Sexual Deviation*. Oxford: Oxford University Press.

Rutter, M. (1979) *Changing Youth in a Changing Society*. London: The Nuffield Provincial Hospitals Trust.

Rutter, M. and Madge, N. (1976) Cycles of Disadvantage: A Review of Research. London: Heinemann.

Saghir, M. and Robins, E. (1973) *Male and Female Homosexuality*. Baltimore: Williams and Wilkins.

Snaith, P. (1983) Exhibitionism : a clinical conundrum. *British Journal of Psychiatry* **143**, 231–5.

Stoller, R. (1968) *Sex and Gender*. London: Hogarth Press.

Sugar, M. (1976) At-risk factors for the adolescent mother and her infant. *Journal of Youth and Adolescence* **5**, 251–70.

Zongker, C. (1977) The self-concept of pregnant adolescent girls. *Adolescence* **12**, 477–88.

Chapter 11

Misuse of Drugs and Other Substances

Categories of dependence

The World Health Organization (1974) has proposed the following categories for the misuse of drugs, and it can serve for the misuse of other chemical substances too.

Drug abuse: Persistent or sporadic excessive drug use inconsistent with or unrelated to accepted medical practice

Drug dependence: A state, psychic and sometimes also physical, resulting from the interaction between a living organism and a drug, characterized by behavioural and other responses, that always includes a compulsion to take the drug on a continuous or periodic basis in order to experience its psychic effects, sometimes to avoid the discomfort of abstinence.

Psychic dependence: A condition in which a drug produces a feeling of satisfaction and a psychic drive, that require periodic or continuous administration of the drug to produce pleasure or to avoid discomfort.

Physical dependence: An adaptive state that manifests itself by intense physical disturbances when the administration of the drug is suspended. The characteristic feature of physical dependence is the development of a physical withdrawal syndrome associated with abstinence from the drug, although the rate and degree of development of physical dependence will be influenced by individual characteristics.

Another important term is *tolerance* : the body's adaptation to the drug by metabolizing it faster, or by the effect the user seeks becoming less readily evoked, so that more of the drug is needed to produce a similar experience.

What is a drug?

As a group, the abused substances defy watertight definition, largely because they tend to be categorized socially rather than chemically. Alcohol, for example, may be variously described as a food, as a socially acceptable psychoactive drink, as a drug of dependence, and, marginally, as a prescribable medicine, appearing in the British National Formulary (the official prescribing guide for doctors and pharmacists) as a 'borderline substance' (British National Formulary, 1987). Correspondingly, the opiate drugs like morphine and diamorphine (heroin) are enormously valuable as prescribed medicine but extremely dangerous as drugs of abuse.

Drugs and other chemicals and substances that are commonly abused include the following:

The opiates and opiate-like drugs:
diamorphine (Heroin)
morphine
methadone
Amphetamines and other stimulants:
amphetamine
methylphenidate (Ritalin)
diethylproprion (Tenuate)
Cocaine
Caffeine
Nicotine and other substances in tobacco smoke
Barbiturates
Benzodiazepines (Librium, Valium)
Phencylidine
Hallucinogens (e.g. lysergic acid diethylamide or LSD)
Cannabis
Alcohol
Industrial solvents

Opiates

The opiates, which include heroin, are powerful central nervous system depressants, hence their calming, anaesthetic and sleep-inducing effects. They are swallowed, smoked ('chasing the dragon'), inhaled ('snorting') or injected into muscles or skin ('skin-popping') or intravenously ('mainlining' or 'fixing'). Heroin has a rapid onset of action and its intravenous injection is particularly associated with a euphoric 'rush' or 'thrill'. The effects of these drugs include constipation, postural hypotension, histamine-release (causing itching), nausea and vomiting and respiratory depression. Overdose can cause death by its effect on the medullary respiratory centre. Death may also occur following allergic reaction to an injection. However, much of the morbidity and mortality is due to secondary effects of the opiate user's life style (this is in contrast to the direct toxic effects of alcohol) e.g. poverty and malnutrition, criminal activities, and the consequences of using dirty needles, e.g. hepatitis, septicaemia, endocarditis and acquired immune deficiency syndrome (AIDS). Withdrawal of the drug causes at first yawning, sweating, muscle and bone pain and anorexia, running of eyes and nose, tremor and gooseflesh, and later agitation, restlessness, diarrhoea and depression (Strang and Connell, 1985; Dusek and Girdano, 1980).

In physical terms withdrawal over a few weeks under cover of the substitute drug methadone (which can also become addictive) is not in itself difficult; the personality and social factors cause the problems.

A narcotic antagonist like naxolone hydrochloride can be rapidly life-saving in opiate overdose. It can precipitate opiate withdrawal symptoms (Strang and Connell, 1985).

Cocaine

Cocaine, which was studied and used with enthusiasm by Sigmund Freud, and was a constituent of the original Coca-Cola, is a powerful, short-acting central nervous system stimulant, now sometimes used in conjunction with heroin. It is also inhaled or injected. Dependence on the drug is primarily psychological and can be very strong. It can cause anxiety states and a paranoid psychotic illness (Jaffe, 1980). Withdrawal of the drug does not cause physical symptoms, but the psychiatric symptoms require minor or major tranquillizers. Cocaine is known as 'coke' or 'snow'.

Amphetamine

Amphetamine, which is swallowed, inhaled or injected, is also a CNS stimulant producing euphoria, disinhibition and excitement, sometimes with intense tingling (a 'buzz') and occasionally orgasm. Hyperactivity may last for several days. Fatigue, depression and sleepiness follow (Connell, 1968) and there may be suicidal ideas. Amphetamine psychosis, described by Connell (1958) is an acute paranoid psychotic state which can develop with prolonged use. It is treated with phenothiazines. If the psychotic state persists it may be due to continued drug use or the independent existence of a psychotic state (see Connell 1968). It is known as 'speed' or 'sulphate'.

Caffeine

Caffeine is a stimulant of the xanthene group, which is present in significant amounts in coffee, tea, chocolate bars, cocoa and some soft drinks, e.g. colas. Whether any children ingest sufficient to cause them mood, behavioural or learning problems does not seem to be well documented. In adults, excessive coffee drinking can cause anxiety, irritability, diarrhoea, cardiac arrhythmias, poor concentration and indigestion. The caffeine content of a cup of coffee varies with how it is made. Dusek and Girdano (1980) give the caffeine content of a cup of (American) coffee as about 100 mg, and point out that 250 mg plus per day begins to cause side- effects, while 20 cups (taken at once!) would constitute a lethal dose of the drug. These authors state that a one ounce chocolate bar contains 20 mg caffeine.

Nicotine

Cigarette smoking begins for social reasons and particularly among adolescents, among whom a greater proportion (according to figures from the United States) are girls (Dusek and Girdano, 1980). The ill effects of smoking are well-established, and more work on the question of teenage smoking and its discouragement is needed.

Barbiturates and benzodiazepines

Barbiturates are now rarely prescribed for young people, in whom they can cause irritability and aggressive behaviour as well as dependence. Their main dangers are from depression of the CNS generally and respiratory depression in particular, a high risk because the respiratory centre may remain vulnerable while the user is tolerant in other respects (Hollister, 1982). Epileptic fits can accompany barbiturate withdrawal.

The same can be true of the withdrawal of the benzodiazepine drugs such as chlordiazepoxide 'librium' and diazepam 'valium'. They are apparently relatively safer by themselves if taken in overdose, but are commonly misused with other drugs, whose effects they potentiate. They should not be prescribed for adolescents while alternative methods of anxiety management are untried, except with great care : low dose, close supervision, close monitoring of beneficial effects and a short period of prescription.

Phencyclidine

Strang and Connell (1985) describe the recent introduction of this veterinary anaesthetic which has become popular among young people in the United States. It is a CNS stimulant and depressant and can produce hallucinations, gross overactivity, paranoid psychosis, catatonic stupor, violence, epileptic fits and bizarre self-injury. The toxic state can be mistaken for schizophrenia. (Luisida and Brown, 1976; Grove, 1979). It is sometimes classed with the hallucinogens. It is known as PCP or 'Stardust'.

Hallucinogens

The best known is lysergic acid diethylamide (LSD) which can also mimic a schizophrenic illness. It produces hallucinations, illusions and mood changes, although these seem to be strongly coloured by the user's personality and expectations. The drug is transient in the body, but lasting mood disorders, psychotic disorders and personality changes have been reported (Sedman and Kenna, 1965; Hatrick and Dewhurst, 1970). 'Flashbacks', brief re-experiences of the 'acid trip' long after the event may happen, and have not been fully explained.

Cannabis

Cannabis (also known as marijhuana, grass, weed, hash, hemp, hay, bhang, ganja, charas etc.) depends for its effect on tetrahydrocannabinol (THC) It is smoked or, in some areas of the world, eaten or drunk. It is very widely used, e.g. by between 3 and 10 per cent of some school populations in Britain (Kosviner, 1976).

A range of chronic psychiatric disorders and ill-effects have been attributed to cannabis use (e.g. psychosis and persistent apathy) and may be due to the predisposition of vulnerable individuals (see Rathod, 1975; Treffert, 1977; Dusek and Girdano, 1980).

Regular use produces tolerance, and a minority develop psychological dependence (Nahas, 1975). In the short term the effects of cannabis include impaired memory and concentration, withdrawn and depersonalized states sometimes accompanied by hallucinations, and fits may be precipitated in people with epilepsy. An acutely disturbed state may take the form of a panic attack or acute psychosis, and should respond to antipsychotic medication. Overdose can cause hypotension, vomiting and coma.

Alcohol

Alcoholism is a complex condition with far-reaching psychological, physical and social consequences, and cannot be discussed here in adequate detail. Alcohol use is increasing among the young and this is accompanied by an increase in alcohol-related problems (Plant, 1987; Ritson, 1981). The abuse of alcohol is associated with delinquent activities, the abuse of other substances, notably solvent abuse and cannabis, poor educational motivation and precocious sexual activity (Jessor and Jessor, 1977) and is sometimes a related factor in sexual abuse (see Chapter 10) and suicide attempts (Hawton *et al.*, 1982).

When consumed, alcohol initially produces relaxation and a slight elevation of mood. Second or third drinks (taking a drink as a single measure of spirits, a glass of wine or a half pint of beer) then begin to affect muscle co-ordination, balance, speech and vision and affect judgement. Major impairment of mental and physical control begins at about a fifth drink. It is likely that for most people skill (e.g. in controlling motor vehicles) begins to be significantly impaired from the second drink onwards. Sufficient alcohol intake leads on to coma and death.

Most people have strong personal views about how much alcohol they can personally manage, and the patient of any age being interviewed by a clinician is likely to play down the amount consumed.

Example 9
Alan is a sixth form student, doing badly, and referred because of anxiety, depression and apathy partly related to his lack of educational progress and partly because of the arguments this causes in the family. He is highly motivated and socially competent in one area, to the relief of his parents : his participation in a pop group that is modestly successful in an amateur way at local dances. He denies heavy drinking but smokes quite a lot and occasionally takes cannabis. Further questioning about his drinking reveals that he sometimes has 'a pint' with the others in his group. It emerges that this is a 'couple' of pints, or sometimes 'a few pints', once or twice a week.

He denies drinking alone, but it emerges that he has trouble sleeping and 'sometimes' takes a few cans of beer home to drink before going to bed.

'How many do you drink to help you sleep?'
'Just one.'
'Only one?'
'Well, sometimes two'
'Have you ever drunk all you've taken home?'
'Not often. Sometimes.'
'How many would that be?'
'Not more than four cans.'
'Big cans or small cans?'
'Big ones.'
'How often do you have to drink that much, say in a week?'
'Only once or twice.'

In fact, Alan was getting through several bottles of cheap wine every week too.

The recognition, assessment and management of alcoholism and drink-related problems is a specialized field. Edwards (1982) provides a comprehensive and helpful guide.

Solvents

Solvents have been abused for nearly thirty years although this has become prominent more recently as a cause for concern (Tolan and Lingl, 1964; Press and Done, 1967; Skuse and Burrell, 1982). The substances involved include toluene, acetone, naphtha (in model-making cement and other glues), benzene (in rubber solutions), acetone and amylacetate (nail polish remover), carbon tetrachloride, trichloroethane and trichloroethylene (typing correction fluids and dry cleaning chemicals), acetone (impact adhesives), benzene and naph-thene compounds (petrol) and fluorocarbon gas (propellants in aero-sols). They are variously sniffed from the bottle or inhaled from a polythene bag, handkerchief or crisp packet or sprayed directly into the mouth.

Like alcohol these chemicals cause central nervous system depres-sion, producing disinhibition, excitement, euphoria, disorientation, blurred vision and dizziness; users will say that they would prefer alcohol if they could get it. The effects wear off quickly but the smell stays on the breath, and a rash around the mouth, sometimes accompanied by boils, may be seen.

Many deaths of children and adolescents abusing solvents have been reported (e.g. Oliver and Watson in Britain (1977) and Bass in the United States (1970)) but there is some disagreement about the degree and nature of the dangers, e.g. when deaths are caused by falling from heights rather than directly due to the substance. Nevertheless reports include death by laryngeal spasm due to aerosol spray (Black, 1982), fits and encephalopathy (King *et al.*, 1981), polyneuropathy (Matsumura *et al.*, 1972), liver disease (Litt *et al.*, 1972) bone marrow disorders, chronic lung injury and renal failure (Watson, 1977, 1980; O'Connor, 1979). Skuse and Burrell (1982) in their study of 45 adolescents (28 boys, 17 girls) reported anorexia, weight loss, nausea and vomiting, cardiac arrhythmias and acute bronchospasm.

In this study most of the young people were found to have conduct or emotional (depressive) problems and delinquency was common among the chronic abusers. Masterson (1979) has stressed the need for community prevention by collaboration between doctors, schools, the police and others, while Strang and Connell (1985) advise that harm could be done by making too much of the problem, and that treatment should be based in the community and child psychiatric services, rather than in special drug dependency clinics.

Drug takers

Oppenheimer has reviewed the characteristics, circumstances and affiliations of young people who abuse drugs (Oppenheimer, 1985) and concluded that there are no features that could be described as typical. She draws attention to the many complex factors such as the considerable variation from culture to culture, and the problems for legislators caused by rapid changes in drug use. Sex differences in adolescent drug users is not so marked as among adults, where males predominate; an exception appears to be in smoking, where in a US study, smoking among males is decreasing while there has been an increase among females (Green, 1979). There is uncertainty whether drug users are influenced by a drug-taking peer group, or seek out such groups; and delinquency appears sometimes to precede drug use and then become a consequence. However, demographic factors may affect both. Some personality factors may be related to drug use, e.g. rebelliousness and extraversion, and some studies report an association between adolescent drug misuse and parental, and particularly maternal, use of drugs and alcohol. (See review by Oppenheimer, 1985.)

Drug problems : notes on management issues

(i)   The motivation of the drug user will have a powerful influence on management, and of course this will not be easy to assess at first. Caution is advised. By the same token it may take time to get an accurate and complete picture of the extent of drug misuse and the problems it is causing. Urine tests to check for the use of drugs may be needed.

(ii)   For younger adolescents experimenting with drugs, attempts should be made to work individually and with the family on wider problems, including the supervision the child gets and the example set by other members of the family.

(iii) For the older adolescent, and the management of opiate abuse, special clinics and sometimes residence in special therapeutic centres (like Phoenix House), are indicated because of the special skills and experience needed in this work. Many such centres adopt quite strict and abstinent regimes, and it is not known how their achievements compare with, for example, the progress of young drug users who break the law and go to prison.

(iv)   The short-term and long-term physical consequences of drug abuse and the dangers of casual or deliberate self-neglect and self-harm need attention, as do the major social problems of the drug user becoming alienated from normal social contacts and identifying strongly with a drug subculture.

References and further reading

Bass, M. (1970) Sudden sniffing death. *Journal of the American Medical Association* **212**, 2075–9.

Black, D. (1982) Misuse of solvents. *Health trends* **14** 27–8.

British National Formulary (1987) London: British Medical Association and the Pharmaceutical Society of Great Britain.

Connell, P.H. (1958) *Amphetamine Psychosis. Maudsley Monograph No. 5.* London: Institute of Psychiatry.

Connell, P.H. (1968) The use and abuse of amphetamines. *The Practitioner* **200**, 234–43.

Dusek, D. and Girdano, D. (1980) *Drugs.* Menlo Park, California: Addison-Wesley.

Edwards, G. (1982) *The Treatment of Drinking Problems : A Guide for the Helping Professions.* London: Grant McIntrye.

Green, J. (1979) Overview of adolescent drug use. *In* Beshner G. and

Friedman, A. (Eds), *Youth Drug Abuse : Problems, Issues and Treatment* pp 17–44. Lexington, Massachusetts : Lexington Books.

Grove, V. (1979) Painless self-injury after ingestion of 'angel dust'. *Journal of the American Medical Association* **242**, 655.

Hatrick, J. and Dewhurst, K. (1970) Delayed psychosis due to LSD. *Lancet* **2** 742–4.

Hawton, K., O'Grady, J., Osborn, M. and Cole D. (1982) Adolescents who take overdoses : their characteristics, problems, and contacts with helping agencies. *British Journal of Psychiatry* **140**, 124–31.

Hollister, L. (1982) Psychotropic drug interactions. In Cohen, S., Buchwald, C., Solomon, J., Callahan, J. and Katz, D. (Eds), *Frequently Prescribed and Abused Drugs : Their Indications, Efficacy and Rational Prescribing*, pp 7–20. New York: Haworth Press.

Jaffe, J. (1980) Drug addiction and drug abuse. In Gilman, A.G. Goodman, L. and Gilman A. (Eds), *The Pharmacological Basis of Therapeutics*, Sixth Edition, pp 535–84. New York: Macmillan.

Jessor, R. and Jessor, S. (1977) *Problem Behaviour and Psychosocial development: A Longitudinal Study of Youth.* New York: Academic Press.

King, M., Day, R., Oliver, J., Lush, M. and Watson, J. (1981) Solvent encephalopathy. *British Medical Journal* **2**, 663–5.

Kosviner, A. (1976) Social science and cannabis use. In Graham, J. (ed), *Cannabis and Health*, pp 343–77. London: Academic Press.

Litt, I., Cohen, M. and Schonberg, S. (1972) Liver disease in the drug-using adolescent. *Journal of Paediatrics* **81**, 2, 238–42.

Luisida, P. and Brown, P. (1976) Clinical management of phencyclidine psychosis. *Clinical Toxicology* **9**, 4, 539–45.

Masterson. G. (1979) The management of solvent abuse. *Journal of Adolescence* **2**, 65–75.

Matsumura, M., Ingue, N. and Ohnishi, A. (1972) Toxic Polyneuropathy due to glue sniffing. *Clinical Neurology* (Tokyo) **12**, 6, 290–6.

Nahas, G. (1975) Marihuana : toxicity and tolerance. In Richter, R. (ed), *Medical Aspects of Drug Abuse*, pp 16–37. Maryland: Harper and Row.

O'Connor, D. (1979) A profile of solvent abuse in school children. *Journal of Child Psychology and Psychiatry* **20**, 365–8.

Oliver, J. and Watson, J. (1977) Abuse of solvents for 'kicks': a review of 50 cases. *Lancet* **1**, 84–6.

Oppenheimer, E. (1985) Drug taking. In Rutter, M. and Hersov, L. (eds), *Child and Adolescent Psychiatry : Modern Approaches*. Oxford: Blackwell Scientific Publications.

Plant, M. (1987) *Drugs in Perspective*. London: Hodder and Stoughton.

Presse, E. and Done, A. (1967) Physiologic effects and community control measures for intoxication from the inhalation of organic solvents. *Paediatrics* **39**, 451–61 and 611–22.

Rathod, N. (1975) Cannabis Psychosis. *In* Connell, P. and Dorn, N. (eds), *Cannabis and Man*, pp 90–104. London: Churchill Livingstone.

Ritson, B. (1981). Alcohol and young people. *Journal of Adolescence*; **4**, 93–100.

Sedman, G. and Kenna, J. (1965) The use of LSD-25 as a diagnostic aid in doubtful cases of schizophrenia. *British Journal of Psychiatry* **111**, 96–100.

Skuse, D. and Burrell, S. (1982) A review of solvent abusers and their management by a child psychiatric out-patient service.*Human Toxicology* **1**, 321–9.

Strang, J. and Connel, P.H. (1985) Clinical aspects of drug and alcohol abuse. *In* Rutter, M. and Hersov, L. (eds), *Child and Adolescent Psychiatry : Modern Approaches*, pp 501–15. London: Blackwell Scientific Publications.

Tolan, E. and Lingl, F. (1964) 'Model psychosis' produced by inhalation of gasoline fumes. *American Journal of Psychiatry* **120**, 757–761.

Treffert, D. (1977) Marihuana use in schizophrenia : a clear hazard. Presented at 130th Annual Meeting of the American Psychiatric Association, Toronto; quoted in Strang and Connell, 1985.

Watson, J. (1977) 'Glue sniffing' in profile. *The Practitioner* **218**, 255–9.

Watson, J. (1980) Solvent abuse by children and young adults. *British Journal of Addictions* **75**, 27–36.

World Health Organisation (1974) Twentieth Report of the Expert Committee on Drug Dependence. *Technicalm Report Series No. 551.* Geneva: World Health Organisation.

Chapter 12

Anorexia Nervosa, Bulimia and Obesity

Anorexia nervosa

Anorexia nervosa is characterized by serious weight loss which is self-induced by food avoidance (especially carbohydrate avoidance) and by exercise, and sometimes compounded by deliberate purging with laxatives, and by vomiting. (See *bulimia nervosa*, below). It is best known as a disorder of adolescent girls and young women, but also occurs in pre-adolescent girls, and in boys and men.

The key psychological feature in all groups is a dread of weight gain and in particular fatness; the intense dieting is undertaken specifically to avoid this. There is no primary revulsion or fear of food as such, and anorexic patients commonly feel hungry, are preoccupied with their preferred diets, and may have eating 'binges'. Crisp (1974) has called the condition adolescent weight phobia.

There are important associated abnormalities of physiological function which vary with the age and sex of the patient (summarized from Russell, 1985):

In postpubertal anorexia nervosa in girls: amenorrhoea.
In prepubertal anorexia nervosa in girls: failure to grow and gain weight at the expected time of the growth spurt (10-14 years), or actual weight loss; delay of menarche; and delayed secondary sexual development.
In boys : delayed growth, immature penis and scrotum and scanty pubic and facial hair. In males who have developed sexually, there is loss of sexual interest and potency.

Accompanying physical features on clinical examination are associated with starvation : a general thinness which may amount to emaciation; cold, red or blue hands, and feet, sometimes with chilblains; a slow pulse (50-60 per minute) although eating can produce tachycardia; and there may be a growth of fine, downy hair (lanugo hair, as in small babies) over the face and back. The patient may weigh as little as four or five stones (56-70 lbs; 25-32 kg). Severe starvation is associated with ankle oedema and blood examination shows low protein levels and electrolyte disturbance (Crisp, 1980).

The condition is, of course, life-threatening when the more severe degree of malnutrition is reached, and death may be due to gradual physical deterioration complicated by hypothermia, hypoglycaemia and infection, or sudden death due to electrolyte (especially potassium) imbalance. The proportion who die has been estimated at 5 per cent, with suicide as the most common cause.

Psychological features include a conviction that he or she will be physically all right whatever the doctor says or the weight charts or mirror shows. Clinically this determination in the face of reality can seem like intense denial, or like an overvalued idea. However, there is evidence that many anorexic patients have a distorted self-image, perceiving themselves as bigger and fatter than they are (Slade and Russell, 1973; Crisp and Kalucy, 1974). This extreme risk-taking behaviour is not perceived as such by the patient; in adolescent girls, overt ideas of suicide or self-neglect are not prominent. On the contrary, they often express satisfaction with life as it looks to them, provided they remain thin. There may be obsessional symptoms, not always related to eating.

Young anorexic patients may also appear at first to be surprisingly compliant. They may be persuaded to accept parental and medical insistence that they are to take part in a weight-gain treatment programme with relatively little fuss, and some progress can be expected for a time. Then as 40 kg is approached it becomes harder to increase the patient's weight. (It is of considerable interest that menstruation usually begins at a body weight of around 46-47 kg). Enquiry is likely to reveal that the patient is going to considerable lengths, in secret, to undermine treatment; for example by extreme exercise, vomiting and purging, secreting weights in clothing, and drinking large quantities of water before being weighed, as well as (or instead of) refusing meals.

Incidence of anorexia nervosa

The disorder is remarkable for its variation in different populations. It is largely a disorder of young women, but about 10 per cent of cases occur in boys and young men (Falstein *et al.*, 1956; Beumont *et al.*, 1972; Hay and Leonard, 1979) and in prepubertal children (Lesser *et al.*, 1960; Blitzer *et al.*, 1961; Warren, 1968; Minuchin *et al.*, 1980).

The annual incidence in Britain is in the range 0.6 to 1.6 per 100,000 of the total population (Kendell *et al.*, 1973). The highest levels are reported in English schoolgirls from the upper socio-economic classes, e.g. 1 in 100 in independent schools (compared with 1 in 300 in state schools) in the studies by Crisp *et al.* (1976), Crisp (1980) and Szmukler (1983). Even higher incidences are found among students of ballet and fashion (Garner and Garfinkel, 1980).

Although the disorder is found in many areas of the world, including Muslim countries and Eastern Europe (Crisp, 1980), it is rare among Asians and seems not to have been reported at all among black people (Halmi, 1974; Halmi *et al.*, 1977; Russell, 1985).

Aetiology of anorexia nervosa

There are many views about the origins of anorexia nervosa. It is likely that more than one factor is influential, and that different combinations of factors operate in different people's cases.

Biological factors include the possibility of genetic influence (Holland *et al.*, 1984), strong evidence for a hypothalamic-anterior pituitary-gonadal disorder (see reviews by Russell, 1977, 1985 and by Garfinkel and Garner, 1982), and Russell (1985) points out the secondary but important influence of malnutrition.

Bruch (1974, 1978) described the psychopathology of anorexia nervosa in primarily individual psychological terms. She emphasized the secondary influence of starvation in producing a light-headed feeling of euphoria which is consonant with the patient's primary aim at achieving autonomy, control and self-expression, having felt frustrated by her parents from achieving these in a more healthy way. Bruch also described the influence of a disturbed body image.

Crisp (1980) describes the condition in terms of psychobiological regression, the patient succeeding in stopping and then reversing the maturation process to avoid anxieties about growing up.

A number of family therapists have described patterns of family interaction which contribute to the problem (although not necessarily 'causing' it in a linear sense), and which can be worked with to produce recovery (e.g. Liebman *et al.*, 1974; Minuchin *et al.*, 1975, 1980; Selvini Palazzoli, 1978). Dare (1983) has reported successful use of family formulations of the problem and family therapy with younger and particularly prepubertal anorexic girls. (Dare, 1983).

Bulimia nervosa

Bulimia nervosa can arise as a development (after a few months or years) of anorexia nervosa, although it sometimes appears to develop without a pre-existing anorectic state. It is not common among younger adolescents. The main clinical feature is intermittent gorging of food followed by self-induced vomiting and purging. The latter is seen in anorexia nervosa too, but is more prominent in the bulimic condition. In bulimia, there may also be a modest weight gain and the resumption of menstrual periods. Russell (1985) describes abrasions of the hand due to repeated self-induced vomiting in some patients, and Szmukler and Russell (1983) describe three diabetic patients with bulimia who mismanaged their diabetes to achieve weight loss.

Outcome of anorexia nervosa

The disorder takes a variable and unpredictable course, but up to half of patients may recover fully and, for example, achieve the same rate of marriage as the rest of the population (Theander, 1970). One quarter improve but have persisting eating or menstrual problems, and a quarter continue in anorexic ill-health with psychiatric problems of varying severity; follow-up studies suggest that 5 per cent develop bulimia, and 5 per cent die from the complications mentioned earlier. (Tolstrup *et al.*, 1982). The condition is difficult to manage, and it has been suggested that the more experienced centres achieve the better results; on the other hand such centres are also likely to attract patients with more entrenched problems.

Anorexia nervosa and bulimia : notes on management

(i)   First establish the diagnosis. For example, gynaecological or metabolic disorders could give a superficial appearance of anorexia nervosa. Depressive or schizophrenic illness could result in anorexic-like attitudes to weight and eating.

(ii)   Establish the authority with which treatment will proceed. It may be the patient's own co-operation (e.g. with an agreed contract – see Chapter 18), by parental authority, or through the informal authority of the medical team. Occasionally compulsory treatment under Section 3 of the Mental Health Act may be justified when life or health is seriously at risk, e.g. through malnutrition or suicide. It could be argued that compulsory treatment is justified if irreversible stunting of growth (e.g. for a prepubertal girl) is being risked; however, parental authority is usually sufficient and more appropriate for adolescents under 16.

(iii)   Most practitioners agree that the first priority is a return to normal weight, with attempts to understand the psychological antecedents of the disorder coming later (see Russell, 1977; Kalucy, 1978; Dally, 1981). In family work, Dare (1983) emphasizes the responsibility of the parents in feeding the son or daughter who is at risk from starving to death. In-patient work requires a friendly but firm and consistent approach by the medical and nursing team, based on trust and confidence. Sympathy with the patient's fears is reasonable, but firmness about weight gain is crucial. Staff should make clear that their aim is for normal weight to be achieved, not to make the patient fat. (See Russell 1985 on in- patient treatment of anorexic patients.)

(iv)   Russell (1985) also stresses that the amount of food needed for weight gain may be underestimated. 7,500 surplus calories are needed for one kilo of weight gain. Treatment should aim to last 4-8 weeks, with 1200-1800 calories per day initially, rising to above that needed for an average adult (3000-4000 calories per day). Caution at first is necessary because of the risk of acute dilatation of the stomach.

(v)   Some workers use graded rewards, including increasing mobility (e.g. progression from bed rest, through confinement to the bedroom, to participation in the life of the ward, etc.) contingent upon weight gain. (Agras and Werne, 1977; Pertschuk, 1977; Kalucy, 1978).

(vi)   Supervision to prevent weight-reduction strategies by the patient is required.

(vii)   Medication (e.g. phenothiazines, antidepressants) no longer has the important part in treatment that used to be suggested.

(viii)   Monitor progress. There should be a weight gain of about 1500-2000 g weekly. In young adolescents pubertal development (Chapter 1) should be assessed, and the monitoring of luteinising hormone (LH) and follicle stimulating hormone (FSH) may be helpful. Russell (1985) gives an account of the monitoring of physical development, and the prediction of stunting by measuring bone age at the wrists : while bone age remains well under 15 years further growth is possible. Endocrine therapy for delayed menstruation is best postponed until maximum height and weight are achieved, especially for those with pre-menarchal onset of anorexia.

(ix)   It is possible for the progress made by an in-patient team to undermine the parents' authority, and thereby threaten the continuation of progress after discharge. For younger adolescents in particular, authority should be explicitly shared between the in-patient team and the parents, and decisions about admission, weekends at home, discharge etc. taken together.

(x)   Further individual or family therapeutic work should be considered once weight gain is achieved and being reliably maintained.

Obesity

Slimness is admired in Western cultures, including among children (Howard *et al.*, 1971; Stunkard *et al.*, 1972) and obese children are stigmatized (Goodman *et al.*, 1963; Maddox *et al.*, 1968; Chisholm, 1978; Tobias and Gordon, 1980). Obese young people may be discriminated against educationally and in employment (Canning and Mayer, 1966, 1967) and it has been shown that obese adolescent girls can show feelings similar to those of racial minority groups (Monello and Mayer, 1963).

Disease is rare as a cause for obesity, and the results of genetic studies uncertain (Hawk and Brook, 1979). The evidence points to environmental factors being strongly influential, and in particular diet, lack of physical activity and patterns of family feeding. More specifically, obesity has been related to lower rates of breast feeding and high starch content in diets. Psychological explanations tend to the notion of feeding by the mother (and later, eating) becoming a substitute for alternative sources of satisfaction and stimulus (e.g. Bruch 1940, 1974). Obese children and adolescents, stigmatized as referred to above, tend towards anxiety, sensitivity and low self-esteem (Kalucy, 1976), and this may reinforce the self-comforting pattern endangering physical health in adult life.

Obesity: notes on management

(i)   Behavioural techniques, (Gross *et al.*, 1976) particularly when persisted with (Stunkard *et al.*, 1980), can be successful.

(ii)   This should be supplemented by counselling or psychotherapy, and social skills training where this may help self-esteem and the challenge of a changed self-perception.

(iii) Family or group work may be helpful in working with problems of motivation, persistence and self-esteem.

(iv) These measures can aid the key treatment, which is *persistence* with a sensible and carefully monitored diet.

References and further reading

Agras S. and Werne, J. (1977) Behaviour modification in anorexia nervosa : research foundations. *In* Vigersky, R. (Ed), *Anorexia Nervosa,* pp 291–303. New York: Raven Press.

Beaumont, P., Beardwood, G., and Russell, G. (1972) The occurrence of the syndrome of anorexia nervosa in male subjects. *Psychological Medicine* **2**, 216–31.

Blitzer, J., Rollins, N. and Blackwell, A. (1961) Children who starve themselves. *Psychosomatic Medicine* **5**, 369–83.

Bruch, H. (1978) *The Golden Cage : the Enigma of Anorexia Nervosa.* London: Open Books.

Bruch, H. (1940) Obesity in childhood III. Physiologic and psychologic aspects of food intake of obese children. *American Journal of Diseases of Childhood* **59**, 739–81.

Bruch, H. (1974) *Eating Disorders : Obesity, Anorexia and the Person Within.* London: Routledge and Kegan Paul.

Canning, H. and Meyer, J. (1966) Obesity : its possible effect on college acceptance. *New England Journal of Medicine* **285** 1402–7.

Canning, H. and Meyer, J. (1967) Obesity : an influence on high school performance. *American Journal of Clinical Nutrition* **20**, 352–4.

Crisp, A. (1974) Primary anorexia nervosa or adolescent weight phobia. *Practitioner* **212**, 525–35.

Crisp, A. (1980) *Anorexia Nervosa : Let Me Be.* London: Academic Press.

Crisp, A. and Kalucy, R. (1974) Aspects of the perceptual disorder in anorexia nervosa. *British Journal of Medical Psychology* **74**, 349–61.

Crisp, A., Palmer, R., and Kalucy, R. (1976) How common is anorexia nervosa? A prevalence study. *British Journal of Psychiatry* **128**, 549–54.

Chisholm, D. (1978) Obesity in adolescence. *Journal of Adolescence* **1**, 177–94.

Dally, P. (1981) Treatment of anorexia nervosa. *British Journal of Hospital Medicine* **25**, 5, 434–40.

Dare, C. (1983) *Individual and Family Psychotherapy in Anorexia Nervosa.* Paper presented at the 10th International Congress of the Association for Child and Adolescent Psychiatry and Allied Professions, Dublin, 1982.

Falstein, E.I., Falstein, E.C. and Judas, I. (1956) Anorexia nervosa in the male child. *American Journal of Orthopsychiatry* **26**, 751–72.

Garfinkel, P. and Garner, D. (1982) *Anorexia Nervosa : A Multidimensional Perspective*, pp 188–213. New York: Brunner Mazel.

Garner, D. and Garfinkel, B. (1980) Sociocultural factors in the development of anorexia nervosa. *Psychological Medicine* **10**, 647–56.

Goodman, N., Richardson, S. Dornbusch, S. and Hastorf, A. (1963) Variant reactions to physical disabilities. *American Sociological Review* **38**, 429–35.

Gross, I., Wheeler, M. and Hess, K. (1976) The treatment of obesity in adolescents using behavioural self-control. *Clinical Paediatrics* **15**, 920–4.

Halmi, K. (1974) Anorexia nervosa : demographic and clinical features in 94 cases. *Psychosomatic Medicine* **36**, 18–26.

Halmi, K., Goldberg, S., Eckert, E., Casper, R. and Davis, J. (1977). Pretreatment evaluation in anorexia nervosa. *In* Vigersky, R. (ed), *Anorexia Nervosa*, 43–54. New York: Raven Press.

Hawk, L. and Brook, C. (1979) Family resemblances of height, weight and body fatness. *Archives of Diseases of Childhood* **54**, 877–9.

Hay, G. and Leonard, J. (1979) Anorexia nervosa in males. *Lancet* **ii**, 574–6.

Holland, A., Hall, A., Murray, R., Russell, G. and Crisp, A. (1984) Anorexia nervosa : a study of 34 twin pairs and one set of triplets. *British Journal of Psychiatry* **145**, 414–19.

Howard, A., Dub, I. and MacMahon, M. (1971) The incidence, cause and treatment of obesity in Leicester school children. *Practitioner* **207**, 662–8.

Kalucy, R. (1978) An approach to the therapy of anorexia nervosa. *Journal of Adolescence* **1**, 197–228.

Kalucy, R. (1976) Obesity : an attempt to find a common ground among some of the biological, psychological and sociological phenomena of the obesity/overeating syndrome. In Hill, O. (Ed), *Modern Trends in Psychosomatic Medicine* **3**, pp 404–429. London: Butterworths.

Kendell, R., Hailey, A. and Babigian, H. (1973) The epidemiology of anorexia nervosa. *Psychological Medicine* **3**, 200–3.

Lesser, L., Ashenden, B., Debuskey, M. and Eisenberg, L. (1960) Anorexia nervosa in children. *American Journal of Orthopsychiatry* **30**, 572–80.

Liebman, R., Minuchin, S. and Baker, L. (1974) An integrated treatment program for anorexia nervosa. *American Journal of Psychiatry* **131**, 432–6.

Maddox, G., Buck, K. and Liederman, V. (1968) Overweight versus social deviance and disability. *Journal of Health and Social Behaviour* **9**, 287–98.

Minuchin, S., Baker, L., Rosman, B., Liebman, R., Millman, L. and Todd,

T. (1975) A conceptual model of psychosomatic illness in children. *Archives of General Psychiatry* **32**, 1031–8.

Minuchin, S., Rosman, B. and Baker, L. (1980) *Psychosomatic Families : Anorexia Nervosa in Context.* Cambridge, Massachusetts: Harvard University Press.

Monello, L. and Mayer, I. (1963) Obese adolescent girls : an unrecognised 'minority' group? *American Journal of Clinical Nutrition* **13**, 35–9.

Pertschuk, M. (1977) Behaviour therapy : extended follow-up. In Vigersky, R. (ed), *Anorexia Nervosa*, pp 305–13. New York: Raven Press.

Russell, G. (1977) The present status of anorexia nervosa. *Psychological Medicine* **7, 363**–7.

Russell, G. (1983) Delayed puberty due to anorexia nervosa of early onset. In Darby, P., Garfinkel, P., Garner, D. and Coscina, D. (eds), *Anorexia Nervosa : Recent Developments in Research*, pp 331–42. New York: Alan R. Liss.

Russell, G. (1985) Anorexia and bulimia nervosa. In Rutter, M. and Hersov, L. (eds), *Child and Adolescent Psychiatry : Modern Approaches*, pp 625–37. Oxford: Blackwell Scientific Publications.

Selvini-Palazzoli, M. (1978) *Self-Starvation : From Individual to Family Therapy in the Treatment of Anorexia Nervosa*, pp 193–201. Translated by Pomerans, A., quoted in Russell, 1985. New York: Aronson.

Slade, P. and Russell, G. (1973) Awareness of body dimensions in anorexia nervosa : cross-sectional and longitudinal studies. *Psychological Medicine* **3**, 188–99.

Stunkard, A., d'Aquilie, E., Fox, S. and Filion, R. (1972) Influence of social class on obesity and thinness in children. *Journal of the American Medical Association* **221**, 579–84.

Stunkard, A., Craighead, L. and O'Brien, R. (1980) Controlled trial of behaviour therapy, pharmacotherapy and their combination in the treatment of obesity. *Lancet* **11**, 1045–7.

Szmukler, G. (1983) Weight and food preoccupation in a population of English schoolgirls. In Bargman, G. (ed), *Understanding Bulimia and Anorexia Nervosa*, pp 21–8. Report of the Fourth Ross Conference on Medical Research. Columbus, Ohio: Ross Laboratories.

Szmukler, G. and Russell, G. (1983) Diabetes mellitus, anorexia nervosa and bulimia. *British Journal of Psychiatry* **142**, 305–8.

Theander, S. (1970) Anorexia nervosa : a psychiatric investigation of 94 female patients. *Acta Psychiatrica Scandinavica Supplement* **214**, 24–31.

Tobias, A. and Gordon, J. (1980) Social consequences of obesity. *Journal of the American Dietetic Association* **76**, 338–42.

Tolstrup, K., Brinch, M., and Isager, T. (1982) *The Copenhagen Anorexia Nervosa Follow-up Study : General Outcome.* The 10th International

Congress of the International Association of Child and Adolescent Psychiatry and Allied Professions, Dublin, 1982.

Warren, W. (1968) A study of anorexia nervosa in young girls. *Journal of Child Psychology and Psychiatry* **9**, 27–40.

Chapter 13

Tics

Tics, and Gilles de la Tourette's syndrome

Tics, particularly as a transient childhood condition, are very common while Tourette's syndrome is relatively rare, and may be extremely disabling.

Example 10
Robert seems at first a very ordinary boy of fifteen, if a little anxious. But every few moments Robert's face contorts and his neck twists in a number of sudden jerks. He answers questions coherently but then suddenly starts noisily clearing his throat and whispering. The psychiatrist leans forward to try to catch what Robert is saying and finds that he is muttering 'fuck ... fuck ... fuck.'

Later, when the interview has progressed and Robert is less embarrassed at being asked about his problems, the psychiatrist tried to find whether the boy's experience is obsessional in type.

'How does each movement begin? Do you feel that it's going to happen?'
'I just find my face or my eye twitching or something.'
'Ever felt inside that it was going to happen, and tried to stop it in some way?'
'No, it's happened by the time I notice it.'
'For example, do you get a funny feeling in your throat and think to yourself
– shall I clear it or can I put up with it for a bit?'
'It just happens. I don't think about it. I'd like not to do it.'
'But can you ever stop them for a moment?'
'I can, but I don't know how.'
'Can you also do one of the movements, if I were to ask you to?'
'Oh yes.'

The above account of the experience of multiple tics is one of several slightly differing descriptions the clinician can get from different patients, and this is part of the puzzle and the problem of these disorders.

Tics are quick, sudden, repetitive, apparently purposeless co-ordinated movements of small groups of muscles; for example they may take the form of an eye-blink, a twist of the neck, or a jerk of the head. Tics may also be vocal, and include offensive utterances (coprolalia) or gestures (copropraxia) which the patient appears not to intend as such, but which do have social meaning.

Tics usually begin in childhood, as a transient condition of children around the age of six or seven (Pringle *et al.*, 1967) and with boys being affected about three times more often than girls. In some children they last longer (Shapiro *et al.*, 1978).

Tourette's (or Gilles de la Tourette's) syndrome is a name given to multiple motor and vocal tics which may include coprolalia and copropraxia, which begins in childhood or early adolescence and follows a lengthy course. In Corbett's study (Corbett *et al.*, 1969) of 73 patients followed up for between one and eighteen years, more than half had improved (and two-thirds of this group had recovered) and none were clearly worse than when first seen.

Corbett (Corbett *et al.*, 1969) and others suggest that Tourette's syndrome is at one end of a spectrum of tic disorders with transient tics of childhood at the other.

Aetiology

Corbett and his colleagues (1969) did not find in their patients problems before the onset of tics, such as behaviour disorders or hyperkinesis, although these have been reported in earlier studies (e.g. Rapoport, 1959; Eisenberg *et al.*, 1959) and possibly indicate a temperamental vulnerability to the later development of tics (Corbett and Turpin, 1985).

Family studies suggest a genetic contribution to aetiology (Wilson *et al.*, 1978; Kidd *et al.*, 1980; Paul *et al.*, 1981) while some families of patients with Tourette's syndrome show a higher than usual incidence of other emotional and behavioural problems (Corbett *et al.*, 1969) and obsessive-compulsive disorder (Montgomery *et al.*, 1982).

Some studies have reported a high incidence (about half) of non-specific neurological disorders such as so-called 'soft' neurological signs such as clumsiness and variable and non-specific EEG abnormalities (Golden, 1977; Shapiro *et al.*, 1978).

The work by Corbett and his colleagues found a normal distribution of intelligence among their 73 patients, although Shapiro's account reported a large number with high verbal/performance discrepancies on IQ testing.

The view has been taken that the syndrome is based on a disorder of dopamine activity in the brain (Snyder *et al.*, 1970) but a number of biochemical studies (reviewed in Corbett and Turpin, 1985) have not confirmed this.

Tics, and Gilles de la Tourette's syndrome: notes on management

(i)   Haloperidol ('Serenace') in low to moderate doses (e.g. 1.5 mg TDS) can be very helpful, although higher doses may be needed in older, bigger adolescents (see Connell *et al.* 1967). Anti-Parkinsonian drugs for dystonic side effects may be needed (Chapter 18). The mechanism of action is not known but appears to be more specific than an anxiolytic effect alone, and may be due to its blocking dopamine pathways in the central nervous system.

Another powerful dopamine blocker is Pimozide ('Orap') and this too may be effective, beginning with small doses, e.g. 4 mg daily, but higher doses may be needed.

(ii) Behavioural methods tend to give only temporary relief, (see Corbett's and Turpin's review, 1985) and include massed practice, self-monitoring and positive reinforcement of tic-free periods. Focussed relaxation (Bliss 1980) and general stress management techniques may be useful (see Chapter 18). At Bethlem one of our patients with Tourette's syndrome benefited from relaxation training and help with the general self-management of his disability, which seemed to contribute to a general increase in confidence and a reduction in the more elaborate and explosive of his tics.

In general, both behavioural and pharmacological methods should be used. Drugs are likely to be helpful, but behavioural methods may (a) be partially helpful in their own right, (b) enable less medication to be used, and (c) increase the adolescent's sense of autonomy, which will help boost morale.

(iii) Psychotherapy and family work cannot be expected to help directly, but should be considered (a) to reduce tension and anxiety, and (b) to help teach the adolescent and the family coping strategies, and ways of coming to terms emotionally with this distressing, embarrassing and often long-lasting condition.

References and further reading

Bliss, J. (1980) Sensory experiences of Gilles de la Tourette's syndrome. *Archives of General Psychiatry* **37**, 1343–7.

Connell, P.H., Corbett, J.A., Matthews, A.M. and Horne, D.J. (1967) Drug therapy in the treatment of adolescent ticquers : a double-blind trial of Diazepam and Haloperidol. *British Journal of Psychiatry* **113**, 375–81.

Corbett, J.A., Matthews, A.M., Connell, P.H. and Shapiro, D.A. (1969) Tics and Gilles de la Tourette's syndrome : a follow-up study and critical review. *British Journal of Psychiatry* **115**, 1229–41.

Corbett, J. and Turpin, G. (1985) Tics and Tourette's syndrome. *In* Rutter, M. and Hersov, L. (eds), *Child and Adolescent Psychiatry : Modern Approaches*, pp 516–25. Oxford: Blackwell Scientific Publications.

Eisenberg, L., Ascher, E.A. and Kanner, L. (1959) A clinical study of Gilles de la Tourette's disease (maladie des tics) in children. *American Journal of Psychiatry* **115**, 715–26.

Golden, G.S. (1977) Tourette's syndrome : the paediatric perspective. American *Journal of Diseases of Children* **131**, 531–4.

Kidd, K., Prusoff, B. and Cohen, D. (1980) Familial pattern of Gilles de la Tourette. *Archives of General Psychiatry* **37**, 1336–9.

Montgomery, M. Clayton, P. and Friedhoff, A. (1982) Psychiatric illness in Tourette syndrome patients and first degree relatives. *In* Friedhoff, A. and Chase, T. (Eds), *Gilles de la Tourette's Syndrome*, pp 335–40. New York: Raven Press.

Paul, D., Cohen, D., Heimbuch, R., Detlor, J. and Kidd, K. (1981) Familial pattern and transmission of Gille de la Tourette's syndrome and multiple tics. *Archives of General Psychiatry* **38**, 1091–3.

Pringle, M., Butler, N. and Davie, R. (1967) *11,000 7 year-olds*. London: Longman.

Rapoport, J. (1959) Maladie des tics in children. *American Journal of Psychiatry* **116**, 177–8.

Shapiro, A., Shapiro, E., Bruun, R. and Sweet, T. (1978) *Gilles de la Tourette Syndrome*. New York: Raven Press.

Snyder, S., Taylor, K., Coyle, J. and Meyerhoff, J. (1970) The role of brain dopamine in behavioural regulation and the actions of psychotropic drugs. *American Journal of Psychiatry* **127**, 199–207.

Wilson, R., Garron, D. and Klawans, H. (1978) Significance of genetic factors in Gilles de la Tourette syndrome : a review. *Behavioural Genetics* **8**, 503–10.

Chapter 14

Autism and Other Major Disorders of Personality Development

The disorders considered in this chapter are:

Autism
Autistic psychopathy (Asperger's syndrome)
Schizoid personality
Borderline personality disorder

They are considered together because unlike many disorders which demonstrate relatively circumscribed symptoms or disabilities against a background of relatively normal, integrated personality development, young people with these conditions show all- pervading problems with their feelings, attitudes and patterns of social behaviour and relationships.

This is the main reason for considering them together. A second reason is the fact that although the typical disorder in each category is unlike the other three, in clinical practice we often see young people whose problems defy precise categorization, and for whom the above list may constitute the differential diagnosis.

A third reason is the possible nosological relationships between the first three disorders; this too is an area of uncertainty and disagreement.

A fifth category of personality disorder, psychopathy (or sociopathy) is not considered fully here; the term tends not to feature in texts on child and adolescent psychiatry, perhaps because it combines imprecision with being something of a pejorative term, and adolescent psychiatrists may prefer not to seriously propose the diagnosis for young people whose personalities are still developing. However, it seems likely that a proportion of those regarded as psychopathic in adult life are recruited from those who showed conduct disorder in childhood, particularly when there was a history of paternal antisocial behaviour (Robins, 1966; Weiner, 1982).

Autism (Kanner's syndrome)

Autism, or early infantile autism, is a condition which can be identified in the first two or three years of life and it tends to be associated with early childhood; however, its handicaps largely persist throughout life and it is therefore a condition of adolescence and adulthood too.

Kanner's epithet for the condition he described was 'extreme aloneness and insistence on sameness' (Kanner, 1943, 1949), a reminder of the essence of the disorder. Autistic children have poor comprehension of gesture and speech, lack imaginative or co- operative play, their attachment to their parents is weak or idiosyncratic (e.g. they tend not to follow their parents about or go to them in greeting or when frightened), some seem not to be able to discriminate between people, and they seem fundamentally to lack the capacity to organize their gaze, speech, gesture, demeanour etc. into a repertoire of social behaviour. They tend to play alone with objects, often in repetitive, stereotyped ways that seem not to amount to imaginative play; they can become aroused, fearful and enraged if their play or other routines are interrupted. They are sometimes overactive. There may be stereotyped movements and mannerisms. Their language development is delayed and seriously impaired, and shows echolalia, pronoun reversal ('you' for 'I'), problems in understanding language and using it imaginatively, and a tendency to make statements rather than engage in conversation. A common problem is that the child persists with questions about a currently preoccupying matter, and cannot be gratified by adults' answers.

The overall effect of this cluster of disabilities on the developing young person is a sadly impoverished personality, no friends, poor emotional contact with his or her parents, idiosyncratic language development and an apparently scanty sense of self, or self-esteem and of imagination about play or work.

There was a time when autistic children were not differentiated from those with mental handicap. Later, autism was regarded as a childhood schizophrenic illness; more recently, it was clearly differentiated from the schizophrenic disorders, (Kolvin, 1971; Rutter, 1972) and classified as one of the psychoses of childhood. Now, it is categorized in DSMIII (Chapter 4) as a pervasive developmental disorder.

The pattern of behaviour as described clearly differs from intellectual retardation (Chapter 6). In fact about three-quarters of autistic children show varying degrees of mental retardation, but the remainder vary from normal to superior intelligence.

The disorder's characteristics differ markedly from those of schizophrenia (Chapter 15), and there is an absence of delusions, hallucinations and thought disorder of the types described in schizophrenia (Rutter and Garmezy, 1983). Further, autism develops in the first 30 months of life, while schizophrenia rarely develops before late childhood. The family pattern is different too, with language, speech and cognitive abnormalities rather than schizophrenic conditions in the wider family (see Rutter's review, 1985). Finally, autism, although its features vary as the child develops, remains substantially present and seriously handicapping throughout life, unlike schizophrenic illness which tends to have its relapses and remissions.

The prevalence of autism is about 3 children in 10,000 (Lotter, 1966, 1967; Gillberg and Schaumann 1982), and it is three times as common in boys as in girls.

Autism in adolescence

About half of autistic children, especially those at the higher levels of intelligence, gain reasonable ability in language by the time adolescence is reached, and by then some have gained a little in their social relationships, beginning with their families, and progressing, later in adolescence, to attempts at peer relationships. Rebelliousness and attempts at independence also occur late in autistic adolescents (Corbett, 1976) and can lead to family strain. Failure to comprehend other people's feelings and intentions and difficulty with both subtle and (to other people) obvious social signals can cause sexually inappropriate behaviour such as genital exposure, sexual touching, masturbation in public and inappropriate comments. Autistic girls who have trouble managing menstruation may be helped by regulatory (hormonal) medication (Corbett, 1976). The general picture even in milder degrees of autism is of gauche social behaviour and odd, inappropriate preoccupations so that social development is beset with difficulties.

By the time adulthood is reached 60 per cent of autistic young people are still too handicapped to be leading anything like an independent life, and most of this group are in residential institutions. A small group, about 10-15 per cent, make a reasonable social adjustment (Lotter, 1978). The better levels of social adjustment are predicted by an IQ of 60 plus, and the best by normal levels of non-verbal intelligence and achievement of reasonable speech by the age of 5 years (Rutter, 1970).

Other developments in adolescence include the onset of fits in about

20 per cent (Deykin and MacMahon, 1979), and in 28 per cent in another study (Rutter, 1970), with the highest levels of epilepsy when there was also severe mental retardation (Rutter, 1983). Some autistic adolescents who were overactive in childhood become underactive in adolescence, and in Rutter's study (1970) 10 per cent showed inertia, loss of language skills and a deteriorating intellectual performance, although there is no definite evidence that this decline generally continues.

Emotional disturbance and depressive states (Gillberg, 1984; Wing and Wing, 1980) occur in some autistic adolescents, perhaps partly related to painful experiences in relationships which they can neither understand nor avoid. Occasionally, autistic adolescents are seen in a turbulent, angry, unhappy, chaotic, psychotic-like state.

The aetiology of autism remains unknown, but the evidence points increasingly towards it being a disorder of cognitive function resulting in inability to comprehend the social and emotional meaning of language. A number of neurological and biochemical abnormalities have been reported in studies of autistic children, but the evidence for a neurophysiological basis for autism, though likely, remains inconclusive.

Autism : notes on management

(i)   Special education, with special attention to language, is of central importance and Bartak and Rutter (1973) have demonstrated the advantage of a well-organized, structured, handicap-focused programme. Autism is relatively rare, and the most progress is likely to be made in the more experienced, specialized educational units.

(ii) Behaviour therapy with the adolescent's social skills as the focus is also important. There should be a clear aim of encouraging such limited but basic skills as pausing to listen to the other person's reply to a question, showing someone else what they are doing and listening for his or her comment, etc. New learning may well not generalize outside the centre or clinic, so home-based social skills teaching with the parents as co-therapists is valuable (Hemsley *et al.*, 1978; Holmes *et al.*, 1982) and this also helps the parent to become the experienced expert in the child's upbringing and training. It is important, however, for the young person not to gain a therapist and lose a parent : the aim should be for the members of the family to enjoy each other's company as well as give the young person the specialized upbringing needed.

(iii) Individual counselling or psychotherapy may be helpful or relatively useless : the young person's capacity to use such work should be the guide. The expression of emotion should be modulated with care : an autistic young person can respond to a clear, firm, friendly instruction to do (or not do) something; but the expression of personal anger, appropriate with other children, is likely to alarm and confuse the autistic boy or girl.

(iv) Family work should be available to aim to relieve distress and help the atmosphere be as conducive as possible to learning new skills.

(v) As with all adolescents with problems, look for and encourage personal strengths and interests. Autistic adolescents can have fun, and many enjoy music and other forms of rhythm.

(vi) Some autistic youngsters are too much for their parents and day schools to handle, and carefully chosen residential care is then appropriate. The National Autistic Society will provide helpful advice. Their (few) special homes, and those of the Rudolf Steiner organization or run on Rudolf Steiner lines can provide a rewarding life for their residents, as well as expert training. The family will need help with their feelings about such a step (Chapter 18).

(vii) Medication (haloperidol or chlorpromazine) has no specific effect on autism, but in some young people for some periods their arousal-lowering effects may be helpful, and for some patients may be the only way to maintain them in a treatment programme. Antidepressants are worth considering for periods of depression and agitation which nothing else alleviates.

Autistic psychopathy (Asperger's syndrome)

The nature of this condition may be understood if it is pointed out that the management needed is much as above, but as for a young person of higher intelligence and with the milder degrees of autistic handicaps.

What Asperger described in 1944, and called autistic psychopathy, was a condition in which there was a marked lack of social skills, little imagination or empathy for others, social isolation, extreme egocentrism and an idiosyncratic restriction of interests to objects, pursuits or hobbies which others could not perceive as rewarding. (A time-consuming preoccupation with the pattern of the national electric grid system was an interest of one patient seen.)

Example 11
Michael, aged 14, is referred to an adolescent unit after several months of treatment at a child guidance unit. For the last two years he has been

increasingly difficult at his school, which is a special centre for children with emotional and behavioural difficulties; he has no language or learning problems. The immediate concern is his unwillingness to co-operate in any aspect of the school programme, academic or social, and he presents a picture of being disruptive, impervious to reason, and unable to accept support from anyone except one female teacher whom he follows around distraught when he does not have her attention. However, when she does spend time with him he does not seem to make progress educationally or in his behaviour, but makes increasing demands, including that she should adopt him. He has no interest or even the most basic skills in contact with other children. His one enthusiasm is for bits of electric gadgets, and he becomes absorbed in taking such devices apart and putting them together again. His room is full of related tools and bits and pieces but he has no special skill and is unwilling or unable to share this interest with others, although he will go on about small points repetitively.

Michael is often distraught, and cries noisily in a bizarre way, standing still and screaming for minutes on end with arms extended and fists clenched; people who try to comfort him are sometimes hugged for a time and then hit. He is quite a big boy and hurts people, for which he will not apologize, returning to a repetitive theme that no one loves him nor ever will, and 'they' or 'you' only want to 'put me away'. But there are times when he can be engaged in something he enjoys, especially during art therapy, and then he laughs noisily, jumping up and down.

He is of normal intelligence and physically well. He has a troubled and disrupted background, and there have been several attempts to work on a family basis which have been abandoned, every direction taken ending with prolonged sessions of Michael being distraught and unable to be comforted. An individual relationship is built up slowly, and seems to provide Michael with some sense of self-esteem and continuity, but no other change is seen, and if the relationship develops beyond Michael simply being pleased to have regular adult attention, it is not apparent. As we get to know Michael his gloomy, empty view of the world emerges : no one loves him, nor ever will, and no one will do anything for him except put him in an institution. His wish is to 'go home' but he and his mother always get into painful fights, which he acknowledges. Nonetheless that remains his ambition : to be at home. A trial period on antidepressant drugs does not help his mood or help him make more use of the individual, group, behavioural and milieu attempts to help him. However, a low dose of trifluoperazine seems to reduce some of his distress and he can then persist longer with the activities he likes. Higher doses don't help.

This patient illustrates the problems of trying to categorize young people who show major problems in their personality development. One or two experienced clinicians conclude that Michael's problem is undoubtedly best described as Asperger's syndrome, or autistic psychopathy, while others suggest he shows an extreme form of emotional immaturity due to his disrupted background, and that he ought to be accessible to psychotherapy in due course. Others diagnose schizoid personality disorder, and others early schizophrenia. At a conference we are asked if we've done copper studies (for Wilson's disease), which we have. Someone suggests that some people are simply 'oddballs'. Our own conclusion is that Michael's problem is best described as Asperger's syndrome, or atypical autism, with his current protracted distress due to the impact of adolescence on a boy with such limited emotional and social resources. He does reasonably well in due course in a therapeutic school, but after a year or two his infrequent but fierce tantrums become too much. He then tries to cut his wrists. Soon after, at age 18, he is the subject of a large case conference where it is concluded that the local adult psychiatric hospital is the only place for him, although it too is unenthusiastic because of staff shortages, and because he is so immature.

Van Krevelen and Kuipers (1962) and Wing (1981) have provided helpful accounts of Asperger's syndrome and both suggest the similarities with autism.

Schizoid personality disorder

The essence of the schizoid personality is the individual's cold, self-sufficient detachment from other people (Gelder *et al.*, 1985) with a preference for introspection and fantasy (ICD 9 – Chapter 4). People with this type of personality tend to be eccentric, without friends and are usually unmarried. Gelder *et al.* (1985) suggest that some people with these traits, detached from social concerns for long periods and able to concentrate on intellectual preoccupations rather than people, can adapt well to some aspects of life, e.g. in the academic world. This picture seems rather removed from the impression of the schizoid child or adolescent as decribed in the child psychiatric literature, where the features described are more as for Asperger's syndrome, above. However, it may be that some schizoid children as they grow up find an acceptable niche in life and become less stormy with less cause for concern; superficially cold, self-sufficient detachment may be one way of adapting to the cluster of psychosocial handicaps that may be common to variants of autism, Asperger's syndrome and schizoid personality. Wolff and Chick (1980), in a series of studies, used the term schizoid personality for the clinical picture of Asperger's syndrome, and demonstrated some similarities not only with autism but, the authors felt, with the spectrum of schizophrenic disorders (see Chapter 15).

The present situation needs further clarification. Autism is quite distinct from schizophrenia; yet there are some young people with chronic and probably lifelong major handicaps of the sort described in this chapter, who show some characteristics of atypical autism on the one hand, and schizophrenia spectrum disorders on the other. Whether the term 'schizoid personality' will remain a useful category for such young people remains to be seen.

Asperger's syndrome and schizoid personality : notes on management

(i) Special educational help is relatively less central in treatment, compared with autism, but the adolescent with Asperger's syndrome or schizoid personality problems will have a number of serious social handicaps, and careful definition of educational and occupational problems and help with a training programme at an appropriate level are important.

(ii) Social and personality factors are more likely to undermine the above efforts than is lack of intelligence or a specific learning problem, and attempts should be made at social skills training and individual counselling. In some young people individual psychotherapy is helpful. It is not always clear whether what such disabled young people most need and can use is psychotherapy, counselling or sustained befriending, and some thought should be given to this question.

(iii) Related to this last point is the question of the social setting in which the boy or girl is most likely to make friendships and achieve self-esteem and skills. More continuity of help, rather than sessional treatment, will be needed for some. Accordingly, one should think in terms of (a) guidance to the family plus a good teaching or training centre plus active help with leisure activities; or (b) residential care and training with the young person based in a therapeutic community (which may also be a school) or a hostel.

Borderline personality disorder

It might be a source of some relief for the reader to learn that borderline personality disorder is quite distinct from the autistic disorders on the one hand and the schizophrenic disorders on the other.

There is, however, a remaining source of confusion in the American usage of this term, which according to DSM III (Chapter 4) seems to incorporate schizotypal personality (superstitious, unrealistic, odd forms of speech) and which they relate to schizophrenic disorders. It will be found that a number of poorly defined personality problems tend to be grouped together within the concept of borderline disorder, e.g. schizoid personality type (Langfeldt 1939), schizotypal borderline configuration (Kety *et al.*, 1971), pseudoneurotic schizophrenia (Hoch and Polantin, 1949), disturbed ego development (Weil, 1953) and symbiotic psychoses of adolescence (Rinsley, 1977). Some use the term 'borderline states', which suggests a period of disorder rather than a personality characteristic.

My own advice is to regard borderline personality disorder as quite distinct from autistic conditions on the one hand and schizophrenic (or schizophrenic-like, or 'schizophreniform' or 'schizoptypal') disorders on the other. Although it does include a range of quite different problems, it is also reasonably stable as a diagnostic category, and there does seem to be some coherence to it as a condition understandable in the terms of ego psychology, as a disorder of ego development.

I consider the diagnosis of borderline personality disorder when a young person presents with a long history of chaotic feelings and behaviour, usually with chaotic family relationships, but with no evidence of an affective or schizophrenic psychosis, and without the striking deficiencies in social skills of the young person with one of the autistic or schizoid conditions.

Example 12: a composite picture of the borderline personality
The presentation may be of primarily awkward behaviour: running away from home; rapid alternation between taking up training or jobs and then abandoning them; similar behaviour with others, sometimes involving fighting and promiscuity; idealistic schemes alternating with despair, with self-injurious or suicidal acts or threats; periods of seeming quite responsible, e.g. about treatment, interrupted by dramatic changes of mind; periods of great sadness, sometimes with anorexia and withdrawal, which may be interrupted by enraged outbursts of surprising ferocity and with poor impulse control; disorganized attempts at being independent, interrupted by episodes of childlike dependence, and angry incomprehension when adults express their own inability to keep up with these fluctuations, which 'proves', the adolescent will say, that the adults 'don't care'. The clinical picture is very much one of childishness with a good deal of anger and sadness, but exaggerated by the fact of the young person's adolescence. It is also rather like a pathological amplification of normal adolescent mixed feelings and behaviour. There are often depressive and sometimes non-schizophrenic psychotic episodes, which are transient, and marked by depression or chaotic rage.

In summary, there are behaviour problems, fluctuating moods, psychotic episodes and seriously impaired social relationships. There may be drug abuse.

The history of such young people is characteristically marked by separations, which may include actual losses (for example by parental death or separation) or equivalent withdrawal of care and attention (for example, through maternal depression). Some accounts describe the family as typically containing a demanding, controlling mother and an absent or passive father. The parents have difficulties in their mutual relationships, cannot set limits consistently, and seem not to know how to provide normal gratification without being over indulgent, or how to encourage the child's independence in a way that works.

Masterson (1980), in a strongly recommended review, suggests that the origins of the disorder lie in the first two or three years of life, with the relationship between mother and child being one where a natural balance between dependence and independence is not achieved. The dynamic model Masterson proposes is one where the mother withdraws support at crucial stages in the child's attempts at self-assertion, so that the developing child has as alternatives either a withdrawn but safe emotional attachment to the mother, or attempts at self- assertion in an atmosphere perceived as unsupporting or hostile. These alternatives are antithetic to normal development, and the adolescent feels this entrapment with anxiety, rage and despair. The developing child's personality development becomes marked by alternation between disabling over-dependence and an equally disabling lack of trust in relationships, including that with the therapist.

Interesting views and accounts of borderline characteristics are found in Schmideberg (1959), Kernberg (1967), Grinker *et al.* (1968), Masterson (1972, 1973, 1980), Perry and Klerman (1978, 1980) and Aarkrog (1981). Snyder *et al.* (1982) review the possible relationships between depressive disorders and borderline personality disorder.

There are many aspects of accounts of the condition's aetiology, and of the clinical presentation, which can be related to the vicissitudes of ordinary development and their exaggeration in the neuroses. Thus Kroll *et al.* (1981) conclude that while there are patients who show the picture described, such features may also be detected in practically all disturbed people who do not show the classical, circumscribed syndromes of schizophrenic, affective or neurotic disorders. My own view is that the disorder can be a feature of other disorders, or a disorder in its own right (analagous, say, to hypertension) and that Weil's term (1953) 'disturbed ego development', although aetiological rather than descriptive, has much to commend it. Despite the problems of precise definition, long-term studies indicate that the disorder does seem to represent a relatively stable category, that the basic problems (though with varying manifestations) persist for many years, and that the psychotic episodes are not acute schizophrenic episodes; nor do borderline patients develop schizophrenia (Aarkrog, 1981).

Borderline personality disorder : notes on management

(i)   Young people with borderline personality disorders are interesting, intermittently articulate and apparently insightful, and often quick to respond rapidly to the clinician, who will often be given the impression that he or she is the first person the patient has met who seems really able to help. Hence caution is indicated, and the inexperienced psychotherapist can rapidly be drawn into a thera- peutic relationship which may look promising but soon becomes therapeutically impracticable. However, individual psychotherapy by a relatively experienced worker and with careful supervision may be helpful. Early consideration should be given to the question : will an attempt be made at time-limited, focussed psychotherapy (for example, on a goal of leaving home); or should long-term work be embarked upon, e.g. for two or three years? There is a place for trying either, and either may prove helpful or disappointing.

(ii) More predictably helpful than psychotherapy is a programme of care in which firm limits are set on behaviour and normal social behaviour consistently expected. In principle this might best be sought in the home, reinforced by family work; in practice family work is often more helpful with the focus on a constructive separation, and more progress made with the adolescent away from home, in a therapeutic milieu. The milieu may need to be highly organized, or one in which there is help and pressure from the community's social expectations. Which is likely to be more helpful is an important decision to be made in assessment for residential care, and will depend on the adolescent's capacity for being able to take some responsibility for putting things right.

(iii) Medication (antidepressants, phenothiazines, haloperidol) should be considered for episodes of severe depression or psychosis. Antidepressants are also worth considering if psychological and social approaches do not make progress in a young person where sadness and self-deprecation is prominent.

References and further reading

Aarkrog, T. (1981) The borderline concept in childhood, adolescence and adulthood : borderline adolescents in psychiatric treatment and five years later. *Acta Psychiatrica Scandinavica Supplement* **293**, 64.

Bartak, L. and Rutter, M. (1973) Special educational treatment of autistic children : a comparative study. I : Design of study and characteristics of units. *Journal of Child Psychology and Psychiatry* **14**, 161–79.

Corbett, J. (1976) Medical management. *In* Wing, L. (Ed), *Early Childhood Autism. Clinical, Educational and Social Aspects*, Second Edition, pp 271–86. Oxford: Pergamon.

Deykin, E. and MacMahon, B. (1979) The incidence of seizures among children with autistic symptoms. *American Journal of Psychiatry* **136**, 1310–12.

Gelder, M., Gath, D. and Mayou, R. (1985) *Oxford Textbook of Psychiatry*. Oxford: Oxford University Press.

Gillberg, C. (1984) Autistic children growing up : problems during puberty and adolescence. *Developmental Medicine and Child Neurology* **26**, 122–9.

Gillberg, C. and Schaumann, H. (1982) Social class and autism : total population aspects. *Journal of Autism and Developmental Disorders* **12**, 223–8.

Gillberg, C, (1983) *Adolescence in Autism : Awakening of Sexual Awareness*. Paper given at the 1983 European Conference on Autism.

Gillberg, C. (1984) Autistic children growing up : problems during puberty and adolescence. *Developmental Medicine and Child Neurology* **26**, 125–9.

Grinker, R., Werble, B. and Drye, R. (1968) *The Borderline Syndrome*. New York: Basic Books.

Hemsley, R., Howlin, P., Berger, M., Hersov, L., Holbrook, D., Rutter, M. and Yule, W. (1978) Training autistic children in a family context. *In* Rutter, M. and Schopler, E. (Eds), *Autism : a Reappraisal of Concepts and Treatment*, pp 378–411. New York: Plenum.

Hoch, P. and Polantin, P. (1949) Pseudoneurotic forms of schizophrenia. *Psychiatric Quarterly* **23**, 248–76.

Holmes, N., Hemsley, R., Rickett, J. and Likierman, H. (1982) Parents as co-therapists : their perceptions of a home-based behavioural treatment for autistic children. *Journal of Autism and Developmental Disorders* **12**, 331–42.

Kanner, L. (1943) Autistic disturbances of affective contact. *Nervous Child* **2**, 217–50.

Kanner, L. (1949) Problems of nosology and psychodynamics of early childhood. *American Journal of Orthopsychiatry* **19**, 416–26.

Kernberg, O. (1967) Borderline personality organisation. *Journal of the American Psychoanalytical Association* **15**, 641–85.

Kety, S., Rosenthal, D. and Wender, P. (1971) Mental illness in the biological and adoptive families of adoptive schizophrenics. *American Journal of Psychiatry* **128**, 307–11.

Kolvin, I. (1971) Psychoses in childhood – a comparative study. *In*

Rutter, M. (Ed), *Infantile Autism : Concepts, Characteristics and Treatment* pp 7–26. London : Churchill Livingstone.

Kroll, M., Sines, D., Martin, K., Lari, S., Pyle, R. and Zander, J. (1981) Borderline personality disorder : construct validity of the concept. *Archives of General Psychiatry* **38**, 1021–6.

Langfeldt, G. (1939) *The Schizophreniform States.* Copenhagen: Munksgaard.

Lotter, V. (1966) Epidemiology of autistic conditions in young children I : Prevalence. *Social Psychiatry* **1**, 124–37.

Lotter, V. (1967) Epidemiology of autistic conditions in young children II: Some characteristics of the parents and children. *Social Psychiatry* **1**, 163–73.

Lotter, V. (1978) Follow-up studies. *In* Rutter, M. and Schopler, E. (Eds), *Autism : A Reappraisal of Concepts and Treatment*, 475–95. New York: Plenum.

Masterson, J. (1972) Treatment of the Borderline Adolescent : A Developmental Approach.

Masterson, J. (1973) The borderline adolescent. *In* Feinstein, S. and Giovacchini, P. (Eds), *Adolescent Psychiatry II : Developmental and Clinical Studies*, 240–68. New York: Basic Books.

Masterson, J. (1980) *From Borderline Adolescent to Functioning Adult : The Test of Time.* New York : Brunner Mazel.

Perry, J. and Klerman, G. (1978) The borderline patient : a comparative analysis of four sets of diagnostic criteria. *Archives of General Psychiatry* **35**, 141–52.

Perry, J. and Klerman, G. (1980) Clinical features of the borderline personality disorder. *American Journal of Psychiatry* **137**, 165–73.

Rinsley, D. (1977) An object relations view of borderline personality. *In* Harticollis, P. (Ed), *Borderline Personality Disorders.* New York: International Universities Press.

Robins, L. (1966) *Deviant Children Grown Up.* Baltimore: Williams and Wilkins.

Rutter, M. (1970) Autistic children : infancy to adulthood. *Seminars in Psychiatry* **2**, 435–50.

Rutter, M. (1972) Relationships between child and adult psychiatric disorders. *Acta Psychiatrica Scandinavica* **48**, 3–21.

Rutter, M. (1983) Cognitive defects in the pathogenesis of autism. *Journal of Child Psychology and Psychiatry* **24**, 513–31.

Rutter, M. (1985) Infantile autism and other pervasive developmental disorders. *In* Rutter, M. and Hersov, L. (Eds), *Child and Adolescent Psychiatry : Modern Approaches*, pp 545–66. Oxford: Blackwell Scientific Publications.

Rutter, M. and Garmezy, N. (1983) Developmental psychopathology. *In*

Hetherington, E.M. (Ed), *Socialization, Personality and Development, Volume 4, Handbook of Child Psychology* Fourth Edition, pp 775–911. New York: John Wiley and Sons.

Schmideberg, M. (1959) The borderline patient. *In* Arieti, S. (Ed), *American Handbook of Psychiatry, Vol. 1*, pp 398–416. New York: Basic Books.

Snyder, S., Sajadi, C., Pitts, W. and Goodpaster, W. (1982) Identifying the depressive border of the borderline personality disorder. *American Journal of Psychiatry* **139**, 6, 814–17.

Van Krevelen, D. and Kuipers, C. (1962) The psychopathology of autistic psychopathy. *Acta Paedopsychiatrica* **29**, 22–32.

Weil, A. (1953) Certain severe disturbances of ego development in childhood. *Psychoanalytic Study of the Child* **8**, 271–87.

Weiner, I. (1982) *Child and Adolescent Psychopathology*. New York: John Wiley and Sons.

Wing, J. and Wing, L. (1980) Provision of services. *In* Wing, L. (ed). *Early Childhood Autism*. Oxford: Pergamon Press.

Wing, L. (1981) Asperger's syndrome : a clinical account. *Psychological Medicine,* **11**, 115–30.

Wolff, S. and Chick, J. (1980) Schizoid personality in childhood : a controlled follow-up study. *Psychological Medicine* **10**, 85–100.

Chapter 15

Schizophrenic Disorders

Introduction: the diagnosis of schizophrenia

Schizophrenia (better termed the schizophrenic group of illnesses) can present with characteristic symptoms that meet quite tight diagnostic criteria, but the clinician will often see adolescents and young adults in whom the diagnosis is suspected, but far from certain.

Some widely-used criteria for the diagnosis were described by Kurt Schneider (1959) as symptoms of the first rank. They are:

(1) Hearing own thoughts spoken aloud.
(2) Hallucinatory voices talking about the patient in the third person (e.g. 'look at her' etc.) and commenting on the patient's appearance, activities, intentions etc.
(3) Somatic hallucinations, particularly of sexual interference.
(4) Thought withdrawal or insertion, i.e. that the patient's thoughts are being taken away, or put into his or her head, from outside.
(5) Thought broadcasting, in which the patient thinks his or her thoughts are broadcast aloud, and can be heard by other people.
(6) Delusional perceptions, i.e. the patient sees something and attributes special meaning to it – for example, a nurse hands the patient a cup of tea and this means that he or she is the object of persecution.
(7) Passivity experiences, i.e. that the patient's thoughts, feelings or actions are controlled by or under the influence of outside agencies, e.g. other people.

The reason why discussion of schizophrenia constantly returns to this list of first rank signs is the long and continuing history of confusion about the disorder. For example, the practitioner will come across people who, despite being apparently well-informed, think schizophrenia refers to having a 'dual personality', or being 'in two minds' about something. Others regard it as generally synonymous with incurable insanity.

There has been muddle and controversy in professional circles too, which may be understood by a brief reference to two strands in the history of the disorder. In the European tradition, and particularly Anglo-German tradition of clinical description, Emil Kraepelin, in his classical description of schizophrenia, emphasized symptoms such as hallucinations, thought disorder and delusions (Kraepelin, 1919). Eugen Bleuler, who was Swiss and influential in America, attempted more to understand and explain the disorder in terms of its psychology, and this school developed in parallel with a new move away from the notion of schizophrenia as a biological disease and towards its being understandable in psychosocial terms (Bleuler, 1911).

This schism resulted in schizophrenia being regarded as a relatively uncommon, quite tightly defined serious illness in Britain, and a more loosely defined, widely diagnosed disorder in some circles in the USA (World Health Organization 1973). Up to the 1960s it seemed that people were being diagnosed as 'schizophrenic' who, today, on both sides of the Atlantic, would be diagnosed as having affective, borderline or neurotic disorders or regarded as simply eccentric. One outcome in the 1960s was the emergence of protest at 'schizophrenic' people being treated as ill when they were really responding in a healthy and natural way to abnormal family or social and cultural circumstances, and who needed not doctors and medication but psychotherapy and social change. It is likely that many troubled people who were the focus of this 'radical psychiatry' movement did indeed need psychotherapy and social change, and moreover were not suffering from schizophrenia.

The diagnosis of schizophrenia

The International Pilot Study of Schizophrenia (World Health Organization, 1973; Carpenter *et al*, 1974) was an attempt to clarify the picture, and the following pattern of symptoms, taken from international surveys, emerged as most likely to discriminate the disorder in a way that could receive clinical agreement in many different countries:

- delusions of control;
- thought insertion, broadcast or withdrawal;
- auditory hallucinations in the third person;

- auditory hallucinations addressing the person, and not apparently based on his or her affective (mood) state.

If such symptoms persist (In DSM III – Chapter 4 – a duration of at least six months is required), and if there is no evidence of a physical illness or toxic state causing the symptoms, the diagnosis of schizophrenia can be made.

This by no means clears up the problems of diagnosis and definition. First, there are special problems of diagnosing schizophrenia in children and adolescents – see below. Second, it is not always easy to rule out a neurological cause. Third, from time to time the clinician will see young people who are grossly disabled by very poor social functioning and lack of personal motivation in any direction and appear ill-definedly ill.

Such people may have superficially reasonable social skills in terms of a quiet courtesy and compliance, but very little capacity for making realistic plans or using help to think up modest goals or attain them. There may be frustrated anger when pushed (for example, to take part in activities or even to get up in the morning) but no other self-assertiveness. This is accompanied by a sense of apathy and emptiness within, but there is no evidence for depression or socially inhibiting anxiety. Often, there will have been many unsuccessful attempts at treatment and rehabilitation, and such adolescents move into young adulthood without training, jobs, friends or recreational interests. They become detached from their families, or live at home in a highly dependent state. Those therapeutic settings which expect some motivation and response from their clientele turn them down, and the risk of a slow downward drift towards vagrancy seems real. The person concerned is not an unconventional 'drop-out' but an unhappy, isolated individual with little apparent internal or external life. There may be occasional psychotic episodes with some of the first rank symptoms, but this is unusual, and the rather unsatisfactory diagnosis of simple schizophrenia may be made on the basis of the chronic, disabling impoverishment described above. Befriending is possible, indeed necessary, but the active therapist or would-be rehabilitator is characteristically frustrated by lack of any 'leverage'.

A schizophrenic illness may however present with florid, clear-cut first-rank symptoms:

Example 13
Carol, who is 16, has always been regarded as a rather isolated girl. Her lack of friends seems due to unpopularity rather than shyness, because she is relatively outgoing in a tense, demanding, idiosyncratic sort of way. However, she has not previously been regarded as unwell.

For about a month she has been increasingly agitated and unhappy, and her mother understands she has developed an intense, unspecified distress related to her last menstrual period. She stops washing, eats and drinks little and her day becomes disorganized : she is up and about in an anxious, restless fashion until late at night, and by day is withdrawn, preoccupied and uncommunicative. She takes to wandering about the house half-clothed, even when there are visitors. One evening there is a disturbing scene when she asks a clergyman – who has visited the family to see if he can help – to take her home with him and when he says no she attacks him violently.

On examination she explains that she was made pregnant by a man, someone whom the vicar knows. She says she wasn't attacked or raped (although in later episodes of distress she screams that she is being raped); rather, she felt 'something come inside her' in the night; it was 'some sort of devil'. When asked if she could have been mistaken, and perhaps had a feeling which was due to some other cause, this is firmly denied. She *knows* she was impregnated by 'something', and there is no question of doubt about it. It has happened several times since. She hears voices describing her as a slut and a prostitute. It doesn't puzzle her that there is no one around when the voices come, and she cannot think of them in terms of imagination or something overheard or misheard: they are real to her. She wanted to have the baby, having been made pregnant, but the voices said she was going to have an abortion, and she knows that the vaginal bleeding she had (on the night her parents found her acutely distressed) was the pregnancy being forcibly terminated. About the vicar, an old friend of the family, she has mixed feelings. She tells a nurse that he sent a devil to rape her; this is something she just 'knows'. On the other hand she also *knows* that he can help her in some way she cannot explain.

Diagnostic problems in childhood and adolescence

There are four major areas of difficulty in diagnosing schizophrenia, particularly in younger or otherwise relatively immature adolescents.

First, however convincing the clinical presentation, it has been shown that young adolescents diagnosed as having a schizophrenic illness are quite likely to be diagnosed with equal certainty as having an affective psychosis next time they become acutely ill, and vice versa (Zeitlin, 1986). In fact, a mixed picture of schizophrenic and affective (manic or depressive) symptoms is not uncommon, and some clinicians then favour using the diagnosis 'schizoaffective illness'.

Second, psychological symptoms are often less well differentiated in the younger age group (about 8 to 12 years) in whom schizophrenic illnesses very occasionally present. This may be partly due to the stage of physiological maturation reached, so that the expression of the disorder is different, or partly due to difficulties in articulating bizarre and frightening experiences. In such young people systematized paranoid delusions are less common, and instead the clinical presentation is dominated by high levels of anxiety, incoherent speech, bizarre grimacing and stereotyped movements, intense preoccupation with inner thoughts and fantasies, poor emotional control with unpredictable outbursts of rage and, sometimes, violence. Social judgement is poor, and there is a diminishing social and academic performance; the overall picture as first presented, may be of antisocial behaviour rather than illness (Weiner, 1982), or there may be a prodromal period of mood disturbance (Eggers, 1978).

Third, Rack (1982) points out that outside European cultures (e.g. in Asia, Africa and the Caribbean) schizophrenic- like transient reactions to stress may occur, and certainly such schizophreniform psychogenic psychotic reactions are seen occasionally in children and adolescents of non-European background.

Fourth, schizophrenic-like conditions may be seen when a child or adolescent is under stress and also has one or more of the following characteristics : low intelligence, relative emotional immaturity, or one of the personality disorders described in Chapter 14. In principle, the child should not be regarded as schizophrenic in the absence of the characteristic symptoms and behaviour described in this chapter; in practice one may be dealing with a distraught child who cannot be comforted nor explain what he or she is feeling, experiencing or thinking. This makes diagnosis difficult, and may last for some time.

Dysmorphophobia

Adolescents sometimes present with the preoccupation that part of their body (e.g. nose, ears, mouth, breasts, buttocks, penis) is too large, small or the wrong shape, or changing shape in some way. Adolescents are commonly self-conscious of their appearance, judgement about the ideal shape of various parts is subjective, and teenagers are indeed going through a period of growth and differential change. Accordingly, it is not always clear whether a 'cosmetic' concern is normal, an overvalued idea or a delusion. In dysmorphophobia, the preoccupation may be either of the latter : a delusion, if there is a conviction beyond all reflection or discussion that there is something wrong with the part of the body concerned; or an overvalued idea, which is a strongly held judgement the patient makes, and which is not so much illogical as something the clinician believes the patient is making too much of. If the idea is truly delusional, the patient may have a schizophrenic illness; more often the wider problem is one of personality disorder or, unusually, depression (Hay 1970).

Aetiology of schizophrenic disorders

There is now no serious doubt that genetic influences play an important part in the aetiology of schizophrenia. This conclusion is based on a number of studies which have demonstrated in the relatives of schizophrenic patients a statistical increase in incidence of the illness as the blood relationship becomes closer. For example, there is a higher incidence in identical twins than in non-identical twins, and a higher incidence in non-identical twins that in other siblings, and so on.

These studies have been confirmed even when children brought up in quite different homes have been studied: the so-called 'adopted away' type of survey. (See, for example, Rosenthal *et al.*, 1971; Gottesman and Shields, 1975; Kety, 1983).

The continuing search for a biochemical cause remains as inconclusive as ever (Matthysse, 1976), and this is true of the idea that an abnormality of dopamine transmission, or of serotonin or methyl metabolism, might underly the disorder.

Several CT (computerized tomography) studies have demonstrated enlarged ventricles in the brains of patients with schizophrenia (Golden *et al.*, 1980; Weinberger *et al.*, 1980) although Benes *et al.*, (1982) found no CT scan abnormality in the brains of eleven adolescents and young adults with schizophrenia. It is doubtful whether a specific organic cause of the disorder is emerging from such studies, although it remains possible that chronic organic brain syndromes may contribute to some forms of the illness.

There have been some interesting prospective studies of the children of schizophrenic women, (Mednick *et al.*, 1974, 1978) since these young people constituted a high risk group, and it was reported that these high risk children showed distinctive physiological reactions to stress and were passive as babies, with a short attention span. These findings, however, have not been confirmed or replicated; for example, the long-term New York study has not found evidence of abnormal autonomic functioning although attentional dysfunction was found (Erlenmeyer-Kimling *et al.*, 1984). These studies do suggest a relationship between these findings, maternal psychiatric disorder and later psychiatric disorder in the child, but there is insufficient evidence of these findings as precursors of schizophrenia (Rutter and Garmezy, 1983).

For many years there have been theories of the family causation of schizophrenia, e.g. the 'double-bind' or contradictory message (Bateson *et al.*, 1956), marital stress and parental irrationality (Lidz, 1958), family mystification and overcontrol, and also disordered communication – e.g. vague, indefinite, loose – in the parents of schizophrenics (Singer and Wynne, 1965). A careful attempt to replicate the findings of the latter researchers did find communication abnormalities of the sort Singer and Wynne described, but they were a function of greater verbosity on the part of the fathers, which was the only confirmed characteristic of parental communication (Hirsch and Leff, 1975).

In an interesting review of these and other family studies, and a report of their own, Blakar and his colleagues found in the families of borderline and schizophrenic patients a failure of communication patterns to change and develop over time, compared with controls. In both groups communication seemed egocentric and inefficient and did not change with experience. Instead, there was a tendency to 'pseudo-dialogue', characterized by a mutual retreat from useful communication in the schizophrenic group, and the use of communication as conflict in the borderline group (Blakar, 1980).

Social causes of relapse in schizophrenia

Although it is uncertain whether family and social factors are among the causes of schizophrenia, they play a part in precipitating it. Several studies of 'life events' have shown that significant social changes are common in the three weeks before the onset of florid symptoms (Brown and Birley, 1968; Birley and Brown, 1970). Over-involvement with highly critical, intrusive relatives who express high levels of emotion ('high EE') is associated with relapse of the illness within months of discharge from hospital (Brown et al., 1962, 1972).

Two factors have been shown to protect against relapse of schizophrenic illness: the regular taking of appropriate medication, and limitation of exposure to high EE relationships (Vaughn and Leff, 1976), while the presence of both protective factors has an additive preventative effect (Leff and Vaughn, 1981). One way of limiting this intense family involvement is by helping the patient and family separate; but Leff and his colleagues have also shown in a controlled trial that educating families about schizophrenia and using family group work to reduce EE where it was high significantly reduce the relapse rate (Leff et al., 1982).

Are there identifiable precursors of schizophrenia?

A number of studies have indicated personality characteristics of children who subsequently develop schizophrenia in adolescence and young adulthood. They include antisocial behaviour confined to the family, a tendency to worrying and depression and overdependence, and unpopularity due to oddness and eccentricity rather than shyness (Robins, 1966; Offord and Cross, 1969; Rutter, 1972; Garmezy, 1974 a, b). These are, of course, very general characteristics, and are precursors, not predictors.

It has already been mentioned that adolescents diagnosed as having a schizophrenic illness may earlier have been diagnosed as having an affective disorder. Many studies show that disorders of mood, conduct and personal relationships are commonly diagnosed in young people who later receive the diagnosis of schizophrenia (Sands, 1956; Symonds and Herman 1957; Warren, 1965 a, b; Masterson, 1967).

Prevalence, course and prognosis

Where reasonably standardized diagnostic criteria are used, the annual prevalence of schizophrenia in different countries is similar at about 2-4 per 1000 of the population (Jablensky and Sartorius, 1975). The incidence in most general (adolescent and adult) populations is just under 1 per cent.

Using quite narrow diagnostic criteria, Manfred Bleuler followed up over 200 patients over 20 years and found that full recovery occurred in 20 per cent, usually in the first two years of continuous illness. Full recovery was unusual after five years of continuous illness. Overall, about one-third made a generally good recovery, and a quarter remained severely disturbed (Bleuler, 1974).

Various attempts have been made to predict the outcome of schizophrenia (see Brockington and Leff, 1978) and the overall conclusion appears to be that caution is advised in trying to predict outcome in the individual patient's case (see account by Gelder *et al.*, 1985). However, there is reasonable agreement that the following factors tend to be statistically associated with a better outlook :

(a) Higher intelligence, normal EEG and late onset (Pollack, 1960; Annesley, 1961).
(b) Acute onset, affective symptoms, affective illness in the family, clear-cut precipitants (Vaillant, 1962, 1964; Stephens *et al.*, 1966; and in a study of 65 adolescents, King and Pitman, 1971).
(c) Higher intelligence, later onset (after 10 years) and secure, friendly personality (Eggers, 1978).

Schizophrenic illnesses : notes on management

(i)   Diagnosis is not straightforward in young people. Bear in mind as alternative or contributory problems: (a) affective illness, (b) the effects of stress on vulnerable personalities, (c) physical disorder, including drug toxic states.

(ii)   In explaining the disorder and its possible outlook to the family, the above uncertainties should be balanced against gloom-laden assumptions of a poor outlook. Adolescent and family should have the situation explained to them, and, at review meetings (Chapter 18), the current position and prospects explained.

(iii) Medication is the cornerstone of effective treatment in the schizophrenic illnesses (Chapter 18). Chlorpromazine or halope-ridol is useful where sedation is particularly important, and thioridazine a good alternative but the dose should not be greater than 600 mg daily (see Chapter 18). Trifluoperazine is useful where the priority is to try to reduce the patient's delusional thinking or distressing preoccupations. Low (i.e. anxiolytic) doses of, for example, trifluoperazine are worth trying when it seems likely that psychogenic influences are particularly important in aetiology. Pimozide is a useful drug, but can cause over-activity. Depot preparations, e.g. fluphenazine, should be considered for long- term use, especially when medication is proving helpful but compliance is a problem. Sulpiride looks promising.

    The right dosage is the dose which produces maximum help with minimum side-effects. Adult-type dosage may be needed. The approach should be to be clear about the goals of drug therapy and monitor the results : each patient's case should be regarded as a therapeutic experiment in this respect.

    Anti-parkinsonian medication (e.g. procyclidine, orphenadrine) should be used if such unwanted effects occur.

(iv) Likely side-effects should be explained to adolescent and parents. The risks of long-term medication (Chapter 18) must be explained too, to parents, but how far to explain long-term low risks to the patient can be a problem. An adolescent of 16, giving his or her own permission for medication, and no longer acutely ill or distressed, should be properly informed to be able to give proper consent; but there may also be the danger of a useful drug being refused because of too much anxiety about a low level of risk. It is a matter for clinical and ethical judgement, and difficult.

(v)   It is always possible to clarify the adolescent's handicaps and the family's actual problems whatever the fine points of diagnostic uncertainty. These handicaps should be the focus of help by counselling, social skills training, occupational therapy and training for leisure, living skills and education or work. Behavioural approaches (Chapter 18) are often helpful. Again, goals should be clear and progress monitored.

(vi)   There is no evidence for family therapy being the useful primary treatment for schizophrenia. However, there is good evidence that work with the family by reducing emotional arousal and critical intrusiveness can reduce the risk of relapse. This work, accompanied by information about the illness in general and the adolescent's problems in particular, is always important. Many families find the National Schizophrenia Fellowship helpful.

(vii) If due to disability and family circumstances it seems that out-patient or day care will not be enough, residential care may be needed. If so, the least institutional, least clinical setting the patient can cope with should be sought, e.g. a supervised hostel or therapeutic community in preference to a hospital. Family work should, then, focus on the issue of separation. However, a period of hospital admission is often needed in practice, especially early in the illness or in acute episodes.

References and further reading

Annesley, P. (1961) Psychiatric illness in adolescence : presentation and prognosis. *Journal of Mental Science* **107**, 268–78.

Bateson, G., Jackson, D., Haley, J. and Weakland, J. (1956) Towards a theory of schizophrenia. *Behavioural Science* **1**, 251–64.

Benes, F., Sunderland, P., Jones, B., LeMay, M., Cohen, B. and Lipinski, J. (1982) Normal ventricles in young schizophrenics *British Journal of Psychiatry* **141**, 90–3.

Birley, J. and Brown, G. (1970) Crises and life change preceding the onset and relapse of acute schizophrenia : clinical aspects. *British Journal of Psychiatry* **116**, 327–33.

Blakar, R. (1980) *Studies of Familial Communication and Psychopathology. A Social-developmental Approach to Deviant Behaviour.* Oslo: Universitetsforlaget.

Bleuler, E. (1911) *Dementia Praecox or the Group of Schizophrenias.* (Translated by J. Zinkin 1950). New York: International Universities Press.

Bleuler, M. (1974) The long-term course of the schizophrenic psychoses. *Psychological Medicine* **4**, 244–54.

Brockington, I. and Leff, J. (1978) Definitions of schizophrenia : concordance and prediction of outcome. *Psychological Medicine* **8**, 387–98.

Brown, G. and Birley, J. (1968) Crisis and life changes and the onset of schizophrenia. *Journal of Health and Social Behaviour* **9**, 203–14.

Brown, G., Monck, E., Carstairs, G. and Wing, J. (1962) Influence of family life on the course of schizophrenic illness. *British Journal of Preventive and Social Medicine* **16**, 55–68.

Brown, G., Birley, J. and Wing, J. (1972) Influence of family life on the course of schizophrenic disorders : a replication. *British Journal of Psychiatry* **121**, 241–58.

Carpenter, W., Strauss, J. and Bartok, J. (1974) The diagnosis and understanding of schizophrenia. I. Use of signs and symptoms for the identification of schizophrenic patients. *Schizophrenia Bulletin* **11**, 37–49.

Eggers, C. (1978) Course and prognosis of childhood schizophrenia. *Journal of Autism and Childhood Schizophrenia* **8**, 21–36.

Erlenmeyer-Kimling, L., Marcuse, Y., Cornblatt, B., Friedman, D., Rainder, J. and Rutschmann, J. (1984). The New York High Risk Project. *In* Watt, N., Anthony, E., Wynne, L. and Rolf, J. (Eds), *Children at Risk from Schizophrenia : A Longitudinal Perspective.*. New York: Cambridge University Press.

Garmezy, N. (1974a) Children at risk : the search for the antecedents of schizophrenia. Part I : Conceptual models and research methods. *Schizophrenia Bulletin* **8**, 14–90.

Garmezy, N. (1974b) Children at risk : the search for the antecedents of schizophrenia. Part II : Ongoing research programs, issues and intervention. *Schizophrenia Bulletin* **9**, 55–125.

Gelder, M., Gath, D. and Mayou, R. (1985) *Oxford Textbook of Psychiatry*. Oxford: Oxford University Press.

Golden, C., Moses, J., Zelazowski, R., Graber, B., Zatz, L., Horvath, T. and Berger, P. (1980) Cerebral ventricular size and neuropsychological impairment in young schizophrenics. *Archives of General Psychiatry* **37**, 619–23.

Gottesman, I. and Shields, J. (1975) *Schizophrenia : the Epigenetic Puzzle*. Cambridge : Cambridge University Press.

Hay, G. (1970) Dysmorphophobia. *British Journal of Psychiatry* **116**, 399–406.

Hirsch, S. and Leff, J. (1975) *Abnormalities in Parents of Schizophrenics*. Institute of Psychiatry, Maudsley Monograph No 22. London: Oxford University Press.

Jablensky, A. and Sartorius, N. (1975) Culture and schizophrenia. *Psychological Medicine* **5**, 113–34.

Kety, S. (1983) Observations on genetic and environmental influences in the aetiology of mental disorder from studies on adoptees and their relatives. *In* Kety, S., Rowland, L., Sidman, R. and Matthysse, S. (Eds),

Genetics of Neurological and Psychiatric Disorders, pp 105–114. New York: Raven Press.

King, L. and Pitman, G. (1971) A follow-up of 65 adolescent schizophrenic patients. *Diseases of the Nervous System* **32**, 328–34.

Kraepelin, E. (1919) *Dementia Praecox and Paraphrenia* (Translated by R. Barclay). Edinburgh: Churchill Livingstone.

Laing, R. (1960) *The Divided Self*. London: Lavistock Publications.

Leff, J. and Vaughn, C. (1981) The role of maintenance therapy and relatives' expressed emotion in relapse of schizophrenia : a two year follow-up. *British Medical Journal* **139**, 102–4.

Leff, J., Kuipers, L., Berkowitz, R., Erberlein-Vries, R. and Sturgeon, D. (1982) A controlled trial of social intervention in the families of schizophrenic patients. *British Journal of Psychiatry* **141**, 121–34.

Lidz, T. (1958) Schizophrenia and the family. *Psychiatry* **21**, 21–7.

Masterson, J. (1967) *The Psychiatric Dilemma of Adolescence*. Boston : Little, Brown and Co.

Matthysse, S. (1976) Schizophrenia : relation to dopamine transmission, motor control and feature extraction. *In* Schmitt, F. (Ed), *The Neurosciences : Third Study*, pp 733–7. Cambridge, Massachusetts: MIT Press.

Mednick, S., Schulsinger, F., Higgins, J. and Bell, B. (1974) *Genetics, Environment and Psychopathology*. New York: Elsevier.

Mednick, S., Schulsinger, F., Teasdale, T., Schulsinger, H., Venables, P. and Rock, D. (1978) Schizophrenia in high-risk children : sex differences in predisposing factors. *In* Serban, G. (Ed), *Cognitive Development of Mental Illness*, pp 168–97. New York: Brunner Mazel.

Offord, D. and Cross, L. (1969) Behavioural antecedents of adult schizophrenia. *Archives of General Psychiatry* **21**, 267–83.

Pollack, M. (1960) Comparison of childhood, adolescent and adult schizophrenics. *Archives of General Psychiatry* **2**, 652–60.

Rack, P. (1982) *Race, Culture and Mental Disorder*. London: Tavistock Publications.

Robins, L. (1966) *Deviant Children Grown Up*. Baltimore: Williams and Wilkins.

Rosenthal, D., Wender, P., Kety, S., Welner, J. and Schulsinger, F. (1971) The adopted-away offspring of schizophrenics. *American Journal of Psychiatry* **128**, 307–11.

Rutter, M. (1972) Relationships between child and adult psychiatric disorders. *Acta Psychiatrica Scandinavica* **48**, 3–21.

Rutter, M. and Garmezy, N. (1983) Developmental psychopathology. *In* Hetherington, E. (Ed), *Socialization, Personality and Social Development, Volume 4, Handbook of Child Psychology*, pp 775–911. New York: John Wiley and Sons.

Sands, D. (1956) The psychoses of adolescence. *Journal of Mental Science* 102, 308–16.

Schneider, K. (1959) *Clinical Psychopathology* (English translation of 1950 edition). New York: Grune and Stratton.

Singer, M. and Wynne, L. (1965) Thought disorder and family relations of schizophrenics : IV. Results and implications. *Archives of General Psychiatry* **12**, 201–12.

Stephens, J., Astrup, C. and Mangrum, J. (1966) Prognostic factors in recovered and deteriorated schizophrenics. *American Journal of Psychiatry* **122**, 1116–21.

Symonds, A. and Herman, M. (1957) The patterns of schizophrenia in adolescence. *Psychiatric Quarterly* **31**, 521–30.

Vaillant, G. (1962) The prediction of recovery in schizophrenia. *Journal of Nervous and Mental Disease* **135**, 534–43.

Vaillant, G. (1964) Prospective prediction of schizophrenia remission. *Archives of General Psychiatry* **11**, 509–18.

Vaughn, C. and Leff, J. (1976) The influence of family and social factors on the course of psychiatric illness : a comparison of schizophrenic and depressed neurotic patients. *British Journal of Psychiatry* **129**, 125–37.

Warren, W. (1965a) A study of adolescent psychiatric in-patients and the outcome six or more years later. I. Clinical histories and hospital findings. *Journal of Child Psychology and Psychiatry* **6**, 1–17.

Warren, W. (1965b) A study of adolescent psychiatric in-patients and the outcome six or more years later. II. The follow-up study. *Journal of Child Psychology and Psychiatry* **6**, 141–60.

Weinberger, D., Bigelow, L., Kleinman, J., Klein, S., Rosenblatt, J. and Wyatt, J. (1980) Cerebral ventricular enlargement in chronic schizophrenia. *Archives of General Psychiatry* **37**, 11–13.

Weiner, I. (1982) *Child and Adolescent Psychopathology*. New York: John Wiley and Sons.

World Health Organization (1973) *The International Pilot Study of Schizophrenia. Volume 1*. Geneva: World Health Organization.

Zeitlin, H. (1986)*The Natural History of Psychiatric Disorder in Childhood*. Institute of Psychiatry, University of London: Maudsley Monographs.

Chapter 16

Depressive and Manic Depressive Illness

Some problems of terminology and classification

The question of depression as a normal or neurotic reaction to circumstances was discussed in Chapter 7. This chapter is concerned with depression as an individual illness with disordered physiology or biochemistry making a significant contribution.

A crucial question for the psychiatrist treating a severely depressed adolescent is whether or not to use medication. On the one hand most states of depression in young people seem understandable in the light of their psychological development and social (e.g. family) situation, so that treatment based on psychological and social principles seems most appropriate. Moreover, drugs are essentially toxic and usually prescribed with some reluctance for young people. Further, prescribing medication when the real problem is to do with personal and family matters is an erroneous distraction that can perpetuate the problem. On the other hand, there is no doubt that antidepressant medication can dramatically improve depressive states that may otherwise be chronic, debilitating and life-threatening.

The complex discussion of whether a depressive state is a psychosocial reaction or an individual biological illness, or how far it is something of both, needs to be simplified to the following key clinical question: in the case of a depressed boy or girl, is there sufficient evidence of a biological (i.e. physical) contribution to the disorder to justify a pharmacological treatment? The answer will usually turn out to be 'no' but the pharmacological treatment of depressed adolescents can occasionally be immensely helpful.

It is largely agreed in general adult psychiatry that medication is more likely to be helpful when depression is accompanied by biological symptoms such as loss of appetite and weight, sleep disturbance, diurnal variation of mood, and psychomotor retardation – physical slowing. It is also considered the appropriate treatment when the depressive state becomes psychotic in type, with delusions of worthlessness, guilt and physical disease or bizarre physical change (a depressed patient may believe his brain has rotted away). The literature and our available knowledge do not make any fundamental distinction between such major depressive psychoses and the relatively less severe biological depressive illnesses, even though the clinical presentation can be very different. Thus the following depressive illnesses are grouped together under the heading Affective Psychoses in the ICD-9 (see Chapter 4) Classification:

Affective Psychoses:
Manic-depressive psychosis, manic type (= monopolar manic illness)
Manic-depressive psychosis, depressed type (= monopolar depressive illness = endogenous depression = psychotic depression)
Manic- depressive illness, with manic and depressive swings of mood.

Under a separate heading in ICD-9 is Reactive Depressive Psychosis, i.e.

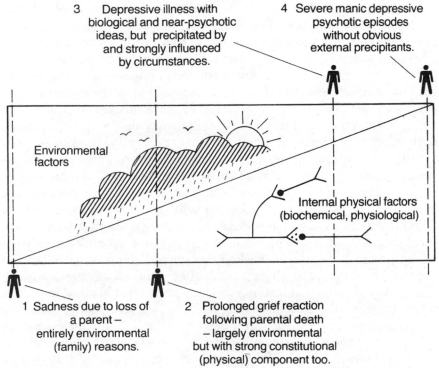

Figure 16.1 Internal and environmental factors in aetiology.

an illness similar to manic-depressive psychosis of the depressive type, but apparently provoked by a recent life experience such as a loss.

It is these disorders, very different in presentation but probably having in common a significant physiological component that are the subject of this chapter.

The relationship between the depressions of Chapter 7, and the depressive or affective illnesses of this chapter, may be summed up simply in Fig. 16.1. Most of the different states of depression are likely to be to varying degrees partly environmental and partly physical in their origins. Some depressive states (on the left of the figure), however, can be regarded as so normal a response to circumstances that for practical purposes a physiological component can be disregarded. And some (on the right) are so grounded in the individual's physiology that he or she becomes ill without any external precipitant beyond the ordinary ups and downs of life.

'Atypical' depression

The problem for child and adolescent psychiatry is how maturational changes affect the experience, physiology and expression of what in adults we call depression. The terms 'atypical' and 'masked' depression and 'depressive equivalents' have been used for children and adolescents who do not appear depressed, but whose behaviour (e.g. misconduct, promiscuity, drug abuse, violence) and experiences (e.g. bereavement, parental neglect) lead the clinician to conclude that they 'ought' to be depressed (see, for example Glaser, 1967; Toolan, 1974; Malmquist, 1971). It can be argued that young people may not become depressed with adult-type symptoms because their perception and experience (emotionally or cognitively) are different from an adult's experience, because their brain neurochemistry has not developed the capacity or vulnerability to show depressive signs, or because their psychosocial expressiveness is immature. Whether what they do express should be called 'depressive' is debatable. Weiner (1982) suggests that it is better to speak of age-related symptoms of depression and secondary reactions to depression rather than 'masked' or 'atypical' depression. Whatever the semantics, however, there is no doubt that *superficially* breezy, noisy, active and excitable youngsters who may seem naughty and impulsive rather than sad may be seen leading high risk, self-destructive lives with little apparent self-regard, and indeed Shaffer (1974) showed that in some young people who committed suicide antisocial behaviour was the problem beforehand. In his review of depression and mania in childhood, Shaffer (1985) concludes that the extent to which we can apply adult concepts of depressive illness to children remains unclear, but that (a) adult-type depressive illness does occur in adolescence, (b) pre-pubertal emotional disorders do seem to differ substantially from adult-type depressive disorders, and (c) the expression of affect (mood) is different at different ages.

Depressive illness

Adolescents may be seen who are tearful, miserable, full of self-blame and ideas of worthlessness and hopelessness and thinking of suicide, who have sleep disturbance and diurnal variation and may be agitated or withdrawn and unable to concentrate; in other words, who present the clinical picture of adult-type depressive illness. However, such symptoms may prove surprisingly transient or situation-dependent. For example, the adolescent may be profoundly withdrawn in school or in the family, but lively, extrovert and mischievous when roaming about with other young people. Correspondingly, relatively limited psychosocial intervention such as one or two supportive conversations, or a single family assessment that demonstrates that seemingly impossible topics can be safely and helpfully opened up, may bring about surprising changes for the better in the young person's mental state.

When such symptoms persist, however, it is very often not clear how best to proceed. The temptation is often to persist with psychotherapy or family therapy, and certainly there sometimes seems to be no option other than continuing exploration and support on an individual or family basis, during which time the adolescent may or may not improve substantially. But it is hard to predict when a primarily psychotherapeutic approach is likely to help severe depressive symptoms. In practice one will find that a particular therapist's style (in some settings there may be a choice) or a particular approach (e.g. through creative work or other activity) enables an adolescent to express angry and sad feelings which may involve the therapist. He may then be able to reflect on feelings and past experiences and begin to widen his or her repertoire of behaviour and responses – to show a capacity to change. From such beginnings an ultimately helpful period of psychotherapy can emerge (see Chapter 18).

The tricyclic antidepressants have a range of uses in children's disorders (see Chapter 18) but they seem much less *predictably* of benefit in depressive illness in adolescents than in adults with similar symptoms. Strober and Carlson (1982) reported the effectiveness of antidepressants in depressive illness (i.e. unipolar illness) in adolescents, but there are few convincing studies of the usefulness of these drugs in this age group. My own impression is that they can be helpful, and sometimes impressively so, and the longer depression persists despite other attempts to help, and the closer the symptoms are to adult-type biological depression, the more one should be prepared to give antidepressant medication a proper trial, i.e.. at adequate dosage for an adequate period. This means increasing the dose (while side-effects are tolerable) and maintaining medication for six weeks to two months before trying an alternative drug. However, it remains quite possible that there is a group of adolescents with severe depression who could be helped more rapidly and effectively by medication than by time-consuming psychotherapeutic and family therapeutic methods, and research which convincingly showed who they are would be valuable.

Manic-depressive illness

When depressive illness as described above recurs, or when there are repeated episodes of mania, the condition is described as manic depressive illness, unipolar type. If both manic and depressive episodes occur, it is described as manic-depressive illness, bipolar type.

Manic depressive illness does occur in adolescence (Anthony and Scott, 1960; Carlson and Strober, 1978; Welner *et al.*, 1979; Rogeness *et al.*, 1982; Gammon *et al.*, 1983) while studies of adults have indicated, restrospectively, that in about a quarter to one-fifth of cases the disorder apparently began in the patient's teens, (Winokur *et al.*, 1969; Carlson *et al.*, 1977; review by Carlson, 1983; Loranger and Levine, 1978). Some studies suggest that the outlook, in terms of frequent episodes of illness and a high incidence of suicide, is particularly poor when bipolar illness has an early onset in adolescence (Olsen, 1961; Welner *et al.*, 1979).

Manic symptoms (and even the somewhat less intense signs of the state known as hypomania) are striking in their florid intensity.

Example 14
John is sixteen, and was on lithium carbonate for his manic-depressive illness when he discharged himself from hospital. He has now been readmitted after several weeks off the drug.

He is in a noisily cheerful state and delighted to be back in the unit, although during the course of the last two hours he has in rapid succession adamantly refused to return to the hospital, then asked to be admitted, then attacked staff who suggested his admission, and finally has been persuaded to come back. Within moments of arrival he has announced that he is going to leave and then, still in his top coat, rushed out to join in a game of football and shake hands with all his old friends. When asked to come off the field to talk to his doctor he asks to have a meal instead. He is soon persuaded to come and see the doctor he knows, and hurries along ahead of the nurses, then breaks off and heads at a trot into school. Here he approaches a member of the domestic staff in conversation about the colour of her hair and becomes enraged when she will not give him a cigarette. He complains bitterly at being slighted and marches briskly about the grounds, scowling, and shouting and punching out at anyone who approaches him.

Eventually he is brought back to the unit by several nurses, detained on a section of the Mental Health Act and sedated. He agrees to accept oral medication; then throws it over a nurse and is given intramuscular chlorpromazine instead. He asks the nurse who injects him to lend him some money for the cinema. When well, John is a mild-mannered, polite and studious boy.

John shows the excitability characteristic of manic and hypomanic states. Sometimes he is briefly sociable in a chaotic, disinhibited sort of way, but there are rapid changes to irritability and anger and back again. He is distractible and his judgement is poor. He cannot sustain attention for long, and there are rapid changes of mind about what he wants to do and to whom he is prepared to respond. He has grandiose ideas about a major national sporting event in which he expects to be given an important role, which (briefly) becomes an urgent reason why he must leave the hospital immediately. He does not show the rapid rhyming and punning speech that some manic patients show. By the time he is becoming calmer it is clear that he is physically near exhaustion, and that a great deal of sadness is near the surface.

Example 15
Louise is seventeen and has had two rather similar episodes, except that in her case restlessness and excitability are not accompanied by violence. During these periods of manic overactivity she is also apprehensive and believes that a number of people in the neighbourhood know 'all about' her, and can read some wicked thoughts other people have put into her mind. She has heard voices talking accusingly about her when there was no one there. What they say confirms her suspicions. Between these periods of illness, some of which are marked more by tears and despair than excitability, she is a really quite well though somewhat solitary and awkward girl. She is diagnosed as having a schizoaffective illness.

The boundaries between manic, schizoaffective and schizophrenic illnesses are not so clear cut, however, in adolescence as they may be in adulthood. For example Zeitlin (1986) has shown that one cannot predict the nature of a second attack from the nature of the first (whether affective or schizophrenic), at least in younger adolescents. Catatonic signs have been shown to be as frequently associated with affective illness as with schizophrenia, in adolescence (Hassanyeh and Davison, 1980). In a prospective study, Strober and Carlson (1982) showed that bipolar (manic and depressive) illness was more likely when the clinical presentation was acute, with psychomotor retardation and with delusions that were congruent with mood; when there was a family history of bipolar illness; and when the response to antidepressants was poor, compared with a unipolar group. A hypomanic response to antidepressant medication is said to be highly predictive of a bipolar illness (Strober and Carlson, 1982; Akiskal *et al.*, 1978).

Lithium carbonate is well established in the treament of affective illness, and is discussed in Chapter 18. It appears to be effective in treating manic-depressive adolescents too (Brumback and Weinberg, 1977; Horowitz, 1977; Youngerman and Canino, 1978).

Are there 'manic-depressive equivalent' disorders?

A number of studies have proposed that there are some disorders of adolescence other than manic depressive illness which respond to lithium. Reports have included its occasional effectiveness in various problems including anorexia nervosa, aggressiveness and hyperactivity (Annel, 1969a, b; Dostal and Zvolsky, 1970; Sheard, 1975; Van Putten and Sanders, 1975; Lena *et al.*, 1977; Reilly, 1977; and Kymissis *et al.*, 1979) and in a patient with anorexia nervosa who had a family history of depressive illness and who made curiously episodic progress during a weight gain programme (Stein *et al.*, 1982). Campbell (1976) found the drug helpful for mentally retarded children with psychotic, aggressive and self-mutilating behaviour, and predicted improvement with lithium when the drug either decreased focal EEG abnormality, or when it increased diffuse slow activity and slowing of the alpha rhythm in normal EEGs.

If lithium is helpful in some of these conditions, it may be because certain episodic conduct problems of adolescence share some physical aetiological factors with manic depressive illness; or, more simply, that lithium can improve or prevent the mood swings in some adolescents which make their other problems worse (Steinberg, 1980). However, as with the tricyclic antidepressants, it is impossible to predict with confidence which adolescents in these 'atypical' categories will respond dramatically to lithium (which some do) and which young people will not be helped at all.

Depressive and manic-depressive conditions: notes on management

(i)   Diagnosis can be a problem. With the exception of severe manic and depressive states, it is not easy to distinguish between the states of distress, sadness and gloom described in Chapter 7 as emotional problems and largely reactive or psychogenic in origin, and the depressive illness that has a strong biological component, and in which medication may be useful. If the most helpful treatment approach is not clear, as will usually be the case, begin with the general approaches that will be useful in any case:

(a)   begin family meetings to explore problems further and to establish rapport and support

(b)   begin individual exploratory interviews with the adolescent to monitor his or her mental state, to get to know the boy or girl at a more 'feeling' level, and to assess the potential helpfulness of such individual sessions

These sessions may or may not proceed to family therapy and/ or individual counselling or psychotherapy, depending on what seems helpful.

(ii)   Assess carefully for suicidal or aggressive feelings, plans or ideas, and remember that general self-neglect and isolation, with the loss of friendships, school time, work and leisure pursuits is also self-destructive in a less dramatic but insidious way. Consider how much supervision is needed for the adolescent's safety (admission to hospital may be needed, but others too can be responsible for the adolescent's safe care).

(iii)   There are three aspects of management that need to be kept carefully in balance:

(a)   The depressed adolescent is likely to have strong feelings of loss and impoverishment and lowered self-esteem. The clinician should help mobilize a sense of being 'looked after' (by family and by therapist) but without undermining self-esteem and autonomy further. She should be expected to play a part in decisions (e.g. about medication); but if she can't, decisions may have to be made for her on the grounds that she is too unwell (i.e. 'being held' *v.* autonomy).

(b)   The patient's sadness may make her feel that nothing can ever get right again, and there will be feelings of weariness and apathy. It helps to make clear that there will be plenty of time, so that the adolescent is given time and space, and the pressure to 'get well' is taken off. Angry and sad feelings will need to be accepted and lived with rather than denied or fought off. But it is also important to avoid the treatment becoming as chronic and hopeless as the disorder. The therapist should be active and optimistic as well as accepting the adolescent and her pain. Beware chronic 'supportive psychotherapy' that may perpetuate a sense of dependence and helplessness (i.e. 'accepting' *v.* 'fighting' depression).

(c) Third, the family dynamic cliché that the individual is expressing the family's sadness is sometimes precisely correct. Look for the family that cannot be gratified even when the adolescent (relieved at outside intervention) shows a little improvement. In such circumstances family therapy should be attempted, and it may have to proceed to dealing with issues of separation and independence for the boy or girl. Sometimes separate work with the parents may be needed. A balance between attending to the needs of the adolescent and the needs of the family (or parents) will be required.

(iv) In monitoring progress, allow for adolescents' capacity for denial and changeability. Profound sadness and apparent cheerfulness at different times and with different people can both be genuine emotions. It is as important to 'give permission' for having a good time (e.g. an outing with an extrovert friend) as it is to encourage the acceptance of feelings of depression.

(v) Lack of changeability may be an indication that the depression is largely 'within' the adolescent, and perhaps has a strong biological component. Persisting sadness with the features described earlier as biological should lead to a consideration of antidepressant medication. This is not in my view incompatible with concurrent psychotherapy or family therapy, but some take the view that prescribing drugs demonstrates that neither patient nor family has a genuine role in therapy. Antidepressants are discussed in Chapter 18.

(vi) Severe, persisting depression which resists all attempts to help may justify the use of electroconvulsive therapy (ECT), but it is rarely needed in adolescence (see Chapter 18).

(vii) Lithium should be used to treat manic states, and to try to prevent the recurrence of manic and severe depressive states. Manic adolescents can be extremely difficult to sedate, and lithium and major tranquillizers may both be needed (see Chapter 18). Manic patients may be suddenly extremely violent.

(viii) Do not underestimate the emotionally draining effect on colleagues and parents of trying to help an intractably depressed patient.

References and further reading

Akisal, H., Bitar, A., Puzantian, V., Rosenthal, T. and Parks, W. (1978) The nosological status of neurotic depression. *Archives of General Psychiatry* **35**, 756–66.

Annell, A. (1969a) Manic-depressive illness in children and effect of treatment with lithium carbonate. *Acta Paedopsychiatrica* **36**, 292–301.

Annell, A. (1969b) Lithium in the treatment of children and adolescents. *Acta Psychiatrica Scandinavica Supplement* **207**, 19–30.

Anthony, E. and Scott, P. (1960) Manic-depressive psychosis in childhood. *Journal of Child Psychology and Psychiatry* **1**, 53–72.

Brumback, R. and Weinberg, W. (1977) Mania in childhood. II, Therapeutic trial of lithium carbonate and further description of manic-depressive illness in children. *American Journal of Diseases of Childhood* **131**, 1122–6.

Campbell, M. (1976) Biological interventions in psychoses of childhood. *In* Schopler, E. and Reichler, R. (Eds), *Psychopathology and Child Development*, pp 243–70. London: Plenum Press.

Carlson, G. (1983) Bipolar affective disorders in childhood and adolescence. *In* Cantwell, D. and Carlson, G. (Eds), *Affective Disorders in Childhood and Adolescence: An Update*, pp 61–83. Lancaster: MTP Press.

Carlson, G., Davenport, Y. and Jamison, K. (1977) A comparison of outcome in adolescent and late-onset bipolar manic-depressive illness. *American Journal of Psychiatry* **134**, 919–22.

Carlson, G. and Strober, M. (1978) Manic-depressive illness in early adolescence. *Journal of the American Academy of Child Psychiatry* **17**, 138–53.

Dostal, T. and Zvolsky, P. (1970) Anti- aggressive effect of lithium salts in severely mentally retarded adolescents *International Pharmacopsychiatry* **5**, 203–7.

Gammon, G., John, K., Rothblum, E., Mullen, K., Tischler, G. and Weissman, M. (1983) Use of a structured diagnostic interview to identify bipolar disorder in adolescent in-patients ; frequency and manifestation of the disorder. *American Journal of Psychiatry* **140**, 543–7.

Glaser, K. (1967) Masked depression in children and adolescents. *American Journal of Psychotherapy* **21**, 265–74.

Hassanyeh, F. and Davison, K. (1980) Bipolar affective psychosis with onset before age 16 years: a report of 10 cases. *British Journal of Psychiatry* **137**, 530–9.

Horowitz, H. (1977) Lithium and the treatment of adolescent manic-depressive illness. *Diseases of the Nervous System* **38**, 480–3.

Kymissis, P., Padrusch, B. and Schulman D., (1979) The use of lithium in cyclical behaviour disorders of adolescence: a case report. *Mount Sinai Medical Journal* **46**, 141–2.

Lena, B., Surtees, S. and Maggs, R. (1977) The efficacy of lithium in the treatment of emotional disturbance in children and adolescents. *In* Johnson, F. and Johnson, S. (Eds), *Lithium in Medical Practice*, pp 79–83 Lancaster: MTP Press.

Loranger, A. and Levine, P. (1978) Age at onset of bipolar affective illness. *Archives of General Psychiatry* **35**. 1345–8.

Malmquist, C. (1971) Depressions in childhood and adolescence. *New England Journal of Medicine* **284**, 887–93 and 955–61.

Olsen, T. (1961) Follow-up study of manic-depressive patients whose first attack occurred before the age of 19 years. *Acta Psychiatrica Scandinavica Supplement* **162**, 45–51.

Reilly, P. (1977) Lithium administration contributing to the management of anorexia nervosa. *Rhode Island Medical Journal* **60**, 419–22, 455–6.

Rogeness, G., Reister, A. and Wicoff, J. (1982) Unusual presentation of manic-depressive disorder in adolescence. *Journal of Clinical Psychiatry* **43**, 37–9.

Shaffer, D. (1974) Suicide in childhood and early adolescence. *Journal of Child Psychology and Psychiatry* **15**, 275–91.

Shaffer, D. (1985) Depression, mania and suicidal acts. *In* Rutter, M. and Hersov, L. (Eds), *Child and Adolescent Psychiatry: Modern Approaches*, 698–719. Oxford: Blackwell Scientific Publications.

Sheard, M. (1975) Lithium in the treatment of aggression. *Journal of Nervous and Mental Disease* **160**, 108–18.

Stein, G., Hartshorn, S., Jones, J. and Steinberg, D. (1982) Lithium in a case of severe anorexia nervosa. *British Journal of Psychiatry* **140** 526–8.

Steinberg, D. (1980) The use of lithium carbonate in adolescence. *Journal of Child Psychology and Psychiatry* **21**, 263–71.

Steinberg, D. (1983) *The Clinical Psychiatry of Adolescence. Clinical Work from a Social and Developmental Perspective*. Chichester: Wiley.

Strober, M. and Carlson, G. (1982) Bipolar illness in adolescents with major depression. *Archives of General Psychiatry* **39**, 549–55.

Toolan, J. (1974) Masked depression in children and adolescents. *In* Lesse, S. (Ed), *Masked Depression*. New York: Aronson.

Van Putten, T. and Sanders, D. (1975) Lithium in treatment failures. *Journal of Nervous and Mental Disease* **161**, 255–64.

Weiner, I. (1982) Child and Adolescent Psychopathology. New York: Wiley.

Welner, A., Welner, Z. and Fishman, R. (1979) Psychiatric and adolescent in-patients: 8-10 year follow-up. *Archives of General Psychiatry* **36**, 698–700.

Winokur, G, Clayton, P. and Reich, T. (1969) *Manic Depressive Illness* St Louis: C.V. Mosby.

Youngerman, J. and Canino, I. (1978) Lithium carbonate use in children and adolescents. *Archives of General Psychiatry* **35**, 216–24.

Zeitlin, H. (1986) *The Natural History of Psychiatric Disorder in Childhood.* Institute of Psychiatry, University of London: Maudsley Monographs.

Chapter 17

Physical and Psychosomatic Problems

Physical disorder in adolescent psychiatry

The physical health of adolescents is relevant to the adolescent psychiatric team in a number of quite different ways:

(a) because all adolescents have a body and, moreover, a developing body and one that they are very aware of;
(b) in residential settings, the ordinary disorders and problems of adolescence (acne, premenstrual tension, headaches, eyesight problems, dental care, cuts and grazes and breakages) need medical and nursing attention from the point of view of prevention and general health care as well as treatment;
(c) some psychiatric problems present with physical consequences : e.g. anorexia, self-neglect or injury, paralyses;
(d) some physical problems present with psychiatric symptoms : e.g disorders of the central nervous and endocrine systems, and infectious and toxic states;
(e) some problems are maintained by the interaction of psychological and physical causes, e.g. poorly controlled diabetes, asthma and some gastro-intestinal disorders, or have both physical and psycho-social consequences, e.g. epilepsy.

A survey of the physical problems encountered in an adolescent psychiatric unit (Steinberg *et al.*, 1988) has shown a high incidence of conditions in all these categories, and included a number of conditions (such as a non-functioning kidney, hypertension, urinary tract infection and a mole needing removal) not apparently related to the psychiatric problem, as well as several that were (such as thyrotoxicosis, intestinal obstruction, cerebral neurodegeneration, dehydration).

What is a psychosomatic disorder?

My own view is that the idea of there being a particular group of psychosomatic disorders is a concept that divides psyche and soma more than it unites them. It grew out of a growing realization of the interaction between psyche and soma in a number of conditions such as asthma or migraine, but an important and developing view of medicine is that there are psychological, social and physical facets to all medical problems and that their interaction needs to be understood from all points of view – in terms of prevention, aetiology, diagnosis, prognosis and treatment. This is the basis of 'whole person' or holistic medicine, and should be fundamental to good practice in medicine generally and in psychiatry in particular.

Thus, any disorder can be usefully seen as psychosomatic, including bones broken in motor cycle accidents (one of the more common adolescent physical problems), lung cancer and schizophrenia. However, in some conditions in some people the physical and the psychological factors (as causes, as consequences or as treatment) are particularly prominent as special problems, and some examples of these clinical situations are considered here.

Is it physical?

One of the most difficult problems for the clinician is the suspicion that an apparently psychological condition may have a definite physical cause. Psychiatric work with adolescents and their families can be very challenging and requires proceeding with authority and confidence. This may be difficult if the clinician has a nagging suspicion that (for example) weight loss, abdominal pains, headaches or poor concentration might be due to undiagnosed physical illness. The mythology of clinical psychiatry is full of two sorts of cautionary tale : the psychiatrist who is shown to have been treating a brain tumour by psychotherapy; and the psychiatrist who diagnoses the physical illness that the referring general physician missed. Neither story is reassuring.

One answer, as implied by some general psychiatric teaching, is for 'every' patient to have a full physical examination. But this seemingly tidy solution does not stand up to scrutiny. What is the place of a physical examination when a misbehaving or school-refusing adolescent and his family are seen? Moreover, many of the physical problems relevant to child and adolescent psychiatry are not identifiable by a single thorough check-up by a general physician, after which the psychiatrist can safely take over. A developmental, longitudinal view is

needed, as in the cases reported by Rivinus *et al.* (1975) and Corbett *et al.*
(1977), where the presence of neurological disease emerged later in
young people who had had entirely psychological symptoms and signs
at the start.

Example 16
Teresa is fourteen, and is at a special school for mildly mentally retarded
children – her IQ is in the high 60s. (According to the old terminology she
would have been regarded as 'ESN' – educationally subnormal.)

She is admitted to an adolescent unit from a general hospital ward where she
has been thoroughly investigated for weight loss, with no physical abnormality
found. She is increasingly withdrawn and nearly mute. She has amenorrhoea.
At the psychiatric unit her mental state is hard to assess, but what she says
reveals no more than that she is anxious and withdrawn, curling away from
the interviewer with a hand held half over her face. Psychological testing is
impracticable. Physical examination reveals no abnormality. The initial differential diagnosis includes depression in an immature girl of relatively low
intellectual ability, hysteria, schizophrenia and anorexia nervosa. Because she
is (a) very unwell and (b) a puzzle she has a CT (computer tomography) scan,
which shows slight degenerative changes and enlarged ventricles. Her past
history is carefully sifted for evidence of progressive intellectual deterioration,
but by all accounts she was functioning at much the same rather poor level,
intellectually and socially, since infancy. She begins to eat, returns to normal
weight, her periods start again and she begins to respond to the unit's social and
educational programme, although she says very little. A repeated CT scan then
reveals further loss of cerebral tissue. The diagnosis is clearly one of the
progressive neurodegenerative disorders, and further investigations for these
are begun.

A very large number of neurodegenerative disorders have been
described. They are rare, and most are at present incurable (Wilson's
disease is an important exception). Their investigation is complex, and
best undertaken in close collaboration with a special centre experienced
in paediatric neurology, not least because the classification and investigation of these disorders is a growing point of research.

Four important examples are hepatolenticular degeneration (Wilson's disease); Huntington's chorea; metachromatic leucodystrophy;
and Addison-Schilder's disease.

Hepatolenticular degeneration (Wilson's disease)
In hepatolenticular degeneration, a disorder of copper metabolism
probably inherited as an autosomal recessive disorder, copper is
deposited in the liver, basal ganglia of the brain and elsewhere. 40 per
cent present with liver dysfunction, 40 per cent with neurological

symptoms and signs (tremor, rigidity, athetosis, dystonia, flapping tremor at the wrists, lack of facial expression, and sometimes fits); and 40 per cent with psychiatric disorder, including school phobia and behaviour problems, (Scheinberg, 1968; Walker, 1969; Bearn, 1972). Depressive, hypomanic and schizophrenic presentations have also been reported (see review by Lishman, 1978). The disorder is one that fluctuates and remits, but death can follow in a few years if the condition is untreated, with the outlook worse the younger the age of onset. Investigation shows a low blood level of the caeruloplasmin, and increased levels of copper in the urine. A brown colouration is seen on slit-lamp examination of the corneal margin, the Kayser-Fleischer ring. Penicillamine, a very toxic drug, can be successful in treatment of the disorder.

Huntington's chorea

Huntington's chorea is inherited as an autosomal dominant disorder with a virtually 100 per cent rate of manifestation. This means that half the offspring of an affected person can be expected to develop the disorder, with the age of onset being usually between 25 and 50, although it can begin in childhood and adolescence. Males and females are equally affected. It may begin with psychiatric symptoms including personality changes, paranoid and depressive symptoms and suicidal acts and schizophrenic symptoms. Physical signs include clumsiness, fidgetiness, dysarthria, facial grimacing and later gross choreiform movement. Global intellectual deterioration develops insidiously. The presentation in children is particularly marked by clumsiness, ataxia, fits and intellectual deterioration. The disorder usually appears after the patient's children have been born, and the emotional, family, marital and ethical problems are severe (Oliver, 1970; Thomas, 1982). In a helpful paper, Martindale and Bottomley (1980) discuss the problems and the possibilities of counselling and other assistance. In particular, the emerging possibilities of predicting the disorder by special investigations has been described by Quinn and Marsden (1984) as 'an ethical minefield'.

Metachromatic leucodystrophy

Metachromatic leucodystrophy is a rare cause of a progressive dementia which can appear after several years of normal development (Corbett *et al.*, 1977). Investigations show metachromatic material in the urine, abnormal arylsulphatase A activity in urine and leucocytes, dilated ventricles on CT scanning, diffuse slow wave activity on EEG, and marked slowing in peripheral nerve conduction.

Addison-Schilder's disease

Addison-Schilder's disease (X-linked adrenoleucodystrophy) is rare, can present with psychiatric symptoms and progressive intellectual deterioration, and there is abnormal adrenalcortical functioning.

The investigation of these disorders is complex and as already mentioned should be undertaken jointly with a specialist centre. Electroencephalographic, electromyographic, biochemical and biopsy methods of investigation are available, but brain biopsy is risky, often unhelpful and is being superseded by other methods. For further reading in this and related areas see Wilson (1972); Brett and Lake (1975); Bolthauser and Wilson (1976); Neville (1979); and Brett 1983).

The general approach to take in these uncertain conditions is to treat current handicaps and work with the patient and family while repeating psychometric investigation and physical investigations at the intervals advised by psychology and neurology colleagues. The work with the family inevitably has to focus on anxiety, uncertainty, loss and fear of loss. Even when deterioration does not lead to death, the changes in the patient represents an experience of severe loss to the parents and siblings, and often such feelings are present in the affected patient too. The eventual transfer of a child who has been the object of a great deal of attention to a long-stay hospital where facilities may well be far poorer is another blow. If the child can be so helped with his or her self-care and behaviour to an extent which makes possible a transfer to a therapeutic community of the Rudolf Steiner sort, this represents some comfort in a sad situation.

Is it psychological?

The physical consequences of psychological functioning may be seen in, for example, anorexia nervosa and obesity (Chapter 12) and hysteria (Chapter 7). Failure to thrive in young children, failure to grow in older children, and delayed puberty in young teenagers have variously been ascribed to psychological and physical causes. Growth hormone deficiency has been found in some young people, and it has been suggested that severe emotional deprivation can produce hypopituitarism and growth retardation (Powell *et al.*, 1967), although dietary insufficiency seems the more likely mediating factor (Rutter, 1981). Small boys with delayed puberty may be seen who eat little, stubbornly resist food, and in many ways present the picture of anorexia nervosa (Chapter 12).

Psychological problems of physical illness

One of the commonest reasons for the admission of adolescents to hospital is road accidents (the other being attempted suicide), and *head injury* and its sequaelae are increasingly serious problems among older children, adolescents and young adults (McCabe and Green, 1987). The latter report describes the serious effects on adolescents' behaviour, mood and self-esteem, and suggests approaches to rehabilitative work with the adolescent and the family.

The management of *diabetes mellitus* in adolescence can be problematic, with rebelliousness about diet, medication and the monitoring of urine causing difficulty and danger (Tattersall and Lowe, 1981). The need for a combination of medical supervision and self-care can feed into the adolescent's mixed feelings about being independent of adults, and when things go wrong the young person's parents are unsure how protective and intrusive to be. In the most worrying situations an angry adolescent, depressed about the illness and dependence on medication, and angry because the parents feel they can 'do nothing right', may resort to neglect of the illness and dangerous misuse of insulin. From the available evidence it should not be assumed that the problems encountered in managing diabetes in adolescents are necessarily primarily psychological or primarily technical. Both factors may well be operating, and the range of types of psychological problem is wide (Gale and Tattersall, 1979; Tattersall, 1981). Taylor (1985), in reviewing the problem, points out that sporadic referral of difficult cases from paediatrician to psychiatrist is likely to prove a poor basis for effective collaborative work, and more regular liaison, e.g. in joint clinics, might be more helpful.

Epilepsy is a condition that causes much anxiety and misunderstanding, and there have been some changes in the terminology used in recent years. Anyone may have a fit, or seizure, if the stimulus is strong enough (as when ECT is given, when an abnormal electric discharge of brain cells is provoked). Some people have a low epileptic or convulsive threshold, i.e. their brain cells readily discharge in this abnormal way for relatively minor reasons, while in others seizures are an indication of major brain disorder. Epilepsy is now categorized into generalized (involving both sides of the brain) and partial seizures. *Generalized seizures* may be:

- tonic-clonic (major fits, or 'grand mal');
- myoclonic (muscle jerks);
- absences (petit mal).

Partial seizures involve only part of the brain, and are subdivided into:

- simple (focal) motor or sensory fits;
- complex, in which there may be complicated sensory or emotional experiences or behaviour.

The associations between epilepsy and emotional and behavioural problems in childhood and adolescence are complicated. There are likely to be: parental anxiety and distress; the adolescent's fears about the disorder and its effect on his self-image and self-esteem; the cerebral effects of the fits (e.g. bizarre experiences or mood changes); the effects on intellectual functioning, for example, of any brain damage associated with the epilepsy; and not least the effect of anticonvulsant medication on cognitive functioning and behaviour. The importance of these quite different effects will, of course, vary from one young person's case to another's.

In general, there is a high incidence of behaviour problems among children and adolescents with epilepsy. In the Isle of Wight study (Rutter *et al.*, 1970) there was a prevalence of epilepsy of 7.2 per thousand among 5- to 14-year-olds, with the incidence of psychiatric disorders (largely mood and behaviour problems) varying from just under 30 per cent to just under 60 per cent depending on the type of epilepsy, with the lower incidence when the epilepsy was of uncomplicated idiopathic (i.e. no obvious cause) in type. A number of studies have drawn attention to the adverse effects of anticonvulsant drugs on children's behaviour (Stores, 1975, 1978) and cognitive performance (Corbett *et al.*, 1985). There have been a number of studies suggesting an association between the type of epilepsy and psychiatric disorder, and particularly between aggressive behaviour and epilepsy originating in the temporal lobe. In his review, Shaffer (1985) concludes that the strongest link between epilepsy and psychiatric disorder, at least in physical terms, is through the presence of brain damage and its severity. The relationship between temporal lobe epilepsy and psychiatric disorder appears complex, and Taylor (1981, 1985) discusses the importance of taking into consideration not only the fact of temporal lobe involvement but the side affected, the time the disorder began, and the sex of the patient. Taylor (1985) also points out the importance of parent-child relationships in the emergence of individual and family problems, quite apart from any precise neurological relationships there may be with mood and behaviour. Aspects of the investigation and managment of epilepsy in schoolchildren is discussed in Ross and Reynolds (1985).

Cystic fibrosis is an inherited disorder occurring in 1-2 per 2000 births, and seriously affects the glands of the gastrointestinal tract and the pancreas, liver and lungs. It is a serious and life-threatening illness but can be helped by complicated and demanding treatment which involves diet, physiotherapy and antibiotics and frequent admissions to hospital. Sexual development may be delayed, pregnancy full of risk and male patients may be sterile. Many studies have described the distress and lowered self-esteem this chronic condition and its treatment cause, especially in the adolescent years (Kellerman *et al.*, 1980; Zeltzer *et al.*, 1980).

Asthma has been regarded as a classic example of a psychosomatic disorder, but although emotional states can play a part in the precipitation of attacks, several studies have shown that the rate of psychiatric problems in asthmatic children is no higher than among those with other physical disorders (Graham *et al.*, 1967). Help with the emotional states that can precipitate asthmatic attacks, particularly when focussed on family anxiety, which may be very high (Lask and Matthew, 1979) can be valuable. Anxiety and misunderstanding may lead to the overuse and misuse of inhaled bronchodilators. It is important to check that the boy or girl knows how to use properly the one prescribed.

Taylor (1985) has helpfully reviewed the problems of *blindness* and *deafness* in young people, pointing out the deficiencies in the research conducted so far, and the need to consider separately children with more than one handicap. In a study that attempted to deal with several of the common methodological problems, Freeman *et al.*, (1975) showed the relatively high incidence (23 percent) of psychological problems among deaf children, with a particularly heavy burden on mothers which might be reduced if help on a family basis were available.

Blind children appear to manage better educationally than deaf children, but Fraiberg (1977) has shown the ways in which blindness from birth affects the proper development of other capacities and skills, e.g. attachment to parents and the handling of objects.

In general, the earlier the onset of deafness or blindness, and the more that it is associated with other individual and family problems, the greater the degree of handicap.

Physical problems in psychiatric practice : notes on management

(i)   Do not jump to conclusions about the psychological or physical origins of a disorder, because the inter-relationships between physical health, mental state and family are likely to be complex.

Thus highly anxious parents may be appropriately so, and competent physical treatment may be the most important need.

(ii)   Chronic, worrying conditions such as asthma or epilepsy can generate understandable and strongly mixed feelings in parents. These may include anger with the unwell child which the parents feel but which puzzles and distresses them, or they may deny it; an angry dependence on the medical and nursing professions, in whose hands they may have had painful and sometimes horrendous experiences; and confused feelings about how much they, the professionals or the adolescent are responsible for the latter's health care. These feelings need understanding and patience on the part of the clinician; the more he or she tackles them the more accumulated bitterness and distress may be felt in return, but in the long run this often leads to constructive work being done.

(iii) Make sure you know what physical disorder you are dealing with, and can handle it. Don't hesitate to ask for advice from other medical colleagues, and you will learn a lot by collaboration with them (and so may they). Psychiatrists are often shy about their general medical skills, sometimes with good reason; remember that even a brain surgeon may not know the latest about many medical conditions.

(iv) As with other complex psychiatric conditions, diagnosis alone is not a sufficient guide to management. Clarify the specific worries, handicaps and problems being experienced by adolescent and family, organize what can be done for each, and monitor progress. Helpful information and commonsense advice may turn out to be missing even when a patient is under the care of a distinguished centre. Counselling and advice about living with and managing a handicap can be invaluable not only for practical reasons but in terms of self-esteem. Some people find self-help groups valuable, and it is worth knowing about them.

(v)   While part of the task is to help the patient face his problems honestly, it is also important to remind him of what he *can* do too. Do not guess which ambitions (those which are frustrated and those which are still feasible) are the most important. The patient's priorities in these respects may be surprisingly different from your own.

(vi) One assumption that may be made, however, unless demonstrated otherwise, is that chronically unwell or disabled adolescents have painfully mixed feelings about their future independence, both wanting to look ahead to living their own lives but not being sure that they will manage it. Parents commonly have corresponding anxieties. These fears can become self-perpetuating in individuals or in families even when, at a rational level, problems are being coped with. In such situations, individual or family therapy may be helpful.

References and further reading

Bearn, A. (1972) Wilson's Disease. *In* Stanbury, J., Wyngaarden, J. and Frederickson, D. (Eds), *The Metabolic Basis of Inherited Disease.* New York: McGraw Hill.

Bolthauser, E. and Wilson, J. (1976) Value of brain biopsy in neurode-generative disease in childhood. *Archives of Disease in Childhood* **51**, 264–8.

Brett, E. (1983) Ed), *Paediatric Neurology.* London: Churchill Livingstone.

Brett, E. and Lake, B. (1975) Reassessment of rectal approach to neuropathology in children. Review of 307 biopsies over 11 years. *Archives of Disease in Childhood* **50**, 753–62.

Corbett, J., Harris, R., Taylor, E. and Trimble, M. (1977) Progressive disintegrative psychosis of childhood. *Journal of Child Psychology and Psychiatry* **18**, 211–19.

Corbett, J., Trimble, M. and Nichol, T. (1985) Behavioural and cognitive impairments in children with epilepsy : the long-term effects of anticonvulsant therapy. *Journal of the American Academy of Child Psychiatry* **24**, 1, 17–23.

Denmark, J., Rodda, M., Abel, R., Skelton, U., Eldridge, R., Warren, F. and Gordon, A. (1979) *A Word in Deaf Ears – A Study of Communication and Behaviour in a Sample of 75 Deaf Adolescents.* London: Royal National Institute for the Deaf.

Fraiberg, S. (1977) *Insights From the Blind.* New York: Basic Books.

Freeman, R., Malkin, S. and Hastings, J. (1975) Psychosocial problems of deaf children and their families : a comparative study. *American Annals of Deafness* **120**, 391–405.

Gale, E. and Tattersall, R. (1979) Brittle diabetes. *British Journal of Hospital Medicine* **22**, 589–96.

Graham, P., Rutter, M., Yule, W. and Pless, I. (1967) Childhood asthma : a psychosomatic disorder? Some epidemiological considerations. *British Journal of Preventive and Social Medicine* **21**, 78–85.

Kellerman, J., Zeltzer, L., Ellenberg, L., Dash, J. and Rigler, D. (1980) Psychological effects of illness in adolescence. I : Anxiety, self-esteem and perception of control. *Journal of Paediatrics* **97**, 126–31.

Lask, B. and Matthew, D. (1979) Childhood asthma – a controlled trial of family psychotherapy. *Archives of Disease in Childhood* **54**, 116–19.

Lishman, A. (1978) *Organic Psychiatry. The Psychological Consequences of Cerebral Disorder*. Oxford: Blackwell Scientific Publications.

McCabe, R. and Green, D. (1987) Rehabilitating severely head-injured adolescents : three case reports. *Journal of Child Psychology and Psychiatry* **28**, 111–26.

Martindale, B. and Bottomley, V. (1980) The management of families with Huntington's Chorea : a case study to illustrate some recommendations. *Journal of Child Psychology and Psychiatry* **21**, 343–51.

Neville, B. (1979) Progressive and static pathology in paediatric neurology. *Medicine* **33**, 1698–701.

Oliver, J. (1970) Huntington's Chorea in Northamptonshire. *British Journal of Psychiatry* **116**, 241–53.

Powell, G., Bradel, J. and Blizzard, R. (1967) Emotional deprivation and growth retardation simulating idiopathic hypopituitarism. I. Clinical evaluation of the syndrome. *New England Journal of Medicine* **276**, 1271–8.

Quinn, N. and Marsden, D. (1984) Movement disorders 2: Chorea, tic and myoclonus. *Hospital Update* September, 750–7.

Rivinus, T., Jamison, D. and Graham, P. (1975) Childhood organic disease presenting as psychiatric disorder. *Archives of Disease in Childhood* **50**, 115–19.

Ross, E. and Reynolds, E. (1985) *Paediatric Perspectives on Epilepsy*. Chichester: John Wiley and Sons.

Rutter, M. (1981) *Maternal Deprivation Reassessed*. Harmondsworth: Penguin Books.

Scheinberg, I., Sternlieb, I. and Richman, J. (1968) Psychiatric manifestations in patients with Wilson's disease. *In* Bergsma, D. (Ed), *Wilson's Disease*. New York: The National Foundation.

Steinberg, D., Bailey, T. and Simanoff, E. (1988) Physical disorders among adolescent psychiatric in-patients. In preparation.

Stores, G. (1975) Behavioural effects of anti-epileptic drugs. *Developmental Medicine and Child Neurology* **17**, 647–58.

Stores, G. (1978) Anticonvulsants. *In* Werry, J. (Ed), *Paediatric Psychopharmacology : The Use of Behaviour-Modifying Drugs in Children*. New York: Brunner Mazel.

Tattersall, R. (1981) Psychiatric aspects of diabetes – a physician's view. *British Journal of Psychiatry* **139**, 485–93.

Tattersall, R. and Lowe, J. (1981) Diabetes and adolescence. *Diabetologia* **20**, 517–23.

Taylor, D. (1981) Brain lesions, surgery, seizures and mental symptoms. *In* Reynolds, E. and Trimble, M. (Eds), *Epilepsy and Psychiatry*, pp 227–41. Edinburgh: Churchill Livingstone.

Taylor, D. (1985) Psychological aspects of chronic sickness. *In* Rutter, M.

and Hersov, L. (Eds), *Child and Adolescent Psychiatry : Modern Approaches*, pp 614–24. Oxford: Blackwell Scientific Publications.

Thomas, S. (1982) Ethics of a predictive test for Huntington's Chorea. *British Medical Journal* **284**, 1383–5.

Walker, S. (1969) The psychiatric presentation of Wilson's disease (hepatolenticular degeneration) with an etiologic explanation. *Behavioural Neuropsychiatry* **1**, 38–48.

Wilson, J. (1972) Investigation of degenerative disease of the central nervous system. *Archives of Disease in Childhood* **74**, 163–70.

Zeltzer, L., Kellerman, J., Ellenberg, L., Dash, J. and Rigler, D. (1980) Psychological effects of illness in adolescents. II Impact of illness in adolescents – crucial issues and coping styles. *Journal of Pediatrics* **97**, 132–8.

Chapter 18

An Outline of Management

Introduction

The task in adolescent psychiatry is to treat disorder and encourage normal development. The education of young people is a further step: its aim, more ambitious than normal development alone, is to draw out (Latin – *educare*) the boy's or girl's potential for a full cultural life.

Management in adolescent psychiatry therefore has two components: the clinical treatment of individual disorder, and working with other people in the care, upbringing and education of adolescents.

The other people involved will usually be the rest of the adolescent's family, and sometimes the teachers at school. In a residential setting such as a children's home, psychiatric unit or therapeutic community a significant part of the care and education will be in the hands of those who maintain the educational and social milieu there.

Management in adolescent psychiatry therefore includes the following areas of work:

- Individual clinical treatments.
- Family work and family therapy.
- The maintenance of settings so that they allow therapeutic change to take place and facilitate care, up-bringing and education.
- Working with other people, including collaborative and consultative work and training.

Except in work with older adolescents, which can certainly proceed entirely on a private basis between clinician and patient as in adult psychiatry, there are almost always other people involved to a degree, and wider considerations than treatment alone. This means that management must be planned with other people – those who have a legal and ethical right to involvement, and those whose skills will be needed. Beginning any form of intervention in adolescent psychiatry requires that this be acknowledged.

Guide to the chapter

This chapter considers management under the following headings:

 (1) Beginning work
 (2) Emergency intervention
 (3) Individual psychotherapy and counselling
 (4) Creative and activity and experiential therapies
 (5) Family work and family therapy
 (6) Medication
 (7) Other physical treatment: health care, diet and ECT
 (8) Behavioural treatments
 (9) Group work and social therapy
(10) Special education
(11) Writing letters and reports
(12) Monitoring progress
(13) Admission to hospital and other residential care
(14) The therapeutic setting
(15) Collaborative and liaison work and teamwork
(16) Consultative work

(1) Beginning work

In Chapter 5, on assessment, the point was made that problems tend to be multiple, hence the key question 'who is concerned about what, and why?'. There is a corresponding question for management: who are the key people needed for the two broad aspects of work (treatment on the one hand, care and education on the other), and what agreements and permissions are needed to proceed?

Authority to proceed is crucial if effective work is to be sustained with problems which may be complex and difficult and with a patient and family who may be ambivalent. The agreement to accept intervention may be the adolescent's own, or it may be a family decision. But there is no point in trying to help with, say, a young person with conduct problems when there is disagreement about the need for help on the part of those whose co-operation is needed:

Example 17
A psychiatrist agrees to see as an emergency a misbehaving boy of fourteen who, the family doctor says, won't go to school and is driving his mother to distraction. The GP asks if urgent admission could be considered. On examination the psychiatrist finds a sullen boy who says he will do as he likes and wants nothing to do with psychiatrists, and in any case is in a hurry because he has to meet some friends in half an hour. His mother is distraught and depressed. The boy's father hasn't come along, partly because he is busy at work, but mainly because he says 'there's nothing wrong with the boy'. It seems he is very strict with his son, while his wife constantly tries to placate him. The boy is anxious to end the session and makes it clear he won't come again. When the boy's mother is asked if she will bring him again but this time with her husband too, she gazes miserably at her son, who is already standing at the door, and says she cannot guarantee that either will come. 'I'm going', says the boy. Slam.

There is no chance of beginning to help in this situation without the parents' insistence that the boy accepts intervention and without their playing a full part in his management, unless the situation is so bad for the boy, the family or everyone that a Care Order is justified. Non-attendance at school can be a reason for seeking a Care Order. If the boy were sixteen the decision to accept or reject psychiatric intervention would be his. He could accept medical authority informally, as people often will choose to accept a professional's or expert's recommendation. Or, if he were seriously mentally ill and his or other people's health or safety were at risk, he could be compulsorily treated under the Mental Health Act 1983. Permission to proceed will therefore require one or all of the following forms of authority:

- The patient's own understanding and agreement: preferable at any age, essential at age 16 plus.
- The parents' clear authority and support, preferable at any age, essential if the patient is under 16 years old.
- Informal medical authority – i.e. acceptance of the recommendation of the psychiatrist as a trusted professional worker.
- Formal medical authority, on the infrequent occasions that a Section of the Mental Health Act is needed.
- The authority of a Care Order, when justified because a boy or girl is beyond parental care and control or whose normal development is being avoidably impaired. Occasionally Guardianship or Wardship proceedings may be appropriate alternatives.

Issues of authority in the care of adolescents, and the importance of distinguishing between treatment, care, control and other issues, are discussed in Bruggen *et al.*, (1973), Lampen (1978), Bruggen (1979), and Steinberg (1981, 1982, 1983).

Agreement to proceed requires clarity on the part of the clinician about what he is proposing, and understanding on the part of the adolescent and family. It is important that they understand what they are accepting, rejecting or negotiating, whether it is a series of family meetings, the prescription of a drug or admission to hospital. Consent has to be informed consent to have any legal, ethical, or therapeutic meaning. It is important to be straightforward. Suppose an acutely psychotic child is being admitted to hospital, and distressed parents have very reluctantly agreed to the child receiving medication; if the psychiatrist thinks an injection against the child's will is likely to be needed too, the matter should not be avoided or fudged but discussed honestly and sympathetically with the parents. Such questions, very likely already in everyone's mind, should not be skirted around in order to spare the clinician's feelings.

The examples given are fairly vivid ones, but the same applies to less dramatic issues. If family meetings are proposed, make sure that everyone knows what is meant by 'the family'. It may or may not include a grandparent who lives upstairs, or an elder brother or sister who is involved in exams.

It is notoriously easy for agreements to get blurred and for management to suffer accordingly. In a particular adolescent's case the clinician may have decided that to help an anxious girl gain confidence it is necessary to help the parents modify their approach to her, and to understand that she is lacking in confidence and self-esteem but not ill. This appears to be agreed by the rather compliant parents at the first meeting. Yet after several sessions have passed without progress it becomes clear that while the overt agreement is that the parents should be taking an active part in the work, the basic assumption that persists is that the girl is 'mental' and it is up to the psychiatrist to 'do something'. 'Isn't there a pill you can give her?'

The psychiatrist should explain his understanding of the nature of the problem and the management needed and check what the adolescent and parents understand. This can usefully lead to agreeing clear methods and goals. In some cases a written contract is useful. This is a statement of who is going to do what, which can be a focus for discussion at a meeting in the near future when progress can be reviewed. It can be useful to fix the date for such a review meeting as part of the plans made at the first interview.

It is important to think ahead. Is the adolescent going to reach the age of sixteen in the near future? This will affect questions of permission. If the help of another agency or department is going to be needed (e.g.

finding the adolescent a different school) is it clear what procedures will
have to be followed and what the time scale will be? Is it clear who will
be responsible for what at different stages? Medical authority may be
appropriate at the beginning, e.g. if a seriously unwell young patient
with anorexia is (on medical advice) being admitted to hospital, but it
may be crucial for a successful discharge not to unwittingly undermine
parental authority and competence. Thus it can be important to make it
clear from the start that (a) the parents' authority is by no means any
the less for deciding to call upon professional help; and (b) when the
acute emergency has passed they will be involved in taking over an
increasing part of the work of ensuring adequate nutrition for their
daughter.

The sharing out of different aspects of the work according to the
ability, skills and responsibilities of those involved is described elsewhere as a consultative-diagnostic approach (Steinberg, 1983) because
it depends upon two things: the disorder (if any) in clinical terms that
the psychiatrist is trained to recognize, and the problems in other
people's terms that the clinical worker can help them clarify for
themselves. 'Other people's terms' might be, for example, the family's
way of coming to a commonsense appreciation of all or part of the
adolescent's problem; a paediatrician confirming the part he and his
department can still play in a diabetic boy's care; or teachers in a school
being helped to differentiate between conduct disorder and simple
misbehaviour (Steinberg, 1986c).

(2) Emergency intervention

The commonest causes of a request for immediate intervention in
adolescent psychiatry, in approximate order of frequency, are:

(a) Adult (parent or professional) anxiety about a further episode of
    disturbed behaviour such as abusiveness or aggressiveness or other
    lack of control against a background of several years of similar
    behaviour.
(b) Similar concern about similar young people, with the additional
    problem of real or threatened self-injury.
(c) An adolescent whose disorder is not acute, but who is 'in the wrong
    place', (e.g. who has taken an overdose and is in a general medical
    bed or an adult psychiatric bed) and the staff have an urgent
    'disposal' problem; or, staff (e.g. in a children's home) who feel they
    can probably manage a difficult young person, but who are unsure
    about the skills required and the responsibilities involved.

(d) The sudden emergence of adult alarm about a disorder which continues gradually to worsen, e.g. further weight loss in a girl or boy with anorexia nervosa.

(e) Suicidal or self-injurious acts or threats with a more recent history, with or without overt evidence of severe depression.

(f) Acute psychosis (manic, depressive or schizophrenic) or severe distress and incapacity of uncertain origin.

It will be clear from this list that the most common (and often most pressing) crisis involves sudden adult concern about a relatively long-standing problem, often of control rather than illness; while the least common emergency is acute individual illness in the adolescent, needing urgent individual treatment. These important considerations affect the way emergencies in adolescent psychiatry are handled.

The request may be for advice, for an urgent out-patient or domiciliary appointment, or for admission to hospital, or at least removal from the present scene. It is helpful for a clinician or team to have available the following general types of response:

(a) Most important, people and time available to discuss the problem (e.g. on the phone) in appropriate detail with the person making the referral, or with any other key person who is taking responsibilities about which he or she is anxious.

(b) Almost as important, the capacity to offer a very early appointment (same day or within a day or two) usually to the adolescent and family, but occasionally as an urgent consultative meeting with the key workers involved with the boy or girl.

(c) Relatively rarely, the availability of immediate admission to a psychiatric unit.

To provide (a) and especially (b) it is crucial for a clinic or unit to be staffed appropriately. An emergency will take time to sort out and resolve, no less than routine appointments, and any expectation that an emergency can somehow be 'squeezed in' to a full clinic, as if the problem could be clarified and dealt with like an acute appendix, is unrealistic. The only way to be able to provide a service that can deal with emergencies is to have the extra resources (i.e. staff time) needed to do so. The same applies to the option of one or two members of the clinical team being able to make urgent visits to the home.

In my experience (Steinberg *et al*. 1981; Steinberg 1982, 1986a) early admission to an adolescent psychiatric unit (e.g. within a few days) is only occasionally needed – for example, half a dozen times a year in a unit taking say 25-35 admissions per year; while immediate admission is indicated even less often. There are three important and different considerations to be borne in mind by anyone developing an adolescent service. First, requests for immediate admission far outnumber either the practical possibilities of admission, or its necessity. Second, adolescent units are not straightforward places to run, and it is crucial to be guided by what the current staff (and, for that matter, patients) can cope with, not by the availability of a 'bed'. Third, the common protestation that it is self-evidently wrong to admit a young person to an adult psychiatric unit in an emergency usually reflects, in my view, either the fact that the adolescent is not acutely mentally ill, or that the adult ward's staffing or resources is such that would make it less than ideal for people of any age. If an acutely ill adolescent needs immediate admission and there is no 'adolescent' place available, I believe that any humane and competent adult admission ward should be able to cope until an adolescent unit, offering a different type of service and necessarily differently organized, can take over.

Responding to emergencies, with the above points in mind, is not fundamentally different from the approach outlined in section 1, a system which can usually be considered and appropriate arrangements made, communication systems permitting, in little more time than it takes to read:

(a) Information: who knows what the problem is? Describe it.
(b) People: see the key people involved – the people in difficulties (usually but not invariably including the adolescent); and key people whom you will want to involve, e.g. the nurse in charge of the unit, or someone who can offer family crisis meetings or initiate action by the social services department.
(c) Identify what, if anything, needs immediate action, e.g. the safe holding of an acutely agitated and distressed young person, or a dose of a sedative.
(d) Having done so, create time and space for a calm appraisal by all concerned of who needs what and who is in a position to provide it. This is the most difficult and the most valuable step, and can convert most crises into problems that can be properly sorted out over a few days or weeks. The skills needed are partly consultative and partly those used in individual and family therapeutic work.
(e) Having helped the key people to extract manageable goals and pieces of work out of what looked like an incomprehensible mess, timetable what needs to be done, monitored and reviewed by when.

Many acute problems in adolescent psychiatry turn out to be crises of the supervision and control of a seriously misbehaving young person, often in circumstances where the adult anger generated is so strong that control becomes confused with punishment, hence the plea for the 'magic' of psychiatry which, it is supposed, will contain the adolescent more kindly. However, if family intervention cannot reassert the lost adult authority that is needed, it may be necessary to seek the help of the social services department. Sometimes a Care Order is needed.

Example 18
A sixteen-year-old girl in a children's home (her eighth 'placement' in as many years) is staying out late, believed to be working as a prostitute, returning to the children's home drunk, getting into fights, and becomes abusive and violent to the staff when they try to help her or control her. She won't talk to her social worker, refuses to see a counsellor, and will not attend a psychiatric clinic. Urgent admission to an adolescent unit is requested on the grounds that she is in need of 'deep psychotherapy'. However true this may be, there is likely to be little chance of the admission lasting 24 hours or any form of psychotherapy getting under way until the authority and control of the adults looking after her is first affirmed and asserted. Many such young people settle remarkably well when such control is asserted, become less distressed, and the usefulness as well as the feasibility of psychiatry or psychotherapy for that boy or girl then becomes more clearly seen.

It is important to acknowledge the anxiety and distress people feel, and indeed affirm their concern (e.g. about serious illness or other risk). It is important not to be remote or appear aloof from this. But at the same time remember that although panic-stricken people may hope that a calm and competent person will take over, sometimes there is also a perverse and only partially conscious impulse to recruit people to their ranks, including yourself, so that *everyone* can say how impossible 'it' is.

Emergencies in adolescent psychiatry are discussed elsewhere (Steinberg, 1987a, 1987c, 1983) and the literature on crisis intervention (e.g. Caplan, 1961; Bruggen *et al.*, 1973; Bancroft, 1979) is instructive.

(3) Individual psychotherapy and counselling

There are no entirely satisfactory definitions of psychotherapy. In their excellent introduction to the subject, Brown and Pedder (1979) distinguish between *general psychotherapy* (the support, encouragement, relief and advice which anyone might offer, and which is integral to good medical and other professional practice) and *special psychotherapy*, which they subdivide into dynamic psychotherapy and behavioural psychotherapy.

They also draw attention to Cawley's useful classification of four levels of psychotherapy (Cawley, 1977):

(1) *General psychotherapy, as above.*
(2) *General psychotherapy* augmented by understanding on the practitioner's part that current feelings and attitudes are influenced, often unconsciously, by past experiences and relationships, and that the reverberations of these past relationships may colour the relationship with the therapist; although this transference is generally not commented on.
(3) *Dynamic psychotherapy* proper in which the transference and the countertransference (i.e. the psychotherapist's feelings) are recognized and worked with.
(4) *Behavioural psychotherapy* which is concerned with the modification of behaviour. This may include complex social behaviour (e.g. the avoidance which is part of phobic disorders) or physical responses (e.g. the physiological aspects of panic attacks) but it does not concern itself with transference or suppositions about unconscious causes and motivation.

In this chapter behavioural psychotherapy is taken to be synonymous with behavioural therapy, and discussed later in section 8.

The term *counselling*, as used by Rogers (1951), refers to a form of psychotherapy in which the counsellor, or therapist, reflects back to the client what he or she is saying and seems to be feeling, thereby acting as a sounding board to aid reflection and the thinking through of issues. Counselling, thus described, can be used with particular objects in view, e.g. to reach personal conclusions about academic or career questions (e.g. Newsome *et al.*, 1975), in helping people with the self-management of every type of problem (general health, sexual, marital etc.) and in a far wider sense as part of the work of the clergy in helping the mentally ill to lead fuller lives in every way, including the spiritual (e.g. Foskett, 1984). It is clear from different accounts of counselling that, depending on the counsellor, it may amount to the giving of information and advice on the one hand, or become indistinguishable from some forms of psychotherapy on the other.

My own view of counselling, particularly in relation to adolescents, is that it differs in three main ways from dynamic psychotherapy: first, there is an agreed focus such as coming to terms with a handicap, or seeing oneself as a person who can make his or her own decisions; second, the 'to and fro' of conversation involves the counsellor being quite directive about the client thinking for himself or herself about practical issues ('what are you going to do then?'); third, while the client is encouraged to explore attitudes and make his or her own decisions, the counsellor also 'feeds' with ideas and information ('Are you going to have a look in the phone book for the Job Centre then? When? How will you know which one is nearest?'). And yet it is informed by an understanding of the unconscious and the unspoken in relationships. For example, a nurse may counsel an awkward and inhibited adolescent about his self-care and appearance, and will need to understand the feelings (on both sides) about being like a big brother or sister or parent to the boy or girl, in order to do enough but not too much. Counselling is an important general skill in work with adolescents, and incorporates Rogerian psychotherapy (Rogers, 1951), informal advice and informa-tion giving, and psychotherapeutic approaches of the sort described in levels (1) and (2) earlier.

Yet another approach to psychotherapy establishes a therapeutic relationship by using largely non-verbal creative and other activities. These *creative and activity therapies* are outlined in Section 4.

Another, *cognitive therapy*, works directly with the patient's thinking and attitudes and idea-related feelings (e.g. 'It's my fault that Dad left home') and facilitates the exploring of alternative views (e.g. see McAdam, 1986). It involves both behavioural approaches to thinking and the counselling end of the psychotherapeutic spectrum, again, like Cawley's level 2 described earlier.

Is it possible to conclude anything about psychotherapy from these very different approaches? In general, it is work in which the practitioner establishes with another person a relationship which provokes reappraisal, modification and sometimes radical change in the way that person thinks, feels and behaves. The 'provocation', the personal impact which promotes reappraisal, may be explicit and direct, or it may be a rather gradually developing process in which the emerging relationship between therapist and patient becomes the vehicle through which the patient becomes a different sort of person.

The latter, dynamic type of psychotherapy is gradual, subtle and complex and an example can only be given here in the form of a brief and over-simplified anecdote:

Example 19
In the course of psychotherapy, a depressed and anxious girl of seventeen shows a recurring pattern: gradual improvement over the course of one or two sessions, in which she becomes quite lively and animated, followed by a withdrawal into apprehension and gloom. The psychotherapist finds himself becoming increasingly annoyed by the way she slips back after apparently making real progress. In supervision he describes how she becomes more attractive company during the periods of improvement, and he finds himself

relaxing, chatting and not working with the same concentration as when she is depressed. The supervisor comments that when she is miserable the psychotherapist behaves like a concerned parent; when she improves, he behaves like a boyfriend. This echoes her history, in earlier childhood, of bickering parents threatening separation who would draw together when she was depressed, and drift apart, with her father taking her out, when she cheered up. Either way she was trapped: while depressed she was gratified and made to feel safe by her parents' joint concern for her; but as soon as she felt better and showed it they parted again, and her father would compete for her company, making her apprehensive and guilty. A pattern of alternating depression and flirtatiousness has marked her relationships with boyfriends, irritates them, and they drift away. The psychotherapist has a number of responses to consider, but one of them is to be more level with her, not be 'seduced' into jolly chats when she seems brighter, and to recognize the insecurity and apprehension behind her more extrovert phases.

In psychotherapy with adults the therapist might make more or less explicit interpretations from time to time, e.g. relating the young woman's behaviour in the sessions to her behaviour towards her father. Carefully chosen interpretations, offered at the right time, can be used in psychotherapy with adolescents, but experience is needed to make an appropriate comment at the right time and in a way that the young person can use. Younger adolescents, and many older adolescents with maturational problems, are likely to be uneasy in individual psychotherapy, feel easily threatened by the intimacy of the session and share with the struggling therapist the ups and downs of feeling sometimes treated like a child and sometimes like an adult. A series of anxiety-laden fantasies, some the product of experience and some the product of childish fantasy approach the surface like sea-monsters only to be submerged again by a variety of quite different evasions and defences. The psychotherapist sees an adolescent who is now breezy and confident, now despairing, now confiding, and now silent through most of the session and then marches out, slamming the door. Next time the psychotherapist is on the receiving end of a tirade of abuse about the uselessness of the sessions in general and the psychotherapist in particular; next time the patient has a comic at hand during the session but nevertheless uses the time well. Near the end the psychotherapist comments on the comic and the patient slams out again, and misses the next two appointments.

However, psychotherapy with adolescents is by no means necessarily stormy. Young people may also politely comply with other people's wishes and the psychiatrist's willingness that they be seen, and there may even be agreement about the nature of the problem; but a sense of focus and engagement in work can readily be lost, leaving therapist and adolescent wondering why they are meeting.

Example 20
Lesley, an eighteen year-old student in residence at university, has major problems in self- esteem. She has few friends and will only involve herself with other people (e.g. tutors, other students, clubs) when she has to. Nevertheless her social skills are quite adequate on such occasions, and she is not socially phobic. She is an adopted daughter and misses home; however, her inhibitions do not seem based on anxiety or depression, but rather on a long-standing dependence on her adoptive parents for motivation, friendship and even ideas. She is relatively unambitious; she does, reasonably competently, what she is asked to. Her teachers are concerned about how little she seems able to use her abilities and the college opportunities. She appreciates being seen by the college counsellor and attends the sessions conscientiously, but nothing seems to happen. The counsellor has been attentive and sympathetic, and more recently angry, but this doesn't shift Lesley's placid and inactive acceptance of the sessions. He proposes ending them, but she says she wants to continue. The counsellor, in some exasperation, points out that although he would like to help, the reason for their meeting remains a complete mystery to him. It is only when this 'mystery' becomes a focus of work, instead of a peripheral hindrance, that useful work begins.

The adolescent psychotherapist has to be adaptable to the varying maturity of his clientele, the very different coping and defensive strategies they employ, and the different levels at which the work needs to be done. For different patients, and at different times with the same patient, he may need to be directive and talkative, or an accepting listener; he may need to tell the adolescent what to do (e.g. behave reasonably) or take a tangential approach to advice ('How do you expect people to react if you carry on like that?'). There are times to tolerate the adolescent's awkwardness or abusiveness and times when he should get annoyed. Sometimes criticism or praise is out of place, and sometimes it is a mistake not to offer it. The therapeutic balance lies somewhere between being yourself as a friendly and mature adult, and being alert to the technicalities of what seems to be going on and how one ought to respond.

In my view three things should guide the relatively inexperienced psychotherapist or counsellor working with adolescents. First, it is almost always a mistake to try to move too far in the adolescent's direction, adopting, or affecting to adopt, adolescent style, jargon and interests; the adolescent wants an adult, if necessary a bit boring and not too far from the stereotype 'grown up', but at least a man or woman who appears not to mind being thirty or forty or whatever. (I say 'almost always' because some younger professionals are genuinely a little 'adolescent' while not losing their competence, and can carry it off successfully.)

Second, the obverse of the above advice, is not to go too far in the other direction. The anxiety generated by some adolescents can make people fall back on where they feel safer, and in some this may be their background in early elementary psychotherapy, e.g. to listen a lot and say little, and to feed back questions with such comments as 'I wonder why you ask?' and other such professional manoeuvres. Similarly, the sudden grasp of what's going on in a baffling situation can lead the therapist to leap prematurely to sharing his exciting discovery with the patient, and even worse to do so in a jargon-laden speech: 'What you're trying to say is that your mother and father have undermined you when they should have been caring, and you've been deprived of the experience of parents acting in a meaningful role towards you.' Such things are said.

Third, supervision is important. Senior psychotherapists are in short supply and if regular, systematic supervision isn't possible, it is particularly important (a) to limit expectations of what can be done, within the broad spectrum of counselling- psychotherapy described above, and (b) to arrange some forum with a more experienced colleague, or a consultative group, where you can think through what is going on with the help of someone who is not so closely involved. In this context it is worth warning of the risks of starting out with relatively unambitious counselling and being pulled unwittingly into a close relationship.

You should always begin psychotherapeutic work with some ground rules about where and when to meet, how to respond if the patient doesn't attend, what the broad aims of the work will be, what sort of approach in general terms you are going to take, and when you are going to stop to review progress.

Wilson (1986), in an informal account of individual psychotherapy in a residential setting, draws attention to the problems encountered when the psychotherapeutic relationship is one among several other relationships (e.g. with nurses, with teachers, with the psychiatrist, with the family and perhaps a family therapist). In such circumstances not everything in the psychotherapy session can be totally confidential (e.g. a threat of suicide), and the adolescent would know he was being treated dishonestly if people pretended it was; yet within this understanding it is possible to define areas of conversation where privacy will be preserved. He also suggests that one should not take too narrow a perspective of who is or is not 'suitable' for psychotherapy:

'I don't claim its total effectiveness in all cases; nor that it should be applied indiscriminately. But I do see it as a very civilized, humane service offered to another human being. Whatever the diagnosis, however disturbed and chaotic some young people are, one assumes there is some rhyme and reason to their mental lives. Psychotherapy, coming out of psychoanalysis, is essentially to do with meaning; trying to construct some sense about a person's behaviour and thoughts. It is something offered to another person, an opportunity, patiently provided, to find some sort of account of himself.' (Wilson, 1986).

I have not seen a comprehensive account of psychotherapy with adolescents that I could unreservedly recommend. Newsome *et al.* (1975) provide an excellent account of student counselling, and Kessler (1979) provides a good, short account of some of the issues and in particular of the style of the therapist, with appropriate warnings. Masterson and Costello (1980) and Adams (1973), although discussing the special situations of borderline and obsessional patients respectively, nevertheless make some valuable points about psychotherapeutic work with adolescents generally. Brown and Pedder (1979) has already been mentioned as a good introduction to psychotherapy generally, as are Malan (1963), Bloch (1986) and Garfield (1980). A systematic and more academic overview is to be found in Wilson and Hersov (1985).

There are many individual approaches, but there are common themes throughout. A good way to be in a position to perceive them and use them is to be familiar with some of the classical psychodynamic writing, among which, in my view, Freud, A. (1966) and Winnicott (1971) are outstanding.

(4) Creative, activity and experiential therapies

Adolescents who find it difficult to use conversation as therapy sometimes seem to find activities such as art, drama and games helpful, and to achieve through them therapeutic goals. This is the basis of play therapy in younger children, where, for example, a small boy or girl expresses through play with the doll's house some anxieties in the home. However, it would be a mistake to suppose that these creative therapies are no more than a vehicle for people who cannot express their feelings in sophisticated words.

The creative and activity therapies are certainly helpful in this respect, but they go well beyond this. The assumption in using such activities is that they not only enable the expression of attitudes and feelings that are difficult or impossible to put into words, but also make possible the discovery of attitudes and feelings of which the individual or the group were not fully aware.

This process of discovery is usually described as self-expressive. Most people experience creative therapies, however, as *novel* modes of expression, previously untried, which manage to help them express feelings which are themselves partly or wholly new. This experience of participating in arts or drama commonly provokes the mixed feelings that something about oneself may be unwittingly revealed (i.e. the process is powerful) but also that it is not really a serious activity (i.e. it is frivolous, foolish or ineffective). It has often been pointed out that the artists in society may attract this dual attitude, that they are at once magical and ridiculous.

Not surprisingly, both the principles and the practice of the creative therapies are highly individualistic. Creative therapy methods include the following themes and practices:

(a) Creative therapies as *activities that enable and enhance full, natural development*, rather than as adjuncts to medical practice (e.g. Warren, 1984). This view is quite common among creative therapists, and places the subject more in the field of health promotion and personal development than as a treatment of disorder – analogous, for example to physical education rather than physiotherapy. The arts are necessary for human life, and good for you, but that does not make it 'therapy'. Waller (1984) discusses this issue, more from the professional practice than the philosophical point of view, and suggests that art therapy and the teaching of art are at the ends of a continuum, overlapping in the middle in special schools where therapeutic skills are used to help the teaching of children.

(b) *Games, exercises, activities and outings* (e.g. camping trips) where adults and adolescents do things together. The shared aims and achievements, the undertaking of real if modest responsibilities, the models for adult behaviour provided by the staff, the sense of a shared enterprise rather than 'being treated', plus the feeling of belonging to a group and some moderate showing-off together provide new experiences and accomplishments and enhanced self-esteem. Page (1986) has described such things in relation to music and dramatic performances with adolescents, though as education rather than therapy.

(c) In *role play*, adopting positions and behaviour which give insight into one's own or another's feelings and behaviour, or which rehearse an interaction in a more constructive way. For example, an adolescent and parent cannot disagree over the smallest matter without becoming enraged, and benefit from role-playing (and thereby rehearsing) having more constructive arguments.

(d) *Psychodrama* is a different technique, and should not be undertaken without an experienced leader. It was developed by Moreno in the 1920s in New York. Using theatrical trappings and Moreno's guidance, people acted (or rather re-enacted) past and current roles, relationships, problems and conflicts rather than simply talked about them. Some people more than others can get deeply involved in their (and other people's) parts, and the skill of the psychodramatist lies in keeping the session in control and on task. The sessions begin with warming-up and simple trust exercises, and not ending without participants being gently extracted from their adopted roles. For an account of a session see Wynn (1986), and for practical guidance see Jennings (1986).

(e) *Art therapy* involves a relationship between art psychotherapist and patient across, or with, art work which the latter produces; the process of creating the painting, sculpture or clay model provides an extra dimension to the relationship. The piece of work acts as a link beween therapist and patient, as a connection between one session and another, and indeed as something tangible developing, when all three things might otherwise , for that patient, be too tenuous and easily lost. The painting also acts as a container for things past, present and future, real, hoped for or feared, and can so to speak wait until patient and therapist are ready to work with them. It is a misconception that the art work is 'interpreted'; rather, the therapist and patient are concerned with their relationship, the process of production (inhibited, frenetic, obsessive, chaotic, destructive and so on), and the patient's efforts to express what he or she is trying to say. It takes courage, commitment, concentration, self-assertion and a balance between disinhibition and discipline to be productive in art, and all these things are capacities with which the adolescent patient may have problems. As in play therapy, the simple ability to lose oneself in pleasure and fun is something many troubled or disabled young people cannot do, and to achieve this is another important component of art therapy.

Art therapy is a young subject, and in practice will be found sometimes as formal, sessional therapy, and sometimes as an available activity to which patients are sent, as if to an institutional social club. It is not the fault of art therapists that it is sometimes used in the latter way. My own experience of art therapy is that many adolescents are comfortable enough with it to explore uncomfortable feelings and topics they can manage in no other way. In the present state of the profession's development art therapists are often allotted a peripheral role; but learning about what they are doing with patients is rewarding, and full of surprises. See Dalley (1984) and Waller and Gilroy (1986) for accounts of art therapy, and Merry (1986) for a contrasting account of art education with adolescents.

Jennings (1985) provides a broad view of the creative therapies, and Dunne *et al.* (1982) provide an interesting account of active, experiential techniques with adolescents.

(5) Family work and family therapy

The term family therapy is often used fairly loosely to include all work with two or more family members. I find it helpful to distinguish between *family work*, i.e. any work done with adolescent and other family members, and *family therapy* in which the patterns of interaction between members of the household, i.e. all the people living together at home, are used in understanding and responding to problems.

Family work therefore includes family therapy, but also includes other approaches such as explaining an adolescent's illness and treatment to parents and siblings, teaching parents behavioural approaches, or holding review meetings to discuss plans and progress.

Gorell Barnes (1985) and Dare (1985) have provided accounts of the development of family therapy which demonstrate its many roots, for example in the child guidance movement (with its focus on the mother and later both parents), in the social sciences, in the various theories about the nature of schizophrenia (see Chapter 15) and in *general systems theory* (von Bertalanffy 1968). The essence of general systems theory is the way parts operate to form a whole: the organization of the parts and their relationships to each other. The systems approach is a familiar one in Medicine (e.g. the amount of insulin needed by a diabetic patient depends on complex interactions between the endocrine system, the diet, the external environment and the psychological state of the patient). Medical thinking and medical science have, however, advanced largely by reductionist approaches e.g. in the biochemical and physiological studies which showed what insulin was, where it came from, what it did and how it could be prepared as a medicine.

In systems theory as applied to the family, an arbitrary (but appropriate) decision is taken to view the problems of childhood and adolescence from the perspective of the family system, as opposed to the perspectives of intrapsychic functioning on the one hand, or the functioning of the whole of society on the other. Thus an adolescent may be anxious, lacking in confidence, misbehaving, depressed or confused because the family as a whole is operating in such a way as to make at least one of its members (the one sent to the doctor) anxious, lack confidence, misbehave, feel depressed or be confused. A sociologist could argue that a family might 'maintain' a child's misbehaviour because of larger socio-economic circumstances and pressures beyond their control; while a scientist or clinician working on an individual basis could point to the cause of the problem being in the child's individual mental or physical health or development. To understand family therapy it is necessary to appreciate that it is a particular approach, a practical perspective, rather than an aetiological model or single form of therapy alone.

Although the origins and maintenance of a problem may be understood from the perspective of the family as a whole, and family therapy may be regarded as the most appropriate response, it may emerge in family therapy that other work is needed as well or instead. Many family therapists take the view that clinical work may proceed more readily from family work to other work, than vice versa.

Example 21
Jackie is referred because of school refusal. She is a very shy girl who is able to say little about her problems. The meeting begins with the parents trying to encourage and cajole Jackie to 'tell the doctor' what the problem is, and they suggest it might be better if she sees the doctor by herself. The family therapist suggests that they try to look at how difficult things are talked about together, and after an uncomfortable and strained period it emerges that the mother is often depressed, and that the father has a serious drinking problem about which he will not seek advice. There is an assumption that 'Jackie doesn't know about it', but both parents agree that over the years she has often been in tears as a result of parental rows about her father coming home intoxicated. It seems that there have been some very frightening and violent disputes, especially in the past, and many were witnessed by Jackie. More recently there have been less rows, but greater distance between the parents. Jackie's school refusal appears to serve two functions: it is one of the few matters about which the parents are jointly concerned – her 'problem' holds them together; it also enables Jackie, who is chronically fearful, fears growing up and fears leaving the parents, to keep an eye on what is going on between them. The family sessions, with the parents openly expressing their concern about each other and Jackie, and with their disputes made more understandable, containable and safer by the family sessions, provide a firm base from which a programme for a return to school (shared by the parents, guided by a behavioural psychologist) is planned. A second treatment approach which emerges after a few sessions is separate marital therapy for the parents. Jackie returns to school, seeming much more relaxed and feeling no longer responsible for keeping the family together. At the session after Jackie returns to school her father and mother announce that he is now going to seek help with his drinking problem.

It is a widely held assumption in family therapy that in a family where one or more members have psychiatric symptoms, the family's dynamic system has reached a homeostatic state to accommodate the symptoms. Correspondingly, the family is not readily able or willing to change its accommodating pattern of behaviour. To do so would perhaps cause too much anxiety, since they have reached a precarious balance. Moreover, it may be more tolerable to face one problem (e.g. school refusal) than another (e.g. 'secret' drinking and marital schism). Further, the family members, enmeshed with each other in this process, will not know how to begin to change. This much appears to be common ground among family therapists.

Techniques for bringing about change in the family owe something to older psychodynamic therapeutic approaches such as helping the family feel safe with the therapist, interpretation etc; and much to active interventions to force change (strategic approaches). The latter interventions are not necessarily overt. For example, family therapists make great play with manipulative techniques such as paradoxical interventions, e.g. prescribing even more of what the family is doing already (perhaps that the whole family should stay in, all the time, for always, with an agoraphobic member). Such paradoxical prescriptions have a founding father in the inventive genius of Milton Erickson (see, for example, Haley 1973, 1976), but in less experienced hands can be as unhelpful as clumsy interpretations. The common aim, whether the technique is instruction, advice, suggestion, interpretation, a comment or a paradoxical intervention, is to destabilize the symptom-maintaining dynamic of the family system.

Dare (1985, 1986) has carefully outlined the practical steps to be taken in family therapeutic work. First, convening a meeting of the whole household and demonstrating his attentiveness to every family member. Second, negotiating for an acceptable account and definition of the problem which includes the effects of the symptom on the others present. Third, facilitating interaction between the family members, with attention to how they function in general, and how each family member manages or has managed life cycle transitions (e.g. adolescence). Drawing up a family tree can be a helpful technique. The family therapist observes how the family members communicate, verbally and non-verbally, what alliances and sub-groups are formed with whom, how support and control is organized, and how these and other modes of functioning relate to the presenting problem but also to other matters. Therapeutic interventions will be broadly as outlined above, within a framework of the therapist directing attention to one issue or another, encouragement, confrontation, setting of tasks and exercises such as sculpting and role-playing. The timetabling of further sessions is important, with wide differences between therapists about the intervals left between sessions, and when to stop.

The problems and opportunities of family therapy when other therapies are being conducted alongside have been discussed by Dare in relation to the work of an in-patient adolescent unit (Dare, 1986). Approaches to family therapy are also described by Bruggen and Davies (1977), Walrond-Skinner (1976, 1978), Skynner 1976), Bentovim *et al.* (1982), Skynner and Cleese (1984), and Barker (1986). The important work of Selvini Palazzoli and her colleagues in the Milan group is described for example in Selvini Palazzoli *et al*, (1978, 1980). The work of this group of therapists in the field of anorexia nervosa is of particular interest (Selvini Palazzoli, 1970, 1974) for the light it throws on family therapy as well as on this disorder. The same applies to the work of Minuchin and his co-workers (e.g. in Minuchin *et al.*, 1980).

Where does family therapy stand in relation to other methods? As all other therapies have done, it is passing through a growth spurt of great excitement, producing charismatic figures whose presence in conferences draws vast crowds, and generating strong feelings among both adherents and antagonists. As the excitement mounts, the elders among its pioneers and protagonists try to make themselves heard, explaining that they perhaps do not have all the answers. The continuing discussion in most of the references given above, and in the interesting Journal of Family Therapy, demonstrates the arguments within the family therapy movement about its achievements, methods and the need for studies of its effectiveness.

In practically all forms of treatment there are convincing arguments for their effectiveness in theory and often enough in terms of results. To take only two examples, medication is enormously effective in schizophrenic illnesses, and behaviour therapy equally so in many disorders involving anxiety-laden habits. Further, as has been mentioned, family therapy is as much a perspective as a treatment, and does not necessarily exclude other methods when they emerge from family assessment and with family understanding and at least some family involvement in the decision. It follows that a whole-family approach to problems appears to be as reasonable as is a whole- person approach; but for reasons of economy, practicality and common sense, we still need to find out which treatment is predictably most helpful for which problem. Here the body of systematically obtained knowledge remains surprisingly scanty, and this is true not only for family therapy.

Table 18.1

Group	Examples	Other names	NB EXAMPLES ONLY of low adult dose
ANTIPSYCHOTIC = neuroleptics; = major tranquillisers	1 Chlorpromazine	'Largactil'	50–100 mg BD or TDS orally
	2 Trifluoperazine	'Stelazine'	2–4 mg BD or TDS orally
	3 Thioridazine	'Melleril'	50–100mg BD or TDS
	4 Fluphenazine Decanoate	'Modecate' (depot injection)	Test dose 12.5 mg i.m. Then 25 mg fortnightly i.m.
	5 Haloperidol	'Serenace'	1–5 mg TDS orally
	6 Pimozide	'Orap'	2–5 mg TDS
	7 Flupenthixol Decanoate	'Depixol' (depot injection)	Test dose 20 mg i.m. Then 20–40 mg i.m. every 2–4 weeks
ANTICHOLINERGIC DRUGS	8 Orphenadrine	'Disipal'	50 mg TDS
	9 Procyclidine	'Kemadrin'	2.5–5 mg TDS
MINOR TRANQUILLISERS	10 Diazepam	'Valium'	2–5 mg BD or TDS
	11 Chlordiazepoxide	'Librium'	5–10 mg TDS
STIMULANTS	12 Methylphenidate	'Ritalin'	(children) 0.25 to 1.0 mg/kg body weight per day
ANTIDEPRESSANTS	13 Imipramine	'Tofranil'	25–50 mg BD or TDS
	14 Amitriptyline	'Tryptizol'	25–50 mg BD or TDS
	15 Clomipramine	'Anafranil'	10–20 mg daily, increased gradually
ANTICONVULSANTS	16 Phenytoin	'Epanutin'	*150 mg BD
	17 Sodium valproate	'Epilim'	*200 mg TDS initially
	18 Carbamazepine	'Tegretol'	*200 mg BD or TDS
LITHIUM SALTS	19 Lithium carbonate	'Priadel'	*250 mg BD or TDS initially

* See literature

Table 18.1

Examples of uses	Some side-effects and other problems (N.B. not a comprehensive list)	Notes
1 Schizophrenic psychoses; severely agitated states	Extrapyramidal symptoms; tardive dyskinesia; drowsiness; depression; hypotension; skin sensitivity; jaundice; neuroleptic malignant syndrome; blood disorders; etc.	Contra-indicated in blood disorders and glaucoma. (NB – anticholinergic drugs can exacerbate glaucoma)
2 Highdose: schizophrenic psychosis low dose: anxiety	Similar to chlorpromazine, but –	Less sedating, extrapyramidal symptoms more frequent.
3 Schizophrenia	Similar to chlorpromazine, and may cause pigmentary retinopathy. See text.	Less sedating, but extrapyramidal symptoms less frequent.
4 Schizophrenia	Similar to chlorpromazine, but –	Long-acting depot preparation given by deep i.m. injection.
5 Schizophrenic psychoses; severely agitated states	Similar to chlorpromazine, but –	Extra-pyramidal symptoms more frequent; hypotension less common. May cause depression.
6 Schizophrenia	Similar to chlorpromazine, but –	Less sedating; less extrapyramidal symptoms; may aggravate depression and epilepsy.
7 Schizophrenia	Similar to chlorpromazine, but –	Less sedating; extrapyramidal symptoms common.
8 Extrapyramidal side-effects of antipsychotic medication	May cause confusion, excitement, euphoria, dizziness, occasionally tachycardia	Avoid abrupt discontinuation of treatment. Avoid in glaucoma, cardiovascular disease, hepatic or renal impairment. May cause urinary retention.
9 Extrapyramidal side-effects of antipsychotic medication	Similar to orphenadrine; may also cause drowsiness	
10 Anxiety states 11	Drowsiness, dizziness, ataxia, confusion. Affects ability to drive, control machinery etc.	Avoid in glaucoma. Avoid prolonged use and abrupt discontinuation.
12 Hyperkinetic syndrome	Sleeplessness, loss of appetite, headache, abdominal pain, anxiety and depression	May affect growth rate and exacerbate tics, stereotypies and epilepsy. Rarely leads to psychosis and abuse.
13 Depression; enuresis	Dry mouth, sedation, blurred vision, constipation, nausea, difficulty with micturition, postural hypotension. arrhythmias, tachycardia, rashes, sweating, tremor, blood disorders.	May precipitate mania, and cause behaviour problems in *children*. Less commonly may cause seizures. Avoid in glaucoma.
14 Depression		
15 Depression		
16 Epilepsy	Nausea, vomiting, tremor, confusion, headache, insomnia, gum hypertrophy, acne	Contra-indicated in the porphyrias. Caution with hepatic impairment.
17 Epilepsy	Nausea, increased appetite, weight gain, hair loss	Can cause thrombocytopaenia and liver failure.
18 Epilepsy	May cause dizziness, drowsiness, gastrointestinal disturbance, rash. Rarely, blood disorders.	Avoid in porphyrias and cardiac conduction abnormalities. Only causes drowsiness as a toxic effect.
19 Manic depressive psychosis	See Table 18.2	Blood level monitoring essential.

(6) Medication

Drugs may be prescribed for adolescents –

(a) because a drug is the most effective treatment, (e.g. using 'neuroleptics' (see Table 18.1) for schizophrenia);
(b) because symptom-suppression is necessary (e.g. using sedation for an outburst of chaotic, violent behaviour);
(c) as a necessary supplement to other forms of management (e.g. when antidepressant medication helps a patient's mood sufficiently for him to take part in psychological and social treatment, or when neuroleptic drugs contain chronically disturbed behaviour sufficiently to enable a boy or girl to be contained in a setting which may prove educational and therapeutic in more positive ways).

The use of drugs by adolescent psychiatrists varies with their clientele, and of course their clientele varies with their interests and willingness to see young people who may need medication. Among some psychiatrists and teams there is an unwillingness to use medication, and there is evidence that quite a high proportion of recruits to training in the field show little interest in this aspect of treatment (Garralda, 1980).

Table 18.1 outlines some of the drugs used more commonly in child and adolescent psychiatry. When using a drug, consider:

(a) The dose that will achieve maximum benefit with tolerable side (unwanted) effects.
(b) The patient's and family's understanding of the effects and side-effects (including dangers) of the drug, and the length of time it may be needed – and hence their informed consent to its use.
(c) Clarity about the goals of using the drug, so that the effects can be monitored and the dose adjusted. For example, medication may be given to contain an aggressive patient with schizophrenia in a rehabilitation programme, but a lower dose may be sufficient if, later, the patient is in a less demanding therapeutic programme. The place of medication in relation to the overall management programme should be clear.
(d) Is the drug being given? Is the drug being taken, in the prescribed dose or at all? Is it being absorbed and achieving therpeutically useful levels in the blood?
(e) Take great care in written prescriptions and in the records of drugs used. In the team, and particularly in residential treatment, make sure all concerned know about what is being given, changes of dose,

how effects are being monitored, and about side-effects and their treatment.

Guidance on the dose of medication is contained in Table 18.1, but it is difficult to give precise advice here because one's adolescent patients vary in weight from that of a quite small child to young people substantially larger than many adults. For a small boy or girl weighing about 30 kilograms (65 lbs) dose, particularly for major tranquillizers (neuroleptics) should be guided by weight. For larger young people, probably weighing 45 kilograms (100 lbs) upwards, begin with the lowest adult dose and increase with caution to the highest adult doses if necessary.

The ANTIPSYCHOTIC DRUGS (also known as major tranquillizers or neuroleptics) include the phenothiazines, e.g. chlorpromazine, trifluoperazine, thioridazine and fluphenazine; the butyrophenones such as haloperidol and pimozide; and the thioxanthenes such as fluphenthixol. All cause sedation, relieve schizophrenic and other psychotic symptoms, have long-lasting effects (several days), cause extrapyramidal (Parkinson's disease-like) symptoms, and cause changes in cerebral excitability, e.g. may cause seizures in high doses. The recently introduced drug sulpiride belongs to the substituted benzamide group, and is said to be less sedating. Neuroleptics may cause the neuroleptic malignant syndrome.

Extrapyramidal symptoms include facial immobility, excessive salivation, general muscle weakness and lack of movement; acute dystonia, which is painless spasmodic contractions of muscle groups, so that there may be tongue protrusion, neck and spinal muscle spasms and oculogyric (eye muscle) crises; akathisia, an agitated, restless state which may resemble what the medication is supposed to be controlling; and tardive dyskinesia, grimacing movements of the face and tongue. This is unusual, develops gradually, may be predisposed to by brain damage, and unlike the other muscular side-effects may be irreversible, although most patients eventually improve months or years after medication stops. Note that although medication should be stopped if tardive dyskinesia develops reducing the drug dosage may initially worsen it (and a dose reduction may have precipitated it). However, the problems of tardive dyskinesia have to be weighed against the problems of the psychotic illness. Note also that anticholinergic drugs (see below) make it worse (see review by Marsden and Jenner 1980). It is possible that sulpiride may be less likely to cause tardive dyskinesia because of its different effect on dopamine systems compared with other major tranquillizers, but it has not yet been used as extensively as the other drugs.

Chlorpromazine can also cause weight gain, skin pigmentation, vulnerability to cold weather (hypothermia and frostbite) and photosensitivity. The latter can be reduced by the use of shade and skin creams like Uvistat. It also interferes with the metabolism in the liver of morphine, pethidine and the tricyclic antidepressants. It may mask pain and fever, expecially in high doses, and may therefore make the diagnosis of physical disorder difficult. It can cause hypoglycaemia, and interfere with aspects of learning, e.g. attention, concentration, reaction time and fine motor skills. Neuroleptics may cause blood disorders.

Thioridazine does not cause photosensitivity, and is less likely to cause extrapyramidal symptoms, but doses above 600 mg daily can cause pigmentary retinopathy and blindness. All the major tranquillizers may cause hypotension and depression, and the phenothiazines (like tricyclic antidepressants) can reduce circulating growth hormone levels and in the long term affect children's growth (Sherman *et al.*, 1971). Tardive dyskinesia apart, the anticholinergic drugs procyclidine or orphenadrine should be used to control substantial extrapyramidal side-effects. They may cause drowsiness, nausea, dry mouth, constipation, urinary difficulties, precipitate acute glaucoma, and in high doses can cause delirium, confusion and hallucinations.

For young people with chronic psychotic illnesses, and especially where compliance with medication is a problem, depot preparations should be considered. They are given by injection every 2-4 weeks, preceded by a test dose. Their convenience of administration should not lead to complacency about wider aspects of management, including attention to such side-effects as those described above, and particularly the onset of depression.

BENZODIAZEPINES are the most widely used anxiolytic (anti-anxiety) drugs in general psychiatry. Well-known examples are *diazepam* and *chlordiazepoxide*. In larger doses they are sedative and hypnotic in effect and they act also as muscle relaxants and anticonvulsants. They are very widely used in the treatment of anxiety states in adults, and among the problems encountered have been psychological dependence and, on withdrawal, anxiety, insomnia and nausea due to physical withdrawal effects or the return of anxiety symptoms. Fast withdrawal from large doses may cause seizures. The benzodiazepines appear also to reduce inhibitions in aggressive people (Salzman *et al.*, 1974) and the possibility of this contributing to child abuse by over-stressed parents should be considered.

A number of studies in children of the use of these drugs have shown no benefit for anxiety states (Lucas and Pasley, 1969) or conduct disorders and hyperactive children in particular may be made worse (Zrull *et al.*, 1964). They are rarely indicated in children and adolescents, but small doses for limited periods may be useful when overwhelming anxiety is preventing a behaviour therapy programme from getting under way.

STIMULANT DRUGS of the amphetamine type, e.g. *methylphenidate* are very rarely used in adolescent psychiatry. In adults they are used for narcolepsy, and in children have a place in the treatment of the hyperkinetic syndrome when other methods prove insufficient by themselves and poor attention span is marked. Anxiety states may be made worse, and schizophrenia, tics, stereoptypies, hypertension and heart disease are contra- indications (see Taylor, 1985). They appear to interfere with growth (Safer and Allen, 1973; Safer *et al.*, 1975).

TRICYCLIC ANTIDEPRESSANT DRUGS such as *imipramine* have been shown to be useful in the treatment of adult-type depressive disorder in children (Petti and Conners, 1983) and there is a possible place for them in the case of school refusal (Gittelman-Klein and Klein, 1971), but the evidence for their effectiveness in mild depressive states is unclear. *Clomipramine* can be effective in obsessional disorders accompanied by depressive symptomatology (Marks *at al.*, 1980).

Imipramine suppresses bed-wetting and is useful for providing temporary relief or when behavioural methods prove inadequate. Its mechanism of action in this condition is unclear, but is not thought to be due to an antidepressant effect (Shaffer *et al.*, 1979; Taylor, 1985).

The tricyclic antidepressants are also used in hyperactivity as an alternative to the stimulants.

Side-effects include drowsiness, dry mouth, constipation, blurred vision, postural hypotension, weight gain, tremor, hypomania, hallucinations and seizures, and they may exacerbate glaucoma. They are cardiotoxic, and overdose is dangerous. They can cause blood disorders.

The use of ANTICONVULSANT MEDICATION such as *phenytoin* and *sodium valproate* in epilepsy is too large and complex a topic for discussion here, although it should be noted that these drugs may cause a variety of emotional, behavioural and learning problems as side-effects, including confusion and psychotic states (Stores, 1975). Stores (1978) concludes that there is insufficient evidence that the anticonvulsant drugs help overactive and aggressive children although this property has been attributed to *carbamazepine* (Remschmidt, 1976).

LITHIUM CARBONATE is well established in adult psychiatry as a drug which helps control manic states and reduces the recurrence of periods of mania and depression (Coppen *et al.*, 1971; Medical Research Council Drug Trials Subcommittee, 1981). It has been shown to be effective in manic-depressive illness in adolescents (Brumback and Weinberg, 1977; Horowitz, 1977; Youngerman and Canino, 1978) and in a variety of other disorders in young people including aggression in intellectually retarded adolescents (Dostal and Zvolsky, 1970), self-mutilation in an

Table 18.2   Side-effects and toxic effects of lithium.

Early side-effects
Nausea
Fine tremor of the hands
Dry mouth
Thirst and polyuria
Loose stools

Toxic effects
Diarrhoea and vomiting
Ataxia, clumsiness
Slurred speech
Muddled thinking

Severe toxicity
Worsening disorientation
Seizures
Drowsiness, coma

autistic child (Campbell *et al.*, 1982), aggressive behaviour (De Long, 1978, Campbell *et al.*, 1982) and in an episodically resistant case of anorexia nervosa (Stein *et al.*, 1982). Are these examples of lithium improving 'atypical' depression as discussed in Chapter 16? Or producing improvement where a mood disorder accompanies another problem? Or an entirely different effect of lithium? There is a case for the carefully monitored use of lithium in some cases of severe, intractable behavioural and other problems when they are clearly episodic and apparently unrelated to external influences, especially when there is a family history of depressive illness, but an adequate large scale study has yet to be done (Steinberg, 1980).

Lithium is a toxic drug whose blood level should be regularly monitored, and kept within the therapeutic range 0.7 to 1.4 milliequivalents per litre (mE/1). It can cause reversible neurological, thyroid and renal disturbance and these functions should be assessed before treatment and checked at intervals. It is unclear whether it causes irreversible renal damage too, but opinion is in general against this being a serious risk. It is also uncertain whether or not lithium given with haloperidol can cause brain damage (for example, see Loudon and Waring, 1976; Thomas 1979). For the time being it is best to avoid giving these drugs together. Lithium may also inhibit bone growth (Birch, 1979). Table 18.2 outlines its side-effects and toxic effects.

Children on *any* long-term psychotropic medication should have regular blood and liver function tests.

(7) Other physical treatment: health care, diet and ECT

Electroconvulsive therapy (ECT) is believed to work in severe depressive illness because of the seizure caused by the passage of electricity through the brain, and not by the current itself. Despite years of controversy there is little doubt of its effectiveness in severe depressive illness (see Royal College of Psychiatrists, 1977; Kendell, 1981). It has also been used in severe episodes of mania, in acute catatonic schizophrenia, and in schizoaffective psychosis where there is severe depression.

It is little used in adolescent psychiatry. At the Bethlem unit, where priority is given to the admission of severely ill young people, many with affective psychoses, it has been found necessary only three times in ten years. It should certainly be considered where profound, disabling depressive illness is accompanied by symptoms which in adults suggest a likely response to ECT (e.g. rapid onset and psychomotor retardation) and where other treatments are not helping. Extremes of distressed agitation and depressive stupor may be seen, and may be life-threatening in severe depressive illness.

Much of the controversy surrounding ECT surrounds its supposedly casually inappropriate use with inadequate explanation and consent. It is fundamental to good practice in adolescent psychiatry to discuss the pros and cons of all treatment fully with patient and family, and with the patient's social worker if there is one. Most child and adolescent psychiatrists will have little recent experience of using ECT, and if in doubt about the need for this treatment should have no hesitation in seeking the opinion of a colleague in adult psychiatry. Having said this, I believe it is the individual consultant's responsibility to decide whether or not to recommend the treatment.

The psychiatrist in a clinical unit, especially one providing residential care, should be aware of the *general health education and needs* of the patients. Concern about the calorie intake of anorexic patients or the results of CT scans should not be at the expense of attention to young patients' nutrition and general health care, including their teeth, eyesight and hearing. This is particularly important for doctors who have long-term patients in their care, but even in short-stay units the medical and nursing staff should work with teachers on health education. The dangers of drug abuse and the risks of venereal disease, including AIDS, should be on the curriculum. The risks of cigarette smoking and the unwise consumption of alcohol should be explained. In this respect the staff should be aware that, for good or ill, they will be seen as models for adult behaviour. Parents should be informed about what is being taught.

Nutrition and fluid balance are of particular importance when a patient is anorexic for any reason, or dehydrated as a result of psychotic, hysterical or organic illness. Manic patients in particular can become steadily dehydrated and exhausted. Whether acutely ill or not, adolescents unwell enough, self-negligent enough or neglected enough to be in hospital should have their heights, weights and development checked and those who stay for months rather than weeks should have these things reassessed at intervals. *Diet, allergy and behaviour problems* are discussed in Chapter 8; see also Taylor (1979).

Clinicians will be very conscious of the need to exclude a physical cause for psychiatric symptoms, as was mentioned in Chapter 5. In addition, on the evidence of a study at the Bethlem adolescent unit, young people with serious psychiatric problems seem, as a group, to have quite a high incidence of major and minor physical conditions, whether directly related to their psychiatric disorder or not (Steinberg *et al.*, 1988).

(8) Behavioural treatments

Behavioural treatment (which is synonymous with behaviour therapy or behaviour modification) is concerned with observable behaviour; the focus of management is what happens, rather than what the unconscious motivation might be. It requires clarity and precision about the goals for change, the methods and the results. Although people can respond to behavioural approaches without realizing it, the essentially straightforward nature of behavioural treatment lends itself to much more complete understanding and therefore informed consent on the patient's part than is the case with dynamic psychotherapy, many strategies in family therapy, and drug treatment.

Behavioural treatment follows four steps:

(a) *Objective definition and description of the problem.* (For example, a 13 year-old boy of low intelligence who throws schoolwork onto the floor in nearly every lesson, becomes disruptive and violent when staff intervene.)

(b) *Functional analysis,* which is a hypothesis to account for the behaviour in terms of what is sufficient and necessary for it to occur and to persist. (For example the boy is at the back of the classroom pretending to tackle work he doesn't understand or enjoy, becomes increasingly unhappy, and his sequence of misbehaviour successively involves the children nearby, then all the children, then the class teacher and then other staff.) The hypothesis is that the boy finds the increasing disruption in the classroom, caused by his mounting misbehaviour, more rewarding in terms of self-esteem and distraction than staying with a task which he finds frustrating and dispiriting.

(c) *A hypothesis about a therapeutic response is set up.* (For example, if the boy had work limited in quantity and quality to what he can manage; is rewarded by the teacher's attention and public praise at frequent intervals for work achieved and for getting on with his work; and if he is at the front of the class close to the teacher and in full view of the other pupils; then many of the contingencies on which his misbehaviour depends will not be occurring.)

(d) *The hypothesis is tested and systematically monitored.* (The above approach works partially. He remains well behaved and attentive to his work for longer periods, but occasionally gets stuck and then becomes very disruptive again. Outside staff still have to be called in to contain him, and it is proposed that the new approach 'isn't working'. Attention is drawn to what is working and what isn't working. He stays at his work three times longer than he did before, and the quality of the work is improving; he no longer flings it away but keeps his work in a folder for next time.)

(e) *Outcome is evaluated and the treatment programme modified accordingly.* (In view of the continuing problems more attention is given to helping him in the areas where he becomes stuck and frustrated; praise is given for his real overall achievement; mild misbehaviour is determinedly ignored but he is timed out' (see below) when he becomes disruptive. This modified approach is said to be 'not working' because there are violent scuffles two or three times a week. However, the progress charts show that his work is objectively improving, he is working for longer than he has ever done before, and at the start there were violent scuffles twice a day. The programme is still more 'finely tuned' to praise his achievement, but the threshold for 'time out' is lowered. Progress is now very marked, but still requires persistence through the one or two disruptive episodes per week. These decline and stop as he finds more achievement in his work).

The above example illustrates only a few behavioural approaches. Others include:

Positive reinforcement: to encourage desired behaviour.

Shaping: the systematic modification of a behaviour programme with very precise observations and timing to bring about progressive improvements which may be modest but which accumulate.

Time out, which is short for 'time out from positive reinforcement': the patient is removed immediately without excitement or comment, and for an agreed few minutes, from the circumstances which, according to the hypothesis, are reinforcing the behaviour. It should be distinguished from *seclusion*, which means nursing an in-patient away from others to avoid dangerous behaviour. However, even a brief period of time out can be interpreted as an infringement of legal rights, and both time out and seclusion require scrupulous attention to legal and ethical requirements and proper prescription and record-keeping. Seclusion is not a behavioural treatment.

Punishment means doing something unpleasant to extinguish undesirable behaviour. It suggests pain and cruelty, is often badly timed, inconsistent, may provide a model of aggressive behaviour, is often used to replace rather than supplement positive reinforcement, and tends not to have lasting effects (Brown and Christie, 1981). Nevertheless, it has a place in work with young people, e.g. requiring adolescents to pay for damage caused to other people's things, or when an immediate effect is crucial as in Corbett's example (1975) where every other method failed to prevent a mentally handicapped child's severely injurious beating of his head against walls.

Desensitization refers to a graded approach, in reality or in imagination, to a feared situation or object while the patient is in a relaxed state, e.g. by being taught relaxation training. The latter may include progressive muscular relaxation and breathing exercises. This approach has proved helpful in a wide range of childhood fears (e.g. see Kondas, 1967, Ballard and Yule 1981).

Modelling, which can helpfully supplement desensitization, enables anxious or socially inhibited children to observe and learn how confident, competent peers and adults deal with various situations (Rachman, 1972).

Self-monitoring, in which the patient charts his or her own progress, can be effective in itself for fears and obsessional symptoms, as well as a record of progress.

Token reinforcement means giving the child a token such as a disc or a gold star for desired behaviour. The tokens are then exchanged for 'back-up reinforcers', e.g. privileges or other treats.

Response prevention is used to prevent undesirable behaviour: a trusted therapist accompanies and firmly stops the patient from carrying out (e.g.) a compulsive act. The principle is that the compulsive act is seen as anxiety-reducing, and therefore rewarding, albeit in a perverse and handicapping way. The reward of the act is therefore prevented. This has been used successfully with severe obsessive-compulsive behaviour in adolescents (Bolton *et al.*, 1983).

The relationship between behaviour modification and other therapies should be clear. For example, the misbehaving child in the classroom needed careful educational reappraisal; he would also have benefited from social skills training, e.g. being taught how to ask a teacher for help if he felt discouraged or unable to understand his work. As discussed below such training could involve rehearsal and therefore role play.

In the treatment programme used with obsessional young people (Bolton *et al.*, 1983, above) the adolescents' families, who had become involved in the obsessive behaviour, were asked to be involved in the treatment, actively (by using response prevention) or passively (by not taking part in the rituals). Experience in trying to engage parents in behaviour modification will often reveal other difficulties: e.g. the parents may be unable to agree on crucial issues, and cannot negotiate about their differences, or cannot assert normal parental authority or sustain difficult approaches without becoming discouraged. The attempt at behaviour therapy may then provide a focus for other work, e.g. over parenting skills or marital conflict. Such problems will often have provided the anxiety which fuels the problem and the combined family therapy and behavioural approach provide an effective dual treatment strategy. It can be helpful to draw up explicit contracts between adolescent, family and therapist about the focus of work and mutually agreed behavioural changes. For example, the parents may agree to not making a major issue out of trivialities if the son or daughter agrees to abide by certain 'house rules' concerning more serious matters. Tharp and Wetzel (1969) have discussed such approaches in the family and elsewhere, and Homme *et al.*, (1970) and Topping (1986) in the classroom. A particularly important aspect of training parents in behavioural management is in its potential for treating at home young people, such as those with autism, who might otherwise require institutional care (see Chapter 14 and Howlin *et al.*, 1973).

Yule (1985) provides a comprehensive review of a wide range of behavioural approaches. Behaviour therapy has often been regarded as rather mechanistic and not very 'human' in its approach, and unable to deal with the 'real' problems. However, there is good evidence that it is effective, it is not incompatible with other strategies to deal with related problems, and the straightforward way it has to be conducted makes it one of the more understandable and accessible forms of psychiatric treatment. Adolescents making progress in behavioural programmes they have helped draw up and monitor rightly feel a boost in self-esteem at their achievement.

(9) Group work and social therapy

The support, expectations and pressures of social groups, both to explore feelings and attitudes and to help modify them, are important components in a wide variety of group and social therapies. These may include anything from small groups of 4-8 participants to large community groups 40 or 50 strong. Groups may be run on a systems approach, on psychodynamic lines or as vehicles for social skills training, role play, psychodrama, behaviour modification or joint learning. Creative, experiential and play techniques can be used. Group work has a number of characteristics that lend themselves to work with adolescents. First, adolescents do seem to learn at least as much from their peers as from adults; certainly they give priority to peer relationships. Second, the wider range of interpersonal permutations of groups, their shifting focus from topic to topic and person to person, the room for changes in depth of participation, all tend to meet adolescents' needs to go through a series of tentative experiments. Third, some adolescents feel so vulnerable in the intimacy of individual psychotherapy or counselling that they cease to use it properly, at least for the more difficult topics.

Example 22
During a small group session with adolescent in-patients there was a great deal of jokey questioning of the staff about their own sexual attitudes and behaviour. The staff found it quite difficult to get the balance right between personal privacy on the one hand and not coming across as stuffy and inhibiting on the other. Partly because of the presence of a rather disinhibited psychotic girl who believed (incorrectly) that she was pregnant, and who found the discussion exciting, the group became aroused and chaotic; there was much testing out of the staff's responses to obscene and infantile joking and gestures. The group's leaders later thought they had handled the group badly, although their supervisors thought they had managed a tricky group well. In the next group (and to the boys' and girls' surprise) the staff invited further exploration of the subject, and a much more thoughtful and reflective session took place, in which a number of sexual misunderstandings and anxieties were discussed constructively.

Adolescent group work is generally regarded as very desirable in principle but extremely difficult in practice, and with considerable uncertainty about the outcome (see, for example, Kraft, 1968; Frank and Zilbach, 1968; Berkowitz, 1972; Meeks, 1974; Abramowitz, 1976; Weisberg, 1979; Heacock, 1980). These papers describe the value of groups in terms of providing for the adolescents a forum in which they can learn new ways of dealing with personal worries and relationships, feel less isolated with their difficulties, and deal with family-type issues which have not been dealt with in work done with the family. Bruce (1975, 1978) has described the group process along lines derived from Winnicott (Chapter 1) as providing a safe 'play area' in which games which are dangerous in fantasy can be played out.

Small groups have been used for some years at the Bethlem adolescent unit (Steinberg *et al.*, 1978; Steinberg, 1987b). They have drawn from the experience of Bruce and others (above), and the groups' leaders have always been expected to follow the policy of allowing plenty of room for experiments and alternative ways of dealing with issues but within firmly set limits maintained by the staff. The group leaders are active and conversational, not passive, and are prepared to take a lead: although taking a lead can sometimes mean that the members of staff require the adolescents to make decisions. Systematic supervision is regarded as essential. Each small group contains young people with quite different capacities and diagnoses, 'problems' in a boy's or girl's participation becoming a focus for the group's work rather than a handicap. In this way we have found small group work as helpful for young people with psychotic illnesses as it has been for bright, articulate and coherent young people (Steinberg, 1985).

(10) Special education

The relationship between psychological problems and problems in educational attainment have been referred to in Chapters 3 and 8. Elsewhere, the relationship between psychiatric practice and education has been described as twofold: on the one hand, educational methods supplement psychiatric care in enabling the enjoyment, sense of achievement and improved self-esteem that goes with new discoveries and new skills in every area – leisure, academic and occupational. Correspondingly, psychiatric treatment of symptoms and disabilities enables young people to take part in such natural, development-enhancing activities (Page, 1986; Merry, 1986; Steinberg, 1981, 1982, 1986a).

The adolescent psychiatrist can be involved with educational methods and the education system in the following ways:

(a) Because of problems arising in schools, for example in attendance or misbehaviour (see Tattum, 1986).
(b) When the psychiatrist contributes to reports which help advise on the most suitable educational setting for a boy or girl. This may be a day or residential school, normal or 'special' in its resources; it may belong to the local authority or be independent; it may have visiting psychiatric, psychological or psychotherapeutic staff who see children on a sessional basis, or it may operate as a therapeutic community; alternatively, it may be highly structured and containing; it may be large or small, nearby or miles away, and it may operate a 52-week year or have long seasonal holidays. All these things need to be taken into account in recommending to an Education Department what to recommend to a child's parents. (N.B. the term school for the 'maladjusted' has been replaced by school for 'emotional and behavioural disturbance', or 'EBD'; and 'delicate' schools by schools for children who show 'failure to thrive', or 'FTT'.)
(c) When remedial teaching is needed for an adolescent's disability, e.g. in reading or writing.
(d) Where psychiatrists and teachers work together in a clinic or unit. (Steinberg 1986b).

It is important to be alert to educational problems in general and literacy problems in particular in adolescence. There is a tendency to associate such problems with younger children, and to assume that people in their mid-teens will have had such areas of difficulty recognized earlier, and adequately dealt with. Often this is not the case, and the help of remedial teachers, occupational therapists, speech therapists and specialist careers advisers is of great importance in helping an adolescent who has multiple disadvantages, or whose mood and behavioural problems arise largely because of educational and occupational handicaps.

See Howlin (1985) for a thorough review of special education in child and adolescent psychiatry.

(11) Writing letters and reports

Psychiatric notes, letters and reports are often long and rambling, and bring in all sorts of peripheral details and notions of aetiology of little use to the recipient. Try to keep in mind what the recipient (GP, magistrate, etc.) needs to know.

A written account of a meeting with a patient should describe:

(a) whom you saw and when;
(b) the presenting problems;
(c) your diagnosis or provisional diagnoses, certainly referring to other axes (e.g. intellectual, psychosocial (see Chapter 4) where relevant;
(d) what you recommend, or (if you are undertaking treatment) what you are going to do: i.e. drugs prescribed, further investigations, appointments made, etc., and what you have explained to the patient and family;
(e) matters to watch out for: e.g. deteriorating mood, side-effects etc.;
(f) whom to contact with queries, if not yourself.

It may take two or three times as long to write a short, helpful report as a long, unhelpful one.

Court reports can be based on the above framework but have a different emphasis: the court will want guidance on how best to proceed: what you think best for a child, for example, or what, if anything, psychiatric help can contribute. You should give your own honest, pragmatic opinion, based of course on your knowledge and experience, but not an abstract thesis on the pros and cons of one or other approach. A statement of alternatives, however, is not unreasonable: for example, that there are two reasonable courses of action but one, on balance, is more likely to help the child than the other.

For some years I have made a practice of never writing anything that I would not wish the patient to see; and I have increasingly been sending copies of my letters to the patient and family.

Confidentiality is important. Doctors may write to each other about their patients without special permission but you must have permission to write to (or contact) anyone else at all. Medical privilege should be modulated by courtesy, and I think it is better to have permission even for writing to medical colleagues. However, if the other doctor has some current clinical responsibility for the patient (e.g. as family doctor, or having admitted them to hospital) I believe he or she should be fully in the picture about clinical matters with or without the patient's consent.

(12) Monitoring progress

This is mentioned as a reminder rather than for discussion. It is very easy for treatment, especially when it involves subjective judgements and complicated aspects of individual and family life, to lose its way and become interminable. However, it is always possible to set goals of some sort and to review at intervals how far they are being achieved, and whether they need modifying or added to from time to time. This can be valuable, (a) to guide thinking and planning in management; (b) to replace swings of optimism and pessimism about progress with somewhat more objective judgement about how things are going; and (c) not least, as a source of 'feedback' for the patient and family, helping them share with the clinician some notion of what is going on and thereby putting their involvement, autonomy and consent to treatment on a realistic foundation.

(13) Admission to hospital and other forms of residential care

Some characteristics of residential units are discussed below (14). There are losses as well as gains for a boy or girl in a move to residential care, whatever the qualities of the new setting. Removal of young people from their families, friends and neighbourhoods respresents a major disruption in their lives, whatever the limitations of their home life, and however benign, competent or indeed necessary is the move. Parents who accept admission of a boy or girl to an adolescent unit may underestimate the extent to which parental authority and family influence can be challenged and undermined by the move, however covertly and unwittingly, or what sort of a 'hole' it may produce in the adolescent's peer relationships and social life. Further, there is social stigma about mental illness, 'special' education or being 'in care'.

The disadvantages of residential care were referred to in Chapter 3, and the problems and sometimes inappropriateness of using various forms of incarceration for young people have been discussed by Milham *et al.*, (1978), Bruggen and Westland (1979) and Milham (1981). The problem is that looking after young people away from home has so many purposes, some of them muddled. It may be seen as a privilege (for example, in the case of the independent public schools in Britain) or as a punishment (as in the use of Detention Centres); it may be seen as a way of plucking a chaotic adolescent from chaotic circumstances in order to 'assess' the boy or girl in a safe and reasonably orderly setting, as in the case of young people's remand and assessment centres. Such places can create much needed security and breathing space, but there are limitations on how far an adolescent can be assessed in isolation in this way. Some social services departments conduct such periods of assessment with the boy or girl being seen on a day basis, or at home.

There is sometimes confusion or uncertainty about the purpose of admission to a special unit. The emphasis may be variously on control and containment; on special education and training; on long term care – 'placement'; or on treatment. It is common for referral to various adolescent services to be an arbitrary business with the referrer not being absolutely clear what the particular setting has to offer (see the National Health Service Health Advisory Service report *Bridges Over Troubled Waters*) and with muddle over what combinations of treatment, training and education, care and control are actually wanted (Steinberg, 1981, 1982). Moreover, different hospital-based adolescent units see their function in different ways, one offering crisis intervention on a social model (e.g. Bruggen *et al.*, 1973), another a general psychiatric service (e.g. Steinberg *et al.*, 1981, Steinberg, 1986a), others a primarily individual dynamic psychotherapeutic approach (Perinpanayagam, 1978) and so on. Numerically the units tend to be few and far between, with the choice for the referrer or 'consumer' of which unit to use limited by geography and sometimes by catchment area designation. For example, much of South East England (the four London Health Regions), with a population of about 13 millions, is served by 8 or 9 units with about 10-24 places each: Hill End and the Northgate Clinic in the North West region (the latter taking only adolescents over 16); Simmons House and Brookside in the North East, and with a new unit opening at Colchester; Beech House and the Bethlem Unit in the South East; Long Grove Hospital Adolescent Unit in the South West; and the Colwood unit in Sussex straddling the South West and South East regions.

Admission to a psychiatric unit may be for the following sorts of reasons (to help distinguish the author's views from others' they are in my own rank order of importance):

(a) to manage acute seriously suicidal behaviour;
(b) to manage acute psychotic illness;
(c) to investigate complex psychiatric or neuropsychiatric problems, e.g. with probable biological, psychological, social and behavioural components;
(d) when 24-hour management is needed, for example in maintaining a behavioural programme, or when psychotherapy seems both appropriate for a particularly vulnerable person but also likely to provoke chaotic behaviour for a time ('acting out').
(e) For closely (24 hour) supervised medical treatment, for example the in-patient treatment of anorexia nervosa or depression, when a number of closely monitored medical and nursing strategies will be tried.
(f) On the rare occasions when a hospital unit can function as a 'neutral' setting, e.g. holding a young person with conduct problems or school refusal resistant to out-patient work, to see whether the additional treatment and containment enables the family to manage after all. The options, clarified from the time of admission, are either

a return home or a move to a longer term setting which will provide residential education, containment or a therapeutic home.

(g) For long term psychotherapy or milieu therapy. I think this is among the less appropriate uses of a hospital setting for adolescents, except where a psychotherapeutic approach is being attempted for an adolescent with complex problems, e.g. with serious depressive symptoms, borderline personality problems and self-injury or self-neglect. These are often the sort of young people who cannot make the type of personal commitment wanted by many therapeutic schools or communities.

(h) For crisis intervention, or assessment of social or family crises or problems of social behaviour, for which in my view a properly staffed social services setting is more appropriate.

In the last twenty years there has been increasing recognition of the skills of professions other than psychiatry and psychiatric nursing, and it is worth remembering what hospital units can uniquely provide: nursing skills around the clock, with medical care as a major contribution and available on a 24 hour basis. This should be borne in mind in using (and planning, and developing) expensive in-patient psychiatric units for young people.

(14) The therapeutic setting

An adolescent unit will tend to have three main functions, one 'looking outwards' to the family and wider relationships of the adolescents, and two which are part of its residential functioning: *specific treatment programmes* and *an educational and therapeutic milieu.*

The latter is always important; a setting in which boys and girls can share responsibility, develop self-esteem, learn appropriate self- control and assertiveness, develop leisure pursuits and enjoy themselves, and work academically and creatively is as important as good food and other physical necessities. A setting whose environment is nurturing, encouraging, creative and educational is crucial for growing young people whatever their specific problems and treatments, just as a clean atmosphere is an essential complement to surgical operations. One without the other is pointless.

To this extent all clinical units for young people should have a generally therapeutic milieu. However, there are a number of important other residential settings where there may be little emphasis on individual treatment programmes, the milieu as a whole providing the therapy. These will not be discussed in detail here, except to stress their importance for adolescents with emotional and developmental needs that cannot be sufficiently met by their families. Some, such as the Henderson Hospital (Whiteley, 1970; Whiteley 1975) Peperharow (Rose, 1986) are primarily psychotherapeutic centres. Others, such as Shotton Hall (Lampen, 1978) are based on schools. Some, for example those run by the Rudolf Steiner organization or run on the philosophy of Steiner look after young people with chronic mental illness and major handicaps. For accounts of therapeutic communities and their development see the above and Jones (1946, 1968); Main (1946); Bettelheim (1950, 1960); Bettelheim and Sylvester (1952); Martin (1962); Docker-Drysdale (1968); Clark and Yeomans (1969); Clark (1977); and Rapoport (1960).

There are many other special centres, some run by the Health Service, some by Social Services Departments and some run by the private sector which may be organized on behavioural lines (e.g. see Bedford and Tennent 1981). Some use a behavioural or therapeutic milieu within a secure setting (e.g. the Youth Treatment Centres; and see Hoghughi, 1978).

Finally, it is important to note recent developments in adult psychiatry in Italy, where radical legislation has been passed in recent years effectively closing down almost all adult mental hospitals and thereby enforcing care in the community. Because of different arrangements for adolescents there it is not clear what impact this approach has had on young people's psychiatric care. Not surprisingly, many accounts of what has become known as the 'Italian Experience' tend to be for or against it. (See Benaim (1983); Jones and Poletti (1985); Papeschi (1985); Sarteschi *et al.*, (1983).)

(15) Collaborative and liaison work and teamwork

To collaborate means to work together. In liaison work there is collaboration between people, teams, organizations or units the focus of whose work is different: for example, liaison between a psychiatrist and a paediatric department (described by Mrazek, 1985). In teamwork, a group of people often of different disciplines, work together with a shared focus, e.g. in a paediatric team or a psychiatric team.

These ways of working are still developing, with much variation in the way terms are used. I would use the word liaison for any work between different units or departments, and the purpose of this partnership may be clinical work, teaching or research. The clinical work may include holding joint clinics, or an open mutual referral system, or one of the clinicians seeing and advising on the other's patients and perhaps taking over their care. Clearly, anything useful for patients, clinicians, trainees, the department and the speciality is admissible within this joint enterprise. What is important is that there should be clarity and agreement about who is offering what. This is discussed further in section 16, below. I would distinguish between these various ways of working jointly and consultative work as described in Section 16.

Teamwork, and particularly multidisciplinary teamwork, is discussed critically elsewhere (see Parry-Jones, 1986; Steinberg, 1986a). The problems of multidisciplinary teamwork include using incompatible models of care, confusion over roles, and disagreement over decision-making and authority. It can also result in large crowds of people being involved in each young person's case. However, these real problems should be set against the importance in child and adolescent psychiatry of using the skills of different professions, whether collaborating within a team or liaising across agencies. There are young people with complex problems who really do need the involvement of, for example, psychiatrist, nurse, psychologist, occupational therapist, teacher and family worker, while proper study and research in the subject as a whole undoubtedly needs the knowledge and collaboration of these and many other specialist workers.

Some of the issues to be aware of when groups of workers of any discipline work together are:

(a) *The importance of clarifying the aims of the organization.* The use of a common term (e.g. adolescent unit or psychiatric unit) may insubstantially cover up the fact that different members of staff have quite different and perhaps unspoken notions of the organization's aims and methods: e.g. as a clinical service, as a crisis intervention team, as a therapeutic community, etc.

(b) *The importance of clarifying lines of authority,* and in particular how decisions are taken. All accounts of successful units for disturbed young people indicate that firm leadership (sometimes as joint leadership, sometimes with a single person in charge) is important. Despite the fact that much of the business of therapeutic communities takes place by free discussion in a circle, I have never heard of a truly democratic one, which in any case is hard to imagine.

(c) *'Communication'* is often blamed when things do not seem right. What is important is to remember the limitations of people's attention and memory on the one hand, and the general uselessness of memoranda and other sheets of paper except to communicate messages. An organization's communication system is always in need of maintenance and repair, and this regular attention rather than a rigid, perfect system should be the aim. As much as possible of the daily flow of information should be incorporated into working procedures that work. Circulating papers and reports that don't have a clear and immediate usefulness wastes people's time and energy.

(d) If 'communication' is the common scapegoat in teams and organizations, then *'staff support'* is a much sought-after panacea. Probably the least useful form of staff support is anything regarded as a 'staff support group' with its unnecessary connotations of helping along the troubled and the disadvantaged. A hard-working staff group whose focus is making sure everyone knows what's going on, and in particular how other people are thinking and feeling, provides essential information (both 'feeling' and cognitive) for maintenance of the homeostasis needed for people to work properly, which includes enjoying their work. Proper supervision of work done and as generous as possible an academic programme are absolute necessities in this field, not luxuries. Senior staff should make sure that the staff's resources (time, energy, material facilities) match what is expected of them; there are times when it is right for a team or organization to stretch itself, and times when it should say no.

(e) People's *roles* should be clear. A psychiatric registrar should be clear about when he is being the clinical psychiatrist in charge of a patient's medication or offering psychotherapy, and when he is the family therapist. A senior nurse on an in-service course should know when she is in charge of the ward and when she is being a trainee. It should be clear whether a specialist in any discipline is in charge and supervising what is happening, and when he or she is acting in a consultative capacity.

Training issues are discussed in Wilkinson (1986) and Angold (1986). Staff groups are discussed in Skynner (1975) and Foskett (1986).

(f) *Research* is quite often regarded as too big and too complicated for most people to undertake. Large-scale research is certainly complex and time-consuming, but it should be within the interests and reach of most people in adolescent psychiatry to approach their work in a spirit of curiosity and enquiry and to undertake at least small projects and studies and present them and write them up for the information of others. Nursing staff in particular develop vast funds of experience and expertise but are often not encouraged or even allowed to do very much with it in this respect.

(16) Consultative work

In section 15, above, a distinction was made between the various forms of collaborative work and *consultative work*, or *consultation*. This distinction is worth preserving because of the special characteristics of consultation as a general technique.

In essence, consultation refers to one professional worker (the consultant) helping another (the consultee) to manage his or her own work. The consultant, as the term is used here, does not take over responsibility for the consultee's patient or client. Thus it is quite unlike what happens when, for example a consultant psychiatrist takes over from a paediatrician the care of an adolescent who has taken an overdose of drugs.

Why should this approach be useful? First, the problems that emerge in the broad field of child health, care and education are not clearly within the province of one particular profession. It would not be feasible, for example, for every child with an emotional problem to be referred to a psychotherapist, every psychiatrically disturbed child to see a psychiatrist, every conduct-disordered child to be seen by a behavioural psychologist and so on. It would not even make sense, because many of these problems are each also within the field of work of teachers, child care workers, family doctors, paediatricians, social workers and others.

When a specialist acts in a consultative capacity he is achieving a number of quite important things: first, the care of the adolescent or family remains with the person who was first involved, and probably knows the situation best. Second, a re- referral to a new person in a new place is avoided. Third, since the aim of consultation is to help mobilize the consultee's own skills and resources – acting as it were as a reminder and facilitator of what he or she in fact can do – the consultee is left in a better position to deal with similar problems in the future. Consultation, therefore, is not only a joint problem- solving exercise but one that should also assist towards the consultee's own skills.

Example 23

A psychiatrist is asked to offer an urgent appointment for a girl in a Children's Home. She is described as being very depressed, is crying a lot, won't attend school or take part in the home's routine, and won't talk to the staff, who are becoming extremely anxious about her. In taking the referral the psychiatrist becomes very aware of the girl's apparent distress and the anxiety of the staff, but it is not clear that there is a psychiatric problem. He suggests meeting the staff instead, and in particular those who know her best and have most responsibility for her and who are anxious about her.

This stage of consultation – identifying whom to meet – is important. For example, it emerges that the head of the home can't get to the first appointment offered; so a new time is made when he can be there.

During the consultation a number of issues are clarified. First, some changes in the staffing and rota arrangements in the children's home have resulted in some distancing between the girl and a member of staff she has always confided in. Second, there have been differences of opinion between staff within the home and outside in the Department of Social Services about whether this home was the right place for her; she was 'sent in', it emerged, without the usual preparatory procedures. Why? Because the head of the home was on leave at the time. The head of the home says that he has always felt a certain amount of resentment about the way this girl was forced on the home. The staff agree that the way their usual approach was by-passed has resulted in some unintended disadvantages for the girl, e.g. the counselling work with her happens not to have had the close attention the head of the home usually offers. The home has always operated its counselling on an informal rather than sessional basis, and this is readily disrupted by changes in staff timetables. But the home is very understaffed, and they could not possibly arrange for more systematic counselling and supervision.

What consultation demonstrates – and it is as much pointed out by the head of the home and by his colleagues as the 'discovery' of the consultant – is that the girl's problems are well within the competence of the children's home team, but a number of personal, inter-professional and organizational issues have got in the way of their working in their usual skilled way. The problems are not for the most part major ones, although the chronic understaffing has been an important factor in making their work vulnerable. The group learn quite a lot from the discussion about how they might usefully look again not only at their work with this girl, but with the other children too. The meeting is consultative, not decision-making: this is for a policy meeting they have once a month, at which they meet members of the local authority department. As a result of the consultative meeting the head of the home has a number of items for the policy meeting agenda, and the staff have some new and useful ideas about their work in general, and about the girl in particular.

The above example demonstrates a number of quite common developments in consultative work, although they are not usually so straightforward nor resolved in one meeting. Note that the focus of the work may be on the behaviour and attitudes of the staff (*consultee-centred* work), on the organization and resources of the setting (*work-centred*) or on the girl (*client-centred*). Correspondingly, the issues that emerge for the consultant and consultees to work with may be to do with the group's social dynamics, the Home's social dynamics, the relationships between staff, and between staff and children, and with the local politics of organization and administration. Moreover, the focus can change during a period of work (Steinberg and Hughes, 1987). The consultant and consultees need to make sure that the work does indeed stay consultative, and not stray into other tempting areas such as psychotherapy or politics; treading this narrow path can be quite difficult. It follows that it is also important to ensure that the consultant's role is understood and agreed: he or she is not a clinician or a supervisor or psychotherapist for this particular work, but a consultant, used in this special sense.

Consultative work may be undertaken as an *ad hoc* response to a particular referral, as in the above example, or on a regular basis with an individual or a group. The focus of its work can be regularly client-centred, or it may be work-focussed, thereby operating as a forum for staff or unit development. Although it has its rules, it is also important that it operates pragmatically and adaptably.

Caplan's two key works (1964, 1970) are important pioneering accounts of consultative work as described here. Work in relation to child and adolescent psychiatry and psychology in various settings is described by Gallessich (1982), Conoley (1981), Conoley and Conoley (1982) and Steinberg and Yule (1985). The consultative approach from a wider perspective and as a potential major influence in psychiatry and related fields is described in Steinberg (1988).

Concluding note

It is appropriate for a book on adolescent psychiatry to end with the above notes on consultation. A recurring theme in the earlier chapters was the breadth of the subject and the enormous range of problems which the practitioner comes across in his or her day-to-day work. One set of questions is about who has the skills for a particular problem. Another set of questions concerns who should have the authority and responsibility to attend to all the problems inherent in human growth, health, education and relationships. It is with these questions that we need to think not only of what psychiatry, say, has to offer compared with psychology, but of the contribution of clinical workers compared with that of all the others who work with young people: teachers, careers specialists, employers and trainers, youth workers, ministers of religion, among many others. We have also to consider how much should be up to people working in these various ways, and how much is up to the adolescent and the family. The consultative approach, with its careful attention to clarifying what is your problem, what is my problem and what is someone else's problem, provides one way into the complex question of who should be doing what for whom, an issue which is never far away in psychiatry and in the care of children and adolescents.

References and further reading

Abramowitz, C. (1976) The effectiveness of group psychotherapy with children. *Archives of General Psychiatry* **33**, 320–6.

Adams, P. (1973) *Obsessive Children: A Sociopsychiatric Study*. London: Butterworth.

Angold, A. (1986) Trainees in the multidisciplinary team: a worm's eye view. *In* Steinberg, D. (Ed), *The Adolescent Unit*, pp 201–8. Chichester: John Wiley and Sons.

Ballard, M. and Yule, W. (1981) A case of separation anxiety treated by *in vivo* systematic desensitisation. *Behavioural Psychotherapy* **9**, 106–10.

Bancroft, J. (1979) Crisis intervention. *In* Bloch, S. (Ed), *Introduction to the Psychotherapies*. Oxford: Oxford University Press.

Barker, P. (1986) *Basic Family Therapy*. Second edition. London: Collins Professional Books.

Bedford, A. and Tennent, T. (1981) Behaviour training with disturbed adolescents. *News of the Association for Child Psychology and Psychiatry* **7**, 6–12.

Benaim, S. (1983) The Italian Experiment. *Bulletin of the Royal College of Psychiatrists*, January, 7–10.

Bentovim, A., Gorell Barnes, G. and Cooklin, A. (1982) *Family Therapy: Complementary Frameworks of Theory and Practice*. London: Academic Press.

Berkowitz, I. (1972) *Adolescents Grow in Groups: Experiences in Adolescent Group Psychotherapy*. New York: Brunner Mazel.

Bettelheim, B. (1950) *Love is Not Enough*. Illinois: The Free Press.

Bettelheim, B. (1960) *The Informed Heart*. New York: The Free Press.

Bettelheim, B. and Sylvester, E. (1952) A therapeutic milieu. *American Journal of Orthopsychiatry* **22**, 314–34.

Birch, N. (1979) Bone side-effects of lithium. *In* Johnson, F. (Ed), *A Handbook of Lithium Therapy*. Lancaster: MTP.

Bloch, S. (1986) *Introduction to the Psychotherapies* Second Edition. Oxford: Oxford University Press.

Bolton, D., Collins, S. and Steinberg, D. (1983) The treatment of obsessive-compulsive disorder in adolescence: a report of 15 cases. *British Journal of Psychiatry* **142**, 456–64.

Brown, B. and Christie, M. (1981) *Social Learning Practice in Residential Child Care*. Oxford: Pergamon Press.

Brown, D. and Pedder, J. (1979) *Introduction to Psychotherapy*. London: Tavistock.

Bruce, T. (1975) Adolescent psychotherapy groups. *Therapeutic Education* **3**, 38–42.

Bruce. T. (1978) Group work with adolescents. *Journal of Adolescence* **1**, 47–54.

Bruggen, P. (1979) Authority in work with young adolescents: a personal review. *Journal of Adolescence* **2**, 345–54.

Bruggen, P., Byng-Hall, J. and Pitt-Aikens, T. (1973) The reason for admission as a focus of work in an adolescent unit. *British Journal of Psychiatry* **122**, 319–29.

Bruggen, P. and Davies, G. (1977) Family therapy in adolescent psychiatry. *British Journal of Psychiatry* **131**, 433–47.

Bruggen, P. and Westland, P. (1979) Difficult to place adolescents: are more resources required? *Journal of Adolescence* **2**, 245–50.

Brumback, R. and Weinberg, W. (1977) Mania in childhood, II: therapeutic trial of lithium carbonate and further description of manic depressive illness in children. *American Journal of Diseases of Children* **131**, 112–6.

Campbell, M., Cohen, I. and Small, A. (1982) Drugs in aggressive behaviour. *Journal of the American Academy of Child Psychiatry*, **21**, 107–17.

Caplan, G. (1961) *An Approach to Community Mental Health*. London: Tavistock.

Caplan, G. (1964) *Principles of Preventive Psychiatry*. London: Tavistock.

Caplan, G. (1970) *The Theory and Practice of Mental Health Consultation*. London: Tavistock.

Cawley, R.H. (1977). The teaching of psychotherapy. *Association of University Teachers of Psychiatry Newsletter*, January, 19–36.

Clark, D. (1977) The therapeutic community. *British Journal of Psychiatry* **13**, 553–64.

Clark, A. and Yeomans, N. (1969) *Fraser House: Theory, Practice and Evolution of a Therapeutic Community*. New York: Springer-Verlag.

Cohen, W. and Cohen, N. (1974) Lithium carbonate, haloperidol and irreversible brain damage. *Journal of the American Medical Association* **230**, 1283–7.

Conoley, J. (Ed) (1981) *Consultation in Schools: Theory, Research, Procedures*. New York: Academic Press.

Conoley, J. and Conoley, C. (1982) *School Consultation: A Guide to Practice and Training*. New York: Pergamon Press.

Coppen, A., Noguera, R., Bailey, J., Burns, B., Swani, M., Hare, E., Gardner, R. and Maggs, R. (1971) Prophylactic lithium in affective disorders: a controlled trial. *Lancet* **i**, 275–9.

Corbett, J. (1975) Aversion for the treatment of self-injurious behaviour. *Journal of Mental Deficiency Research* **19**, 79–95.

Dalley, T. (1984) *Art as Therapy*. London: Tavistock.

Dare, C. (1985) Family therapy. *In* Rutter, M. and Hersov, L. (Eds), *Child and Adolescent Psychiatry: Modern Approaches*, pp 809–25. Oxford: Blackwell Scientific Publications.

Dare, C. (1986) Family therapy and an adolescent in-patient unit. *In* Steinberg, D. (Ed), *The Adolescent Unit*, pp 83–95. Chichester: John Wiley and Sons.

De Long, G. (1978) Lithium carbonate treatment of selective behaviour disorders in children suggesting manic-depressive illness. *Journal of Pediatrics* **93**, 689–94.

Docker-Drysdale, B. (1968) Residential treatment of 'frozen' children. *In* Docker-Drysdale, B., *Therapy in Child Care*. London: Longman Green.

Dostal, T. and Zvolsky, P. (1970) Anti-aggressive effect of lithium salts in severely mentally retarded adolescents. *International Pharmacopsychiatry* **5**, 203–7.

Dunne, C., Bruggen P. and O'Brian C. (1982) Touch and action in group therapy of younger adolescents. *Journal of Adolescence* **5**, 31–8.

Foskett, J. (1984) *Meaning in Madness*. London: SPCK.

Foskett, J. (1986) The Staff Group. *In Steinberg, D. (Ed), The Adolescent Unit*, pp 169–78. Chichester: John Wiley and Sons.

Frank, M. and Zilbach, J. (1968) Current trends in group therapy with children. *International Journal of Group Psychotherapy* **18**, 447–60.

Freud, A. (1966) *Normality and Pathology in Childhood*. London: Hogarth Press.

Gallessich, J. (1982) *The Profession and Practice of Consultation: A Handbook for Consultants, Trainers of Consultants and Consumers of Consultation Services*. London: Jossey-Bass.

Garfield, S. (1980) *Psychotherapy: An Eclectic Approach*. Chichester: John Wiley and Sons.

Garralda, H.E. (1980) Trainees' attitudes in child psychiatry. *Bulletin of the Royal College of Psychiatrists* February, 26–7.

Gittelman-Klein, R. and Klein, D. (1971) Controlled imipramine treatment of school phobia. *Archives of General Psychiatry* **25**, 204–7.

Gorell Barnes, G. (1985) Systems theory and family theory. *In* Rutter, M. and Hersov, L. (Eds), *Child and Adolescent Psychiatry: Modern Approaches*, pp 216–29. Oxford: Blackwell Scientific Publications.

Haley, J. (1973) *Uncommon Therapy: The Psychiatric Technique of Milton H. Erickson, MD*. New York: W.W. Norton.

Haley, J. (1976) *Problem-Solving Therapy*. San Fransisco: Jossey- Bass.

Heacock, D. (1980) *A Psychodynamic Approach to Adolescent Psychiatry*. New York: Marcel Dekker.

Hoghughi, M. (1978) *Troubled and Troublesome: Coping with Severely Disordered Children*. London: Andre Deutsch.

Homme, L., Casanyi, A., Gonzales, M. and Reichs, J. (1970) *How to Use*

Contingency Contracting in the Classroom. Champaign, Illinois: Research Press.

Horowitz, H. (1977) Lithium and the treatment of adolescent manic-depressive illness. *Diseases of the Nervous System* **38**, 480–3.

Howlin, P., Marchant, R., Rutter, M., Berger, M., Hersov, L. and Yule, W. (1973) A home-based approach to the treatment of autistic children. *Journal of Autism and Childhood Schizophrenia* **3**, 308–336.

Howlin, P. (1985) Special Educational Treatment. *In* Rutter, M. and Hersov, L. (Eds), *Child and Adolescent Psychiatry: Modern Approaches*, pp 851–70. Oxford: Blackwell Scientific Publications.

Jennings, S. (1985) *Creative Therapy*. Banbury: Kemble Press.

Jennings, S. (1986) *Creative Drama in Group Work*. London: Winslow Press.

Jones, K. and Poletti, A. (1985) Understanding the Italian Experience. *British Journal of Psychiatry* **146**, 341–7.

Jones, M. (1946) Rehabilitation of Forces neurosis patients to civilian life. *British Medical Journal* **1**, 533–5.

Jones, M. (1968) *Social Psychiatry in Practice: The Idea of the Therapeutic Community*. Harmondsworth: Penguin Books.

Kendell, R. (1981) The present status of electroconvulsive therapy. *British Journal of Psychiatry* **139**, 265–83.

Kessler, E. (1979) Individual psychotherapy with adolescents. *In* Novello, J. (Ed), *The Short Course in Adolescent Psychiatry*. New York: Brunner Mazel.

Kondas, O. (1967) Reducton of examination anxiety and 'stage fright' by group desensitization and relaxation. *Behaviour Research and Therapy* **5**, 275–81.

Kraft, I. (1968) An overview of group therapy with adolescents. *International Journal of Group Psychotherapy* **18**, 461–80.

Lampen, J. (1978) Drest in a little brief authority: controls in residential work with adolescents. *Journal of Adolescence* **1**, 163–75.

Loudon, J. and Waring, H. (1976) Toxic reactions to lithium and haloperidol. *Lancet* **ii** 1088.

Lucas, A and Pasley, F. (1969) Psychoactive drugs in the treatment of emotionally disturbed children: haloperidol and diazepam. *Comprehensive Psychiatry* **10**, 376–86.

Main, T. (1946) The hospital as a therapeutic institution. *Bulletin of the Menninger Clinic* **10**, 66–70.

Malan, D. (1963) *A Study of Brief Psychotherapy*. London: Tavistock.

Marks, I., Stern, R., Mawson, D., Cobb, J. and MacDonald, R. (1980) Clomipramine and exposure for obsessive-compulsive rituals. *British Journal of Psychiatry* **136**, 1–25.

Marsden, C.D. and Jenner, R. (1980) Pathophysiology of extrapyramidal side-effects of neuroleptic drugs. *Psychological Medicine* **10**, 55–72.

Martin, D. (1962) *Adventure in Psychiatry: Social Change in a Mental Hospital.* Oxford: Bruno Cassier.

Masterson, J. and Costello, J. (1980) *From Borderline Adolescent to Functioning Adult: The Test of Time.* New York: Brunner Mazel.

McAdam, E. (1986) Cognitive behaviour therapy and its application with adolescents. *Journal of Adolescence* **9**, 1–15.

Medical Research Council Drug Trials Subcommittee (1981) Continuation therapy with lithium and amitriptyline in unipolar depressive illness: a controlled clinical trial. *Psychological Medicine* **11**, 409–16.

Meeks, J. (1974) Adolescent development and group cohesion. *In* Feinstein, S. and Giovacchini, P., *Adolescent Psychiatry Volume III.* New York: Basic Books.

Merry, J. (1986) Art in the education of the disturbed adolescent. *In* Steinberg, D. (Ed), *The Adolescent Unit,* pp 43–51. Chichester: John Wiley and Sons.

Milham, S. (1981) The therapeutic implications of locking up children. *Journal of Adolescence* **4**, 13–26.

Milham, S., Bullock, R. and Hosie, K. (1978) *Locking Up Children: Secure Provision within the Child Care System.* Farnborough: Saxon House.

Minuchin, S., Rosman, B. and Baker, L. (1980) *Psychosomatic Families: Anorexia Nervosa in Context.* Cambridge, Massachusetts: Harvard University Press.

Mrazek, D. (1985) Child psychiatric consultation and liaison to paediatrics. *In* Rutter, M. and Hersov, L. (Eds), *Child and Adolescent Psychiatry: Modern Approaches,* pp 888–99. Oxford: Blackwell Scientific Publications.

Newsome, A., Thorne, B. and Wyld, K. (1975) *Student Counselling in Practice.* London: University of London Press.

Page, D. (1986) Music in the education of the disturbed adolescent. *In* Steinberg, D. (Ed), *The Adolescent Unit,* pp 35–42. Chichester: John Wiley and Sons.

Papeschi, R. (1985) The denial of the institution: a critical review of Franco Basaglia's writings. *British Journal of Psychiatry* **146**, 247–54.

Parry-Jones, W.L. (1986) Multidisciplinary teamwork: help or hindrance? *In* Steinberg, D. (Ed), *The Adolescent Unit* pp 193–200. Chichester: John Wiley and Sons.

Perinpanayagam, K. (1978) Dynamic approach to adolescence: treatment. *British Medical Journal* **1**, 563–6.

Petti, T. and Conners, C. (1983) Changes in behavioural ratings of depressed children treated with imipramine. *Journal of the American Academy of Child Psychiatry* **22**, 355–60.

Rachman, S. (1972) Clinical applications of observational learning, imitation and modelling. *Behaviour Therapy* **3**, 379–97.

Rapoport, R. (1970) *Community as Doctor: New Perspectives on a Therapeutic Community*. London: Tavistock.

Remschmidt, H. (1976) The psychotropic effect of carbamazepine in non-epileptic patients. *In* Birkmayer, W. (Ed), *Epileptic Seizures – Behaviour – Pain*. Berne: Hans Huber.

Rogers, C. (1951) *Client-Centered Therapy*. Boston, Massachusetts: Houghton, Mifflin Co.

Rose, M. (1986) The design of atmosphere: ego-nurture and psychic change in residential treatment. *Journal of Adolescence* **9**, 49–62.

Royal College of Psychiatrists (1977) Memorandum on the use of electroconvulsive therapy. *British Journal of Psychiatry* **131** 261–72.

Safer, D. and Allen, R. (1973) Factors influencing the suppressant effect of two stimulant drugs on the growth of hyperactive children. *Paediatrics* **51**, 660–7.

Safer, D., Allen R. and Barr, E. (1975) Growth rebound after termination of stimulant drugs. *Journal of Paediatrics* **86**, 113–16.

Salzman, C., Kochansky, G., Shader, R., Porrino, L., Harmatz, J. and Swett, C. (1974) Chlordiazepoxide-induced hostility in a small group setting. *Archives of General Psychiatry* **31**, 401–5.

Sarteschi, P., Cassano, G., Mauri, M. and Petracca, A. (1983) Current status of psychiatric care in Italy. *In Psychiatry, Human Rights and the Law*. Cambridge: Cambridge University Press.

Selvini-Palazzoli, M., Boscolo, L., Cecchin, G. and Prata, G. (1978) *Paradox and Counter-Paradox*. New York: Aronson.

Selvini-Palazzoli, M., Boscolo, L., Cecchin, G. and Prata, G. (1980) Hypothesising circularity-neutrality: three guidelines for the conductor of the session. *Family Process* **19**, 3–12.

Selvini-Palazzoli, M. (1970) The families of patients with anorexia nervosa. *In* Anthony, E. and Koupernick, C. (Eds), *The Child in His Family, Volume 1*, pp 319–32. Chichester: John Wiley and Sons.

Selvini-Palazzoli, M. (1974) *Self Starvation*. London: Human Context Books.

Shaffer, D., Stephenson, J. and Thomas, D. (1979) Some effects of imipramine on micturition and their relevance to its antienuretic activity. *Neuropharmacology* **18**, 33–7.

Sherman, L., Kim, S., Benjamin, F. and Kolodny, H. (1971) Effects of chlorpromazine on serum growth hormone concentration in man. *New England Journal of Medicine* **284**, 72–74.

Skynner, R. (1975) The large group in training. *In* Kreeger, L. (Ed), *The Large Group* pp 227–51. London: Constable.

Skynner, R. and Cleese, J. (1984) *Families and How to Survive Them*. London: Methuen.

Skynner, R. (1976) One Flesh — Separate Persons. London: Constable.

Stein, G., Hartshorn, S., Jones, J. and Steinberg, D. (1982) Lithium in a case of severe anorexia nervosa. *British Journal of Psychiatry*, 140, 526–528.

Steinberg, D. (1980) The use of lithium carbonate in adolescence. *Journal of Child Psychology and Psychiatry* 21, 263–71.

Steinberg, D. (1981) *Using Child Psychiatry*. London: Hodder and Stoughton.

Steinberg, D. (1982) Treatment, training, care or control? The functions of adolescent units. *British Journal of Psychiatry* 141, 306–9.

Steinberg, D. (1983) *The Clinical Psychiatry of Adolescence* Chichester: John Wiley.

Steinberg, D. (1985) Psychotic and other severe disorders in adolescence. *In* Rutter, M. and Hersov, L. (Eds), *Child and Adolescent Psychiatry: Modern Approaches*, pp 567–83. Oxford: Blackwell Scientific Publications.

Steinberg, D. (1986a) Developments in a psychiatric service for adolescents. *In* Steinberg, D. (Ed), *The Adolescent Unit: Work and Teamwork in Adolescent Psychiatry*, pp 209–21. Chichester: John Wiley and Sons.

Steinberg, D. (1986b) (Ed), *The Adolescent Unit: Work and Teamwork in Adolescent Psychiatry*. Chichester: John Wiley and Sons.

Steinberg, D. (1986c) Psychiatric aspects of problem behaviour in schools: a consultative approach. *In* Tattum, D (Ed), *Management of Disruptive Pupil Behaviour in Schools*, pp 187–205. Chichester: John Wiley and Sons.

Steinberg, D. (1987a) Emergencies in adolescent psychiatry. *Practical Reviews in Psychiatry*, series 2, no. 4.

Steinberg, D. (1987b) Innovation in an adolescent unit: the introduction of small group work. *In* Coleman, J. (Ed), *Working with Troubled Adolescents: A Handbook*. London: Academic Press.

Steinberg, D. (1987c) Management of crises and emergencies. *In* Hsu, L.K.G. and Hersen, M. (Eds), *Recent Developments in Adolescent Psychiatry*. New York: John Wiley and Sons.

Steinberg, D., Bailey, A. and Simanoff, E. (1988) Physical disorders among adolescent psychiatric in-patients. In preparation.

Steinberg, D. (1988) *Interprofessional Consultation*. (In preparation.) Oxford: Blackwell Scientific Publications.

Steinberg, D. and Hughes, L., (1987) The emergence of work-centred problems in consultative work. *Journal of Adolescence* 10, 309–16.

Steinberg, D., Galhenage, D.P.C. and Robinson, S.C. (1981) Two years' referrals to a regional adolescent unit: some implications for psychiatric services. *Social Science and Medicine* 15E, 113–22.

Steinberg, D., Merry, J. and Collins, S., (1978) The introduction of small group work to an adolescent unit. *Journal of Adolescence* 1, 331–44.

Steinberg, D. and Yule, W., (1985) Consultative Work. *In* Rutter, M. and Hersov, L. (Eds), *Child and Adolescent Psychiatry: Modern Approaches*, pp 914–26. Oxford: Blackwell Scientific Publications.

Stores, G. (1975) Behavioural effects of anti- epileptic drugs. *Developmental Medicine and Child Neurology* **17**, 647–58.

Stores, G. (1978) Anticonvulsants. *In* Werry, J. (Ed), *Paediatric Psychopharmacology: the use of behaviour modifying drugs in children*. New York: Brunner Mazel.

Tattum, D. (1986) *Management of Disruptive Pupil Behaviour in Schools*. Chichester: John Wiley and Sons.

Taylor, D. (1985) Psychological aspects of chronic sickness. *In* Rutter, M. and Hersov, L. (Eds), *Child and Adolescent Psychiatry: Modern Approaches*, pp 614–24. Oxford: Blackwell Scientific Publications.

Taylor, E. (1979) Food additives, allergy and hyperkinesis. *Journal of Child Psychology and Psychiatry* **20**, 357–63.

Taylor, E. (1985) Drug treatment. *In* Rutter, M. and Hersov, L. (Eds), *Child and Adolescent Psychiatry: Modern Approaches*, pp 780–93. Oxford: Blackwell Scientific Publications.

Tharp, R. and Wetzel R. (1969) *Behaviour Modification in the Natural Environment*. London: Academic Press.

Thomas, C. (1979) Brain damage with lithium and haloperidol. *British Journal of Psychiatry* **134**, 552.

Topping, K. (1986) Consultative enhancement of school-based action. *In* Tattum, D. (Ed), *Management of Disruptive Pupil Behaviour in Schools*, pp 31–50. Chichester: John Wiley and Sons.

von Bertalanffy, L. (1986) *General Systems Theory*. New York: George Brazillier.

Waller, D. (1984) A consideration of the similarities and differences between art teaching and art therapy. *In* Dalley, T. (Ed), *Art As Therapy*, pp 1–14. London: Tavistock.

Waller, D. and Gilroy, A. (1986) Art Therapy in Practice. *In* Steinberg, D. (Ed), *The Adolescent Unit*, pp 53–63. Chichester: John Wiley.

Walrond—Skinner, S. (1976) *Family Therapy – the treatment of natural systems*. London: Routledge and Kegan Paul.

Walrond-Skinner, S. (1978) Indications and contra- indications for the use of family therapy. *Journal of Child Psychology and Psychiatry* **19**, 57–62.

Warren, B. (1984) (Ed) *Using the creative arts in therapy*. London: Croom Helm.

Weisberg, P. (1979) Group therapy with adolescents. *In* Novello, J. (Ed), *The Short Course in Adolescent Psychiatry*, pp 172–84. New York: Brunner Mazel.

Whiteley, J. (1970) The response of psychopaths to a therapeutic community. *British Journal of Psychiatry* **116**, 517–29.

Whiteley, J. (1975) The large group as a medium for sociotherapy. *In* Kreeger, L. (Ed), *The Large Group: Dynamics and Therapy*. London: Constable.

Wilkinson, T. (1986) Education for nurses: support, supervision, training. In Steinberg, D. (ed) *The Adolescent Unit* pp 155–67. Chichester: John Wiley.

Wilson, P. (1986) Individual psychotherapy in a residential setting. *In* Steinberg, D., *The Adolescent Unit*, pp 97–111. Chichester: Wiley.

Wilson, P. and Hersov, L. (1985) Individual and group psychotherapy. *In* Rutter, M. and Hersov, L. (Eds) *Child and Adolescent Psychiatry: Modern Approaches*, pp 826–838. Oxford: Blackwell Scientific Publications.

Winnicott, D. (1971) Contemporary concepts of adolescent development and their implications for higher education. *In* Winnicott, D., *Playing and Reality*. London: Tavistock.

Wynn, B. (1986) Creative Therapy. *In* Steinberg, D. (Ed), *The Adolescent Unit, pp 73–82*. Chichester: John Wiley.

Youngerman, J. and Canino, I. (1978) Lithium carbonate use in children and adolescents. *Archives of General Psychiatry* **35**, 216–24.

Yule, W. (1985) Behavioural Approaches. *In* Rutter, M. and Hersov, L. (eds), *Child and Adolescent Psychiatry: Modern Approaches*, pp 794–808. Oxford: Blackwell Scientific Publications.

Zrull, J., Westman, J., Arthur, B. and Rice, D. (1964) A comparison of diazepam, d-amphetamine and placebo in the treatment of the hyperkinetic syndrome in children. *American Journal of Psychiatry* **120, 590**-1.

Index

Aarkrog, T., 174
Abramowitz, C., 249
Accident proneness, 116, 205
Ackner, B., 94, 95
Acquired Immune Deficiency
    Syndrome (AIDS), 11, 142, 243
Acton, W., 24
Adams, P., 96, 229
Addison-Schilder's disease, 208
Adjustment reaction, 102
  in management, 103
Admission to hospital, 221–3, 253–4
Adolescence, 1–16
Adolescent services, 25–6, 252–5
Adoption, 41
Aetiology, see Causes of disorder
Affective illness, see Depressive
    disorders
Age difference, 1–3, 9, 54
Agras, S., 155
Agras, W., 93
Akisal, H., 198
Albert, N., 103
Alcohol, 141, 145–6
  Example 9, 145, 244
Allen, R., 241
Amitriptyline, 236–7, 263–4
Amphetamine, 142
Amphetamine-like drugs, 120, 236–7,
    241
Amphetamine psychology, 142
Angold, A., 257
Anorexia Nervosa, 151–4
  in boys, 151–3, 208
  incidence, 152–3
  management, 154–6
Anticonvulsant drugs, 241
Anthony, E., 127, 196
Antidepressants, tricyclic, 126,
    195–6, 236–7, 241
Antipsychotic drugs, 120, 200,
    239–41
Anxiety states, 92–4
  management, 93–4
Aries, P., 27
Art education, 232

Art therapy, 231–2
Arson, see Fire setting
Asperger's syndrome, see Autistic
    psychopathy
Aspirin, 92
Assessment, see Clinical assessment
Association for Child Psychology &
    Psychiatry, 25
Association for the Psychiatric Study
    of Adolescence, 25
Attachment, 36–7
Attempted suicide, Example 2, 84–5,
    90–91 and see Suicide
Attention deficit disorder, 115 and see
    Hyperactivity
Attitudes, adolescents', 44
Authority, 58, 89, 218–19, and
    Example 17, 218
Autism, 40, 80, 165–9
  compared with other disorders,
    166–7
  description, 166–7
  in adolescence, 167–8
  management, 168–9
  prevalence, 167
Autistic psychopathy, 165, 169–71
  Example 11, 169–71
  management, 172

Bancroft, J., 223
Barbiturates, 143–4, 210
Barker, P., 12, 27, 235
Bass, M., 147
Bateson, G., 184
Bearn, A., 207
Beck, A., 103
Bedford, A., 24, 255
Bed-wetting, see Eneuresis
Beech House, 23
Beginning clinical work, 217
Behaviour disorder, 112 and see
    Conduct disorder
Behaviour, parental, 38–40
  Example 17, 218.
  therapies, 244–8
  systematic approach 244–5

Bell, D., 131
Bell and pad, 126
Bellman, M., 127
Belson, W., 44
Benaim, S., 100, 255
Benes, F., 184
Bentovim, A., 126
Benzodiazepines, 89, 94, 143–4,
   236–7, 240
Bereavement, 37
Berger, M., 35
Berkowitz, I., 249
Berney, T., 89
Bethlem Royal Hospital, 23, 61
Bettelheim, B., 255
Beumont, P., 153
Beveridge Report, 24
Birch, N., 242
Birley, J., 185
Blakar, R., 40, 185
Bleuler, E., 180
Bleuler,M., 186
Blindness, 211
Bliss, J., 163
Bloch, S., 229
Blos, P., 4, 11
Bolthauser, E., 208
Bolton, D., 96, 97, 247
Bond, M., 100
Borderline disorder, 40, 173–5
  personality, Example 12, 173
  management 175
Boston Habit Clinic, 22, 24
Bottomley, V., 207
Bowlby, J., 36, 105
Brain damage, 34
Brayman, A., 90
Brett, E., 35, 208
Bridges over troubled waters, see
  Health Advisory Service Report
Brittain, C., 38
Brockington, I., 186
Brody, S., 44
Brook, C., 156
Brooke, E., 90
Brown, D., 8, 223, 229
Brown, G., 37, 185
Brown, J., 5
Brown, P., 144
Bruce, T., 249
Bruch, H., 153, 156
Bruggen, P., 11, 21, 24, 219, 223, 253
Brumback, R., 241
Bulimia nervosa, 154
  management, 154–6

Caffeine, 143
Campbell, M., 198, 241, 242
Campos, J., 36
Canino, I., 198, 241
Cannabis, 144–5
Canning, H., 156
Cantwell, D., 116
Caplan, G., 223
Caplan, H., 99, 260
Carbamazepine, 241
Care and control, parental, 38–9
Care order, 223
Carlson, G., 195, 196, 198
Carpenter, W., 180
Case presentation, outline, 71–2
Causes of disorder, 30–49, 71
Cawley, R., 224, 225
Cheetham, J., 135
Chess, S., 93
Chicago Juvenile Psychiatric Clinic, 24
Chick, J., 171
Chilman, C., 11
Chisholm, D., 156
Chlordiazepoxide, 236–7, 240
Chlorpromazine, 187, 239–40
Christie Brown, J., 58, 131, 133
Chromosomes, 33–4
Chronic illness, 187, 188, 208, 211,
  212
Cigarette smoking, 143, 147, 243
Clark, A., 255
Classification, 50–56
  multi-axial, 51–52
Cleese, J., 12, 235
Clinical assessment, 57–72, 91,
  104–5, 195
Clomipramine, 97, 236–7, 241
Cobb, J., 95
Coca-Cola, 142
Cocaine, 141, 142
Cognitive therapy, 225
Coleman, J., 13, 38, 82
Collaborative work, 255–7
Compulsory treatment, see Mental
  Health Act
Conduct disorders, 111–23
  causes, 116–17
  classification, 112
  definition, 112, 113
  Example 5, 17, 111–12, 218
  management, 119–21
Confidentiality, 59, 251
Conger, J., 38
Connell, P., 142, 163
Conoley, C., 260

Conoley, J., 260
Connors, C., 241
Consent, age of, 135, 219–20, see also
    Authority
Consultation, 19
Consultative work, 258–60
    Example 23, 258–9
Contraceptives, 135
Coppen, A., 241
Coprolalia, 162
Copropraxia, 162
Corbett, J., 98, 99, 162, 163, 167, 210
Costello, J., 229
Counselling, 223–9
    Example 20, 227
    types, 223–4
Court reports, 251
Courts, 120
Cox, A., 39
Creative therapies, 229–32
Criminal behaviour, adolescent see
    Delinquency
    parental, 39–40
Crises, 223 and see Emergency
    intervention
Crisis, definitions, 8
Crisp, A., 151, 152, 153
Cross, L., 186
Culver, K., 119
Cystic fibrosis, 210–11

Dalley, T., 232
Dare, C., 12, 13, 153, 155, 232, 234,
    235
Davies, G., 11, 235
Davison, K., 196
Deafness, 211
Death, 208 and see Suicide;
    Attempted suicide
    parental, 37
Dehydration, 244
Delamater, A., 101
Delinquency, 9, 39–40, 54, 111–23
    definiton, 112
    management, 119–21
    statistics, 117
de Mause, L., 27
Dependance on drugs, see Drug
    misuse
Depersonalisation, 94–5
    management, 95
Depot medication, 187
Depression,
    assessment of, 104–5

in children and adults 194–5
'atypical', 104–5, 194–5
'endogenous', 103, 193
management, 106, 199–200
medication in, 195–6
'reactive', 103–7
Depressive disorders, 85, 103–6,
    192–203
    equivalents, 104–5
Desensitisation, 246
Detention centres, 252
Developmental concepts, 32, 79–80
    disorders, definition, 79–80
    pervasive, 165, 186
Development emotional, 4–6
Dewhurst, K., 144
Deykin, E., 168
Diabetes mellitus, 154, 209
Diagnoses, frequency of, 53, 253
Diagnosis, clinical, 31, 53, 71 and see
    Clinical assessment
Diagnostic and Statistical Manual
    (DSM), 8, 50
Diazepam, 236–7, 240
Diet in Anorexia nervosa, 151
    hyperactivity, 116, 243
Diet in obesity, 156
'Disclosure', 137
Divorce, 134 and see Family factors
Docker-Drysdale, D., 255
Done, A., 146
Dostal, T., 198, 241
Dramatherapy, see Creative therapies
Drug abuse WHO definitions, 140
    definition of, 141
    misuse, 140–50, 173
Drugs of abuse, classification of, 141
    prescibed, see Medication
Drug problems, management, 148
    takers, characteristics of, 147
Dubowitz, V., 101
Dunne, C., 232
Dusek, D., 142, 143, 144
Dysmorphophobia, 97–8, 183

East London Child Guidance Clinic,
    23
Ebels, E., 35
Echolalia, 166
Eclecticism, 22 and see Holistic
    approach
Educational issues in psychiatry, 81,
    113, 249 and see Reading skills,
    Schools
Educational psychologist, 20, 58

Education Welfare Officer, 58
Edwards, G., 146
Ego development & borderline
    personality, 173
Eggers, C., 183, 186
Eisenberg, L., 93
Elective mutism, 80 – 1
    management, 80 – 1
Electro-encephalograms (EEG), 70,
    98, 162, 186, 198, 207
Electroconvulsive therapy (ECT), 209,
    243
Emergency intervention, 60, 220 – 23
    Example 18, 223
Emotional disorders 84 – 109
    classification, 85, 86 – 7
Emotional expression ("EE"), 185
Encopresis, 126 – 129
    management, 127 – 8
Enuresis, 80, 124 – 6
    Example 7, 125
    management, 125 – 6
Epilepsy, 34, 144, 145
    in adolescence, 210
    classification, 209 – 10
    and medication, 210
    and psychiatric disorder, 210
Erickson, M., 234
Erikson, E., 5, 8, 11
Erlenmeyer-Kimling, L., 184
Ethical problems, 137, 207 and see
    Authority; Confidentiality,
    Privacy
Evans, J., 24
Exhibitionism, 133 – 4
Experiential therapy, see Creative
    therapies

Falchikov, N., 44
Falstein, E., 153
Family in clinical assessment, 59,
    60 – 63
Family development, 11 – 13
    factors in aetiology, 36 – 42, 116,
        134
    in schizophrenia, 185
    therapy, 232 – 5
        Example 21, 233 – 4
        in school, refusal, 89
    work 232
Farrell, C., 13
Farrington, D., 40, 118, 119
Feminine boys, 130 – 31
Fire-setting, 119
Fisher, P., 90

'Flashbacks', 144
Fluphenazine, 187, 236 – 7, 239
Fluphenthixol, 236 – 7, 239
Food additives, 116
Foskett, J., 257
Fostering, 41
Fraiberg, S., 211
Framrose, R., 24
Frank, M., 248
Freeman, R., 211
Freud, A., 5, 8, 11, 229
Freud, S., 4, 23, 142
Froebel, F., 23
Fundudis, T., 80
Furnham, A., 43

Gabrielson, I., 135
Gale, E.,209
Gallessich, J., 260
Games, children's 230
Gammon, G., 196
Garfield, S., 229
Garfinkel, B., 153
Gath, A., 34
Geller, M., 87, 93, 171, 186
General Systems Theory, 12
Genetic factors, 33 – 4
Gibson, C., 135
Gillberg,C., 167, 168
Giller, H., 10, 40
Gilles de la Tourette's syndrome, see
    Tourette's syndrome
Gillick, Victoria ('Gillick case'), 135
Gilroy, A., 232
Girdano, D., 142, 143, 144
Gittelman Klein, R., 89, 241
Glaser, K., 104, 194
Glaucoma, 241
'Glue-sniffing', see Solvent abuse
Golden, C., 184
Golden, G., 162
Goodwin, J., 136
Gordon, J., 156
Gorrell-Barnes, G., 12, 232
Gottesman, I., 33, 184
Graham, P., 9, 13, 35, 52, 211
Green, D., 209
Green, R., 130, 131
Grinker, R., 174
Group work, 248 – 9
    Example 22, 248
Growth, physical, 1 – 3, 14
Growth retardation, 208

Haley, J., 234

Halmi, D., 43, 153
Haloperidol, 162–3, 187, 236–7, 239
Hassanyeh, F., 197
Hatcher, S., 135
Hatrick, J., 144
Hawk, L., 156
Hawton, K., 90, 145
Hay, G., 183
Hazell, N., 40, 41
Heacock, D., 249
Health Advisory Service (HAS), 253
    Report 26–7
Health education, 243
Hechtman, L., 116
Hemsley, R., 168
Hepatoventricular degeneration
    (Wilson's disease), 34–5
Herman, M., 186
Heroin, see Opiates
Hersov, L., 41, 86, 87, 88, 101, 229
Hinde, R., 12
Historical milestones, 24
History of child and adolescent
    psychiatry, 22–5, 27
History-taking, see Clinical
    assessment
Hoch, P., 173
Hodgman, C., 90
Holding, T., 90
Holinger, P., 90
Holistic practice, 22, 26, 205
Hollister, L., 143
Homosexuality, 131, 133
Hormonal changes, 1–3
Horowitz, H., 198, 241
Hospital admission, see Admission to
    hospital
Howard, A., 156
Howlin, P., 247, 250
Hughes, L., 259
Huntington's Chorea, 207
    and counselling, 207
Hyatt-Williams, A., 11
Hyperactivity, 114–17, 241
    in adolescence, 116, 117
    causes, 116–17
    definition, 114 and see Attention
        deficit disorder
    and diet, 116
    hyperkinesis, Example 6, 114
Hyperkinetic syndrome, 114
Hypochondriasis 97–9
    management, 98–9
Hysteria, 99–102
    epidemic, 100

management of, 102
    Example 4, 101
Hysterical conversion symptoms
    99–100
    management of, 100–101

Illness behaviour, 99
Imipramine, 89, 126, 236–7, 241
Incest, 99, 136, and see Sexual abuse
Inheritance of disorder, see Genetics
Intellectual quotient (IQ), 69, 76, 77
Intellectual retardation, see Mental
    retardation
Intelligence and autism, 166–7
International Classification of
    Diseases (ICD), 8, 50, 51
International Pilot Study of
    Schizophrenia, 180
Institutional care, consequences of,
    41–2
Isle of Wight Study, 9, 96, 210
'Italian experience', the, 255

Jattensley, A., 186
Jennings, S., 231
Jense, G., 135
Jessor, R., 118, 145
Jessor, S., 118, 145
Jones, K., 255
Jones, M., 255
Journal of Adolescence, 25
Journal of Child Psychology &
    Psychiatry, 25
Journal of Family Therapy, 235
Judge Baker Guidance Centre, 22, 24

Kalucy, R., 152, 155
Kanner, L., 166
Katon, W., 43
Kaufman, I., 13
Kayser-Fleischer ring, 207
Kellaher, L., 13
Kellerman, J,. 211
Kendell, R., 153
Kenna, J., 144
Kent Family Placement Project, 41
Kernberg, O., 174
Kessler, E., 229
Kety, S., 173, 184
King, L., 186
King, M., 147
Kirman, B., 34
Klein, D., 89, 241
Klein, M., 5
Klerman, G., 174

Klinefelter's syndrome, 3, 34
Kolvin, I., 80, 126, 166
Korchin, S., 36
Kraepelin, E., 180
Kraft, I., 248
Kringlen, E., 96
Krupinski, J., 52
Kuipers, C., 171
Kymissis, P., 198

Lake, E., 208
Lampen, J., 219, 255
Langfeldt, G., 173
Language in autism, 166
    borderline disorder, 185, 250, 251
    schizophrenia, 185–6
Larson, L., 38
Lask, B., 211
Lavik, N., 43, 52
Leese, S., 90
Leff, J., 185, 186
Legal issues, 58, 137 and see
    Delinquency, Courts, Court
    reports
Lena, B., 198
Lesbianism, 131, 133
Leslie, S., 43, 52
Lesser, L., 153
Letters, writing, 250–1
Levine, P., 196
Levine, R., 100
Lewis, D., 116
Lewis, N., 119
Liaison work, 255–7
Lidz, T., 184
Lingl, F., 146
Lipsedge, M., 43
Lishman, A., 35, 207
Lithium, 198, 200, 241–2
    toxicity, 236–7, 242
Littlewood, R., 43
Long Grove Hospital, 23
Loranger, A., 196
Lothstein, L., 133
Lotter, V., 167
Loudon, J., 242
Lowe, J., 209
Luisida, P., 144
Lumsden Walker, W., 90

MacMahon, B., 168
Maddox, G., 156
Madge, N., 9, 40, 113
Main, T., 255
Malan, D., 229

Malmquist, C., 194
Management, clinical, outline,
    216–69
Manic-depressive illness, 196–8, 244
    'equivalents',198
    Example 14, 196–7
    management, 199–200
Marital discord, see Family factors,
    Divorce
Marks, I., 87, 93, 97, 241
Marriage in adolescence 134–5
Marsden, D., 207
Martin, D., 255
Martindale, B., 207
Matsumura, M., 147
Masterson, G., 146, 186
Masterson, J., 174, 229
Masturbation, 13
Matthysse, S., 184
Maudsley Hospital, 24, 27
Mayer, I., 156
McAdam, E., 225
McCabe, R., 209
McClure, 90
McEvedy, C., 100
McGuffin, P., 33
Medication, 89, 97, 135, 163, 185, 187,
    195–6, 198, 200, 238–43
Mednick, S., 184
Meeks, J., 249
Mental Deficiency Acts, 24
Mental disorder, parental, 39
Mental handicap, 26, 73–7
    Example 1, 73–4
Mental Health Act 1983, 24, 73, 197
Mental retardation, 73
    and brain disorder, 79
    categories, 76–7
    and psychiatric disorder, 77
Mental subnormality, 73
Mental Treatment Act, 24
Merry, J., 232, 249
Metachromatic leukodystrophy, 207
Methylphenitate, see Amphetamine-
    like drugs
Meyer, A., 23
Meyer, J., 156
Mikkelsen, E., 124
Milham, S., 27, 252
Miller, E., 23
Minuchin, S., 153, 235
Mittler, P., 40
Modelling, 246
Mohr, P., 100
Monello, L., 156

Monitoring progress, 251–2
Montessori, M., 23
Montgomery, M., 162
Morgan, H., 90
Moss, P., 100
Mrazek, D., 136, 265
Mrazek, P., 136
Multi-axial diagnosis, 51–2, 73
Music education, 230

Nahas, G., 145
Narcolepsy, 241
Nasogastric feeding, 101
National Autistic Society, 169
National Society for the Prevention of
    Cruelty to Children, 24
Neurodegenerative disorder, 34, 205,
    208
    Example 16, 206
Neurodevelopment, see Paediatric
    neurology
Neuroleptics, see Antipsychotic drugs
Neurological factors, 34–5
Neurologist-psychiatrist liaison, 209,
    213
Neurology reading list, 35
Neville, B., 35, 208
Newman, O., 118
Newsome, A., 224, 229
Nicotine, 143
Night alarm, see Bell and pad
Noe, J., 139
Normality, 14, 103, 113, 126
Nursing, psychiatric, 27
Nutrition, 244

Obesity, 156
    management, 156
Obsessive compulsive disorders,
    95–7, 241
    Example, 3, 95–6
    management, 95–7
O'Connor, D., 147
Offord, D., 186
Oliver, J., 147, 207
Olness, K., 128
Olsen, T., 196
Opiates, 141–2
Oppenheimer, E., 147
Organisation of work, 221, 253–4,
    255–7 and see Staff management
Orphenadrine, 236–7, 240
Orris, J., 118
Outings, children's, 230
Overactivity, 114 and see
    Hyperactivity

Overdose, see Attempted suicide,
    Suicide

Paediatric neurology, 35
Paediatric-psychiatrist liaison, 208,
    209, 213, 255 and see
    Hypochondriasis, Hysteria,
    Physical health
Page, D., 230, 249
Papeschi, R., 255
Paracetamol, 92
Parental behaviour, 38–40
Parental feelings in physical illness,
    208, 211–12
Parker, G., 41
Parry-Jones, W., 24, 38, 135
Patient, becoming a, 19–20
Pauls, D., 162
Pavlov, I., 23
Pedder, J., 8, 223, 229
Perinpanayagam, K., 24, 253
Perry, J., 174
Pertschuk, M., 155
Petti, T., 241
Phencyclidine, 144
Phobias, prevalence, 93
Phobic states, 92–3
    management, 93–4
Physical disorder in clinical
    assessment, 65, 69, 70
Physical examination, 69, 70
Physical health, 93, 97, 100, 101, 127,
    133, 141–7, 152–7, 168, 184,
    204–15, 239–41, 243
Piaget, Jean, 3
Pimozide, 162, 187
Pitman, G., 186
Pittman, F., 90
Plant, M., 43, 145
Poisons Information Services, 92
Polantin, P., 173
Pollack, M., 186
Pollitt, J., 96, 97
Pop concerts, epidemic hysteria in, 100
Porteous, M., 43
Potteti, A., 255
Powell, G., 208
Poznanski, E., 93
Pregnancy in adolescence, 134–5
Press, E., 146
Pringle, M., 162
Privacy, 59
Probation officer, 58, 120
Problem clarification, 30–31, 53, 113,
    187–8, 208

Problems, frequency of, 53, 253
Procyclidine, 236–7, 240
Promiscuity, 134
Prosser, H., 41
Pseudopsychosis, hysterical, 43
Psychiatric disorders, prevalence, 19
Psychiatry, adolescent, 17, 22–5
Psychodrama, 231
Psychodynamic theory, 4–6, 6–8
Psychological assessment, 69–70,
    208, 244–5
Psychological development, 3–6
Psychological tests, 69–70
Psychosis cannabis, 144
Psychosis, psychogenic, 183
Psychosomatic disorders, 204–15
    definition, 205
    management, 211–12
Psychotherapy, 223–9
    with adolescents, 227–9
    definition and classification 223–4
    Example 19, 225–6
Puberty, 1
Punishment, 246
Pyne, N., 24, 54

Quay, H., 126
Quinn, N., 207
Quinton, D., 41, 43

Racial prejudice, adolescents', 44
Rack, P., 183
Rapoport, R., 255
Reading skills, 111, 113, 116, 120
Reid, J., 81
Reilly, P., 198
Referral process, 19–21
Remschmidt, H., 241
Reports, writing, 250–51
Research, 257
Residential care, 252–5, and see
    Institutional care, Therapeutic
    milieu, Admission to hospital
Response prevention, 246
Rinsley, D., 173
Ritson, B., 145
Rivinus, T., 99
Robins, E., 131
Robins, L., 40, 86, 113, 118
Rogers, C., 224, 225
Role play, 230–31
Rooth, F., 134
Rorschasch test, 69–70
Rose, M., 255
Rosenthal, D., 184

Ruff, G., 36
Russell, G., 153, 154, 155
Russell, J., 41
Rutter, M., 9, 10, 11, 13, 37, 40, 43,
    52, 79, 92, 96, 103, 113, 117, 124,
    127, 166, 167, 184, 210

Safer, D., 241
Saghir, M., 131
Sainsbury, P., 90
St. Ebba's Hospital, 23
Sands, D., 23, 186
Sarteschi, P., 255
Sartorious, N., 186
Schaumann, H., 167
Scheinberg, I., 207
Schizoaffective illness, 197–8
    Example 15, 197–8
Schizoid personality, 171–2
    management, 172
Schizophrenia, 33–40, 179–91
    aetiology, 184–5
    diagnosis, 179, 180, 182–3
    Example, 13, 181–2
    management, 186–8
    medication, 187
    precursors of, 185–6
    Prognosis, 186
    relapse and the family, 185
    'simple', 181
Schizotypal personality, 172, 173
Schmideberg, M., 174
Schmitt, B., 88
Schneider, K., 179
    Symptoms of first rank, 179
Schools, epidemic hysteria in, 100
    influence of, 42, 81
School non-attendance, classification,
    87
Schools Psychological Service, 89 and
    see Educational psychologist
School refusal, 87–90
    Example 21, 233–34
    management, 89–90
Scott, P., 196
Seclusion of patients, 246
Sedman, G., 95, 144
Self-monitoring, 246
Self-poisoning, see Attempted suicide;
    Suicide
Selvini-Palazzoli, M., 153, 235
Separation, 36–7, 89, 130, 131
Sex differences, 10, 54, 130, 131, 147
Sexual abuse, 99, 136
Sexual behaviour in autism, 167

Sexual development, 1–3, 13, 130–9, 210
  parental anxiety, 130–31
  prediction of, 130–1
Sexual identity, 130–31
Sexual problems, management, 137
Shaffer, D., 35, 90, 124, 194, 241
Shapiro, A., 162
Sheard, M., 198
Shorvon, H., 95
Singer, M., 184–5
Skynner, R., 12, 89, 235, 257
Skuse, D., 146, 147
Slade, P., 152
Slater, E., 99
Smayling, L., 81
Smith, L., 126
Smoking, see Cigarette smoking
Snaith, P., 134
Snyder, S., 163, 174
Social development, 13
Social therapy, 248–9
Socio-cultural influences, 43
Soiling, see Encopresis
Solvent abuse, 146–7
  physical effects, 146–7
Special education, 249–50 and see
  Educational issues in
  psychiatry
Sphincter training in encopresis, 128
Staff groups, 257
  management, 200, 253–4, 255–7
'Staff support', 257
Stein, G., 198, 242
Steinberg, D., 10, 17, 21, 22, 24, 37,
  51, 54, 60, 101, 102, 198, 204, 219,
  220–21, 242, 249, 253, 256, 259,
  260
Steiner, R., 23, 208, 255
Steiner, Rudolf, 169
Stephens, J., 186
Stern, R., 95
Stewart, M., 119
Stimulant drugs, 241 and see
  Amphetamine-like drugs
Stoller, R., 133
Stores, G., 210, 241
Strachan, J., 119
Strang, J., 142
Straughan, J., 81
Stress, acute reaction to, 102–3
  management, 103
Stunkard, A., 156
Sturm und Drang movement, 10
Substance misuse, 140–50

Suicide, 90–92
  risk, management of, 91–2
  prediction, 91
Sulpiride, 187
Supervision, 228, 257
Sylvester, E., 255
Symonds, A., 186
Szmukler, G., 153, 154

Tanner, J., 3
Tattersall, R., 209
Tattum, D., 250
Taylor, D., 209, 210
Taylor, E., 114, 115, 116, 244
Teamwork., 255–7
Telephone, work on the, 221
Temperamental vulnerability, 93
Temperament, definition, 35
Tennent, G., 24, 255
Tharp, R., 247
Theander, S., 154
Thematic Apperception Test (TAT), 69
Therapeutic milieu, 254–5
Thioridazine, 236–7, 239
Thomas, A., 93
Thomas, S., 207
Tics, 161–4
'Time Out', 246
Tizard, B., 41
Tobias, A., 156
Token reinforcement, 246
Tolan, E., 146
Tolerance of drugs, 140
Tolstrup, K., 154
'Tomboys', 130–31
Toolan, J., 194
Topping, K., 247
Tourette's syndrome, 161–4
  aetiology, 162–3
  description, 161–2
  Example 10, 161–2
  management, 163
  outcome, 162
Tranquillizers, major, see Anti-
  psychotic drugs
Tranquillizers, minor, see
  Benzodiazepines
Tranquillizing medication, 120, 187,
  236–7, 239–40
Transcultural influences, 43–4, 183
Transexualism 131–3
  Example 8, 131
Treatments, range of, 21
Trifluoperazine, 170, 187

Triseliotis, J., 41
Truancy, 87
Turle, G., 23
Turmoil, adolescent, 8–9
Turner's syndrome, 3, 34
Turpin, G., 162, 163
Tyrer, P., 22, 90
Tyrer, S., 90

Vaillant, G., 186
Vandalism, 118–19
Van Eerdewegh, M., 37
Van Krevelen, D., 171
Vaughn, C., 185
Von Bertalanffy, L., 12, 232

Walker, S., 207
Waller, D., 230, 232
Walrond-Skinner, S., 235
Waring, H., 242
Warren, B., 230
Warren, W., 23, 27, 90, 186
Watson, J., 23, 147
Wechler Adult Intelligence Scale
    (WAIS), 69
    Intelligence Scale for Children
    (WISC), 69
Weil, A., 173
Weinberg, W., 241
Weinberger, D., 184
Weiner, I., 104, 183, 144
Weisberg, P., 249
Weiss, G., 116
Wells, P., 24, 25
Welner, A., 196
Werne, J., 155

Werry, J., 126
West, D., 40, 116, 117, 118
Westland, P., 21
Wetzel, R., 247
Wexler, L., 90
Whiteley, J., 255
Wilkinson, T., 26, 257
Willerman, L., 116
Williams, M., 44
Wilson, J., 208
Wilson, P., 228, 229
Wilson's Disease (hepatolenticular
    degeneration), 34–5, 206–7
Wing, J., 168
Wing, L., 168, 171
Winnicott, D., 5, 11, 229, 249
Winokur, G., 196
Wolff, S., 117, 171
Wolkind, S., 37, 41, 43
Wright, H., 81
Wynn, B., 231
Wynne, L., 184–5

X-linked adrenocorticodystrophy, see
    Addison Schilder's disease

Yeomans, N., 255
Youngerman, J., 198–241
Youth Treatment Centres, 255
Yule, W., 79, 247, 260

Zeitlin, H., 182, 197
Zeltzer, L., 211
Zongker, C., 135
Zvolsky, P., 198, 241